DISORDERS OF
PERIPHERAL NERVES

CONTEMPORARY NEUROLOGY SERIES AVAILABLE:

Fred Plum, M.D., *Editor-in-Chief*
J. Richard Baringer, M.D., *Associate Editor*
Sid Gilman, M.D., *Associate Editor*

DISORDERS OF PERIPHERAL NERVES

Herbert H. Schaumburg, M.D.

Professor and Vice Chairman
Department of Neurology
Associate Professor of Pathology (Neuropathology)
Medical Director, Institute of Neurotoxicology
Albert Einstein College of Medicine
Bronx, New York

Peter S. Spencer, Ph.D., MRCPath.

Associate Professor of Neuroscience and Pathology
Director, Institute of Neurotoxicology
Albert Einstein College of Medicine
Bronx, New York

P. K. Thomas, M.D., D.Sc., F.R.C.P.

Professor of Neurology
University of London at
The Royal Free Hospital
School of Medicine
and The Institute of Neurology
Queen Square, London, England

 F. A. DAVIS COMPANY • PHILADELPHIA

Library of Congress Cataloging in Publication Data

Schaumburg, Herbert H.
  Disorders of peripheral nerves.

  (Contemporary neurology series; 24)
  Includes bibliographical references and index.
  1. Nerves, Peripheral—Diseases. I. Spencer, Peter S.
II. Thomas, P. K. (Peter Kynaston), 1926–
III. Title.
RC409.S33   1983   616.8'7   82-22143
ISBN 0-8036-7732-4

PREFACE

"Disease of the peripheral nervous system stands as one of the most difficult subjects in neurology. Since the structure and function of this system are relatively simple, one might suppose that our knowledge of its diseases would be complete. Such is not the case. At present a suitable explanation cannot be offered in about 40 percent of patients who enter a general hospital with a peripheral nerve disease (usually of chronic progressive type) and the pathological changes have not been fully determined in any one of them. Moreover, the physiologic basis of many of the neural symptoms continues to elude experts in the field."*

The authors do not dispute this unhappy state of affairs, although the figure of 40 percent can perhaps now be improved upon by intensive investigation in special centers.† However, it is our conviction, supported by years of undergraduate medical teaching and experience with individuals outside the neurosciences, that a working knowledge of the common peripheral neuropathies can be mastered by any motivated physician.

This volume evolved from the primary author's 1972 syllabus for the undergraduate and graduate courses on peripheral nerve disease at the Albert Einstein College of Medicine. The favorable reception accorded the syllabus, and increasing requests for its enlargement, indicated the need for a concise, elementary monograph on peripheral neuropathy intended for individuals engaged in the practice of general medicine and neurology. Drs. Spencer and Thomas agreed to collaborate in this endeavor; their abundant, scholarly contributions to this volume have justified the decision to challenge the considerable obstacles posed in creating an international, multiauthored text.

---

*ADAMS, RD AND VICTOR, M: *Principles of Neurology,* ed 2, McGraw-Hill, New York, 1981.
†DYCK, PJ, OVIATT, KF AND LAMBERT, EH: *Intensive evaluation of unclassified neuropathies yields improved diagnosis.* Ann Neurol 10:222, 1981.

We are pleased to acknowledge the following individuals who assisted us in this project: Monica Bischoff, Laurell Edwards, Elaine Garafola, Larry Markowitz and Patricia Vacchelli. We are especially grateful to Dr. Webb Haymaker for allowing us to reproduce his diagrams of peripheral nerves and their segmental innervation.

Dr. Sylvia Fields, Mr. Richard Heffron and their editorial and publishing staff at F.A. Davis have generously offered expert guidance and encouragement.

Contents

Chapter 1

BASIC CONCEPTS AND TERMINOLOGY

DEFINITION OF THE PERIPHERAL NERVOUS SYSTEM (PNS)

The PNS may be defined as those portions of motor neurons, autonomic neurons, and primary sensory neurons that extend outside the central nervous system (CNS) and are associated with Schwann cells or ganglionic satellite cells. The concept of a separate peripheral nervous system is obviously artificial, since the cell bodies of many PNS motor neurons lie within the CNS and some peripheral sensory neurons have extensive central projections. The justification for this concept stems from several notions, two of which are especially relevant to this book: one is the predilection for many diseases primarily to affect the PNS, and the other is its ability to regenerate.

The PNS, so defined, usually includes the dorsal and ventral spinal roots, spinal and cranial nerves, dorsal root and other sensory ganglia, sensory and motor terminals, and the bulk of the autonomic nervous system.[1] The connective tissue and vasculature of peripheral nerve have several unique features, including the perineurial and blood-nerve barriers, and play a major role in PNS disorders. Lymphatic vessels are present in the epineurium but not within the fascicles. The salient components of a peripheral nerve are illustrated in Figures 1 to 4.

RELATIONSHIPS FUNDAMENTAL TO AN UNDERSTANDING OF DISEASE OF MYELINATED PERIPHERAL NERVE FIBERS

Neuron cell body and axon. The axons of peripheral nerve, despite their occasional great length, are simply cytoplasmic extensions of the nerve cell bodies. PNS axons derive most of the proteins essential for maintenance and function from the nerve cell body. Structural components, organelles,

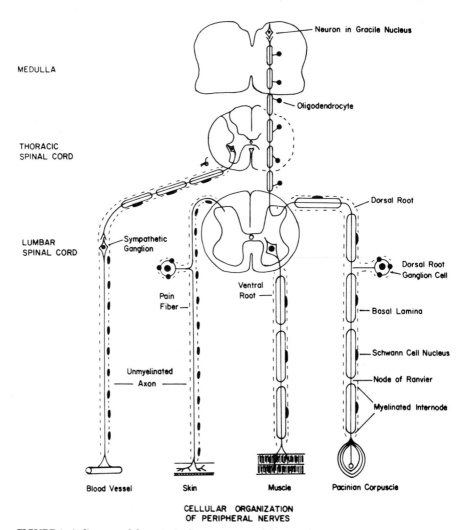

FIGURE 1. A diagram of the principal components of the peripheral nervous system.

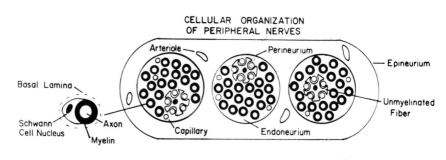

FIGURE 2. A diagram of a peripheral nerve in cross section. The nerve contains three fascicles. The figure on the left represents a high magnification of a myelinated axon in cross section.

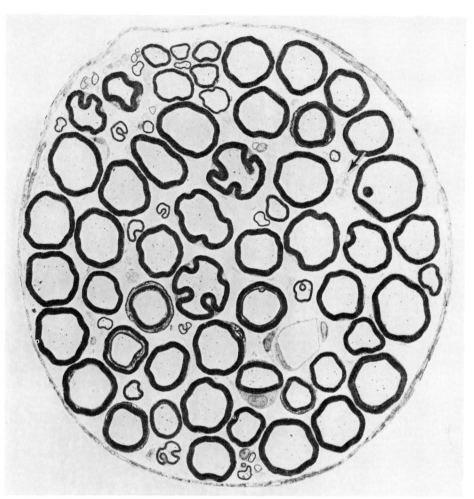

FIGURE 3. Cross section of one fascicle of a peripheral nerve showing myelinated and unmyelinated (arrow) fibers. (From Weinberg, HJ and Spencer, PS, *Studies on the control of myelinogenesis, I. Myelination of regenerating axons after entry into a foreign unmyelinated nerve.* Journal of Neurocytology, 4:395, 1975, with permission.)

nutrients, and metabolic products are transported at several velocities, some in both directions, along the axon.[2] This system renders the axons exquisitely vulnerable to any failure of the anabolic machinery in the cell body, allows viruses and toxins a conduit from the periphery to the CNS, and may be a means of communication of messages (e.g., signals for regeneration, trophic factors) between the ends of the axon and the nerve cell body.[3]

In general, injury to the distal portion of the axon does not result in permanent damage to the nerve cell body; the latter undergoes transient swelling and breakdown of endoplasmic reticulum (chromatolysis), but usually survives and supports regeneration of the damaged axon.[4] The converse is not true; severe damage to the nerve cell body or disruption of proximal axonal integrity results in rapid degeneration of the entire distal portion (see later discussion of Wallerian Degeneration).

Axon, Schwann cell and myelin. Schwann cells envelop axons to form unmyelinated and myelinated fibers surrounded by a basal lamina. PNS myelin is derived from the Schwann cell and is dependent both on the

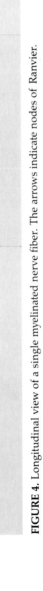

FIGURE 4. Longitudinal view of a single myelinated nerve fiber. The arrows indicate nodes of Ranvier.

Schwann cell itself and the axon for its continued integrity. A single Schwann cell occupies each myelinated internode, almost never associating itself with more than one axon.[5] Death of the axon results in the prompt breakdown of myelin but not the Schwann cell. The opposite is not true; loss of myelin does not usually result in disruption of the axon. This principle is of fundamental importance to an understanding of PNS disorders. An axon denuded of several segments of myelin simply awaits Schwann cell division and remyelination before resuming normal impulse conduction.[6]

Axon and end organ. The effect of axonal transection on muscle is dramatic. Within months the muscle undergoes severe denervation atrophy and will not recover unless reinnervated.[7] This loss of the normal "trophic" effect of nerve on muscle is widely accepted. Less certain are the other alleged trophic functions of nerve for skin, blood vessels, and subcutaneous tissue. Prolonged denervation results in changes of these tissues (red skin, ulcers) sometimes attributed to loss of maintenance function provided by the nerve fiber. Such changes may merely represent the effects of trauma and autonomic dysfunction on these tissues.[8]

Wallerian degeneration and axon regeneration. The morphologic events following a focal crush injury to peripheral nerve are depicted in Figure 13 in Chapter 2. Transection of a nerve fiber results in total degeneration of the axon(s) and myelin distal to the site of injury (Wallerian degeneration.)[9] Within four days the entire distal axon and myelin become fragmented and electrical conduction ceases. The nerve cell body undergoes a chromatolytic reaction, and subsequently, regenerating axonal sprouts emerge from the injured axons at the site of injury. By one week, the distal Schwann cells have divided and are arranged in columns inside their tubes of basal lamina. If regenerating axons reach one of these Schwann cell columns they can regenerate steadily towards the terminal and be myelinated by the waiting Schwann cells. Injuries that do not disrupt connective tissue continuity of a nerve (closed injuries) often have a good prognosis, since regenerating axons usually arrive at their former peripheral terminations, guided by the pre-existing Schwann cell columns. Injuries that transect fascicles or the entire nerve, such as knife wounds, are frequently associated with ineffective or aberrant regeneration. Many sprouting axons may never reach the distal stump, but grow in an aberrant fashion (see Figure 14 in Chapter 2) or a random tangled fashion (traumatic neuroma).

CURRENT CLINICAL TERMINOLOGY

(1) *Neuropathy (peripheral neuropathy).* This is a general term for any disorder—infective, toxic, metabolic—affecting peripheral nerve. It replaces the older term 'peripheral neuritis.'

(2) *Polyneuropathy (symmetrical polyneuropathy).* This term designates a generalized process producing widespread and bilaterally symmetrical effects on the peripheral nervous system. It may be motor, sensory, sensorimotor, or autonomic in its effects, and proximal, distal, or generalized in its distribution.

(3) *Focal or multifocal neuropathy.* These terms indicate local involvement of one or more individual peripheral nerves and are equivalent to the more cumbersome terms 'mononeuropathy' and 'multiple mononeuropathy' ('mononeuropathy multiplex').

(4) *Small-fiber neuropathy*. These are neuropathies in which there is a predominant disturbance of small myelinated and unmyelinated fibers characterized by diminished pain and temperature sensation, often with spontaneous pain and autonomic involvement. There is relative preservation of muscle strength, tendon reflexes, and sensory modalities subserved by the larger myelinated fibers (touch-pressure, vibration, joint position.)

(5) *Large-fiber neuropathy*. Neuropathies that predominantly affect the larger myelinated fibers are characterized by loss of position, vibration and touch-pressure sensibility, tendon areflexia, and lower motor neuron involvement. Sensory ataxia and pseudoathetosis may be prominent if muscle power is preserved.

(6) *Certain symptoms and signs* associated with peripheral nerve disease have, by common usage, acquired varied connotations. These terms are best avoided unless carefully defined. Simple descriptions of patients' complaints are more meaningful than casual use of terms such as 'dysesthesia' (abnormal spontaneous sensations), 'hypoesthesia' or 'hypesthesia' (decreased sensitivity), and 'hyperesthesia' or 'hyperpathia' (increased sensitivity, usually with an unpleasant quality).

REFERENCES

1. CARPENTER, MB: Human Neuroanatomy, ed 7, Williams & Wilkins, Baltimore, 1976.
2. OCHS, S AND WORTH, RM: *Axoplasmic transport in normal and pathological systems.* In WAXMAN, SG (ed): Physiology and Pathobiology of Axons. Raven Press, New York, 1978.
3. SPENCER, PS AND SCHAUMBURG, HH: *Pathobiology of neurotoxic axonal degeneration.* In WAXMAN, SG (ed): Physiology and Pathobiology of Axons. Raven Press, New York, 1978.
4. PRICE, DR AND PORTER, KR: *The response of ventral horn neurons to axonal transection.* J Cell Biol 53:24, 1972.
5. BERTHOLD, C-H: *Morphology of normal peripheral axons.* In WAXMAN, SG (ed): Physiology and Pathobiology of Axons. Raven Press, New York, 1978.
6. RAINE, CS: *Pathology of demyelination.* In WAXMAN, SG (ed): Physiology and Pathobiology of Axons. Raven Press, New York, 1978.
7. SUNDERLAND, S: Nerves and Nerve Injuries, ed 2, Churchill Livingstone, Edinburgh, 1978.
8. THOMAS, PK: *Clinical features and differential diagnosis.* In DYCK, PJ, THOMAS, PK AND LAMBERT, EH (eds): Peripheral Neuropathy Vol 1, WB Saunders, Philadelphia, 1975, p 495.
9. DONAT, JR AND WIŚNIEWSKI, HM: *The spatio-temporal pattern of Wallerian degeneration in mammalian peripheral nerves.* Brain Res 53:41, 1973.

Chapter 2

ANATOMICAL CLASSIFICATION OF PNS DISORDERS

The authors currently endorse an anatomical classification of disorders (Table 1) of the PNS based on whether the condition is characterized by generalized symmetrical or focal involvement.[1] This simple classification stresses the site of apparent primary pathologic change.* For example, although demyelination is a feature of uremic neuropathy, it is clearly secondary to changes in the axon, and uremic neuropathy is considered as an axonopathy.

SYMMETRICAL GENERALIZED NEUROPATHIES (POLYNEUROPATHIES)

Distal axonopathy (central-peripheral distal axonopathy, dying-back neuropathy)

GENERAL. This is the most common morphologic reaction of the PNS and CNS to exogenous toxins, and probably also underlies many metabolic and hereditary neuropathies.[2] The biochemical mechanisms and pathophysiology of distal axonopathy are poorly understood.

HYPOTHETICAL MECHANISM. Initially, a metabolic abnormality occurs throughout the axon. Failure of axon transport results in degeneration of vulnerable distal regions of long or large-diameter axons.[3] Degeneration appears to advance proximally towards the nerve cell body (dying-back) as long as the metabolic abnormality persists; its reversal allows the axon to regenerate along the distal Schwann cell tube to the appropriate terminal. An identical sequence usually occurs simultaneously in the distal ends of long CNS axons (e.g., dorsal columns), although regeneration is less effec-

*Experimental studies with toxic agents suggest that while the initial site and pattern of damage usually are constant for a given substance, sometimes these may vary according to the rate or route of intoxication.

TABLE 1. Anatomic Classification of Peripheral Neuropathy

Two overall types—	1. Symmetrical generalized 2. Focal and multifocal

1. Symmetrical Generalized Neuropathies (Polyneuropathies)

Distal Axonopathies	Toxic—many drugs, industrial and environmental chemicals Metabolic—uremia, diabetes, porphyria, endocrine Deficiency—thiamine, pyridoxine Genetic—HMSN II Malignancy associated—oat-cell carcinoma, multiple Myeloma
Myelinopathies	Toxic—diphtheria, buckthorn Immunologic—acute inflammatory polyneuropathy (Guillain-Barré) chronic inflammatory polyneuropathy Genetic—Refsum disease, metachromatic leukodystrophy
Neuronopathies somatic motor	Undetermined—amyotropic lateral sclerosis Genetic—hereditary motor neuronopathies
somatic sensory	Infectious—herpes zoster neuronitis Malignancy-associated—sensory neuronopathy syndrome Toxic—pyridoxine sensory neuronopathy Undetermined—subacute sensory neuronopathy syndrome
autonomic	Genetic—hereditary dysautonomia (HSN IV)

2. Focal (Mononeuropathy) and Multifocal (Multiple mononeuropathy) Neuropathies
   Ischemia—polyarteritis, diabetes, rheumatoid arthritis
   Infiltration—leukemia, lymphoma, granuloma, Schwannoma, amyloid
   Physical injuries—severence, focal crush, compression, stretch and traction, entrapment
   Immunologic—brachial and lumbar plexopathy

tive.[4] The distal vulnerability of these axons is an enigma. Two important determinants are distance from the cell body and fiber diameter.

Cardinal Pathologic Features (Fig. 5)

(a) Initial distal axonal change may be both multifocal and characteristic of the disorder (swelling, atrophy, organelle accumulation and so forth.)[5]

(b) Eventual axonal disintegration resembles Wallerian degeneration; the myelin sheath breaks down concomitantly with the axon. Secondary demyelination and remyelination may occur more proximally, where the axon is still intact.

(c) Distal muscles undergo denervation atrophy.

(d) Nerve cell chromatolysis may occur in severe cases.

(e) Schwann cells and basal lamina tubes remain in distal nerves and facilitate appropriate peripheral regeneration.

(f) Astroglial proliferation, triggered by distal axonal degeneration, may impede regeneration in CNS. Transsynaptic degeneration may occur in specific sensory systems, for example, the gracile nucleus.

Clinicopathologic Correlation

(a) Gradual insidious onset: Chronic metabolic disease or prolonged, low-level intoxication usually produce prolonged subclinical disease with signs and symptoms gradually appearing later.

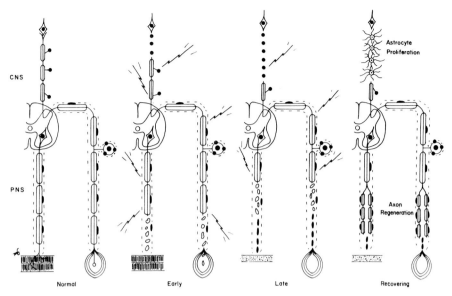

Astrocyte
Proliferation

Axon
Regeneration

| Normal | Early | Late | Recovering |

TOXIC DISTAL AXONOPATHY

FIGURE 5. A diagram of the cardinal pathologic features of a toxic distal axonopathy. The jagged lines (lightning bolts) indicate that the toxin is acting at multiple sites along motor and sensory axons in the PNS and CNS. Axon degeneration has moved proximally (dying-back) by the late stage. Recovery in the CNS is impeded by astroglial proliferation.

(b) Initial findings frequently in the lower extremities: The distal axonopathy hypothesis states that large and long axons are affected early; thus the fibers of sciatic nerve branches are especially vulnerable.

(c) Stocking-glove sensory and motor loss: Axonal degeneration commences distally and slowly proceeds towards the neuron cell body, resulting in *symmetrical, distal* clinical signs in the legs and arms. The earliest symptoms are usually sensory: toe-tip sensations of tingling or pinprick are common initial complaints. The pattern of sensory loss is depicted in Figure 6.

(d) Early and symmetrical loss of ankle jerks: the axons supplying the calf muscles are of extremely large diameter and are among the first affected.

(e) Moderate slowing in motor nerve conduction: In contrast to the demyelinating neuropathies, where the motor nerves or roots are diffusely affected, many motor fibers are intact proximally in the axonal neuropathies and motor nerve conduction velocity may therefore appear normal or only slightly slowed despite clinical signs of neuropathy. Exception: Severe impulse slowing accompanies distal axonopathies in which the axon swells and demyelinates focally.

(f) Normal CSF protein level: Since the pathologic changes are usually distal and the nerve roots spared, most patients with axonal neuropathies have a normal or only slightly elevated CSF protein value.

(g) Slow recovery: Since axonal regeneration (in contrast to remyelination) is a very slow process, proceeding at a rate of 2 to 3 mm per day, recovery may take many months, several years, or never completely occur. Function is restored in reverse order to the sequence of loss.

(h) Signs of CNS disease: This has been encountered in individuals *recovering* from certain toxic neuropathies. Most toxic central-peripheral distal axonopathies are characterized by tract degeneration of the distal extremities of long, large diameter fibers in the CNS *pari passu* with changes in the

ANATOMICAL
CLASSIFICATION
OF PNS
DISORDERS

9

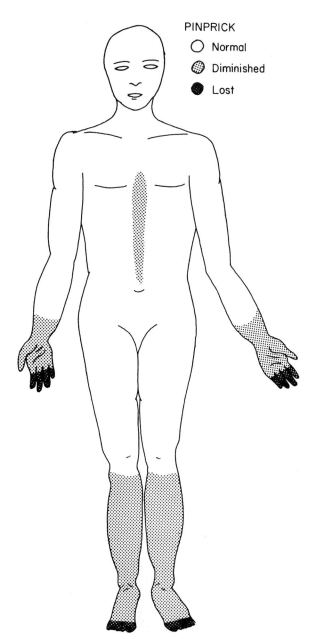

FIGURE 6. Stocking-glove pattern of sensory loss in an advanced stage of distal axonopathy. The area of diminished sensation over midthorax ("cuirass distribution") reflects involvement of distal ends of intercostal nerves.

PNS. Thus, the clinical signs of degeneration in the corticospinal and spino-cerebellar pathways are usually not prominent features early in the illness. However, on recovery from the neuropathy, the patient may manifest hyperreflexia, Babinski responses, and a stiff-legged, ataxic gait.[2]

Myelinopathy

10 **GENERAL.** The term *myelinopathy*, when applied to the PNS, refers to conditions in which the lesion *primarily* affects myelin or the myelinating

(Schwann) cell. Thus, the proximal segmental demyelination that accompanies many axonal disorders is *not* evidence of a primary myelinopathy. Stated another way, segmental demyelination (internodal loss of myelin) is not always synonymous with myelinopathy.

The Guillain-Barré syndrome, an immune-mediated inflammatory, demyelinating neuropathy, is the only frequently encountered disease that primarily affects PNS myelin (see Chapter 3). Toxic and infectious myelinopathies (see Chapter 11, 12, and 16) and hereditary disorders of Schwann cell lipid metabolism (see Chapter 9), are rare. The sequences of morphologic change operant in several myelinopathies have been thoroughly studied and are, in general, well understood. The enzymatic abnormalities in several of the hereditary conditions have been elucidated (see Chapter 9).

HYPOTHETICAL MECHANISMS. It is generally held that the segmental demyelination of spinal roots and nerves in the Guillain-Barré syndrome results from an immune-mediated attack on PNS myelin.[6] The precipitating event or antigen is not known, but the subsequent pathologic events mirror those of experimental allergic neuritis, a condition produced in animals by immunization against peripheral myelin.[7]

The segmental demyelination of diphtheritic neuropathy reported results from toxic inhibition of Schwann cell synthesis of myelin constituents.[8] By contrast, most well studied myelinopathies appear to be characterized by a primary attack on the myelin itself. The Schwann cell perikaryon survives in most of these conditions and retains the ability to divide and form new myelin.

Cardinal Pathologic Features (Fig. 7)

(a) Primary destruction of the myelin sheath occurs, usually leaving the axon intact.

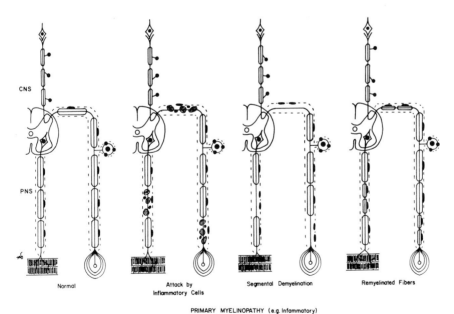

Normal   Attack by Inflammatory Cells   Segmental Demyelination   Remyelinated Fibers

PRIMARY MYELINOPATHY (e.g. Inflammatory)

FIGURE 7. A diagram of the cardinal pathologic features of an inflammatory PNS myelinopathy. Axons are spared as is CNS myelin. Following the attack, the remaining Schwann cells divide. The denuded segments of axons are remyelinated, leaving them with shortened internodes.

(b) Often begins at nodes of Ranvier.

(c) Spinal roots are usually heavily involved, but destruction also affects multiple sites in nerve.

(d) The Schwann cell divides and remyelinates the axon to form short internodes of thin myelin.

(e) Muscle often does not undergo denervation change, but may undergo disuse atrophy if paralysis is prolonged. Axonal loss may occur in primary demyelinating disorders and is occasionally profound. The explanation for this is unclear.

(f) Should *repeated* demyelination occur, Schwann cells divide again, and some of the daughter cells are unable to find a segment of axon to surround. They become detached and form a thin layer around the fiber. The Schwann cells may form multiple rings ("onion bulbs") around the axon.

Clinicopathologic Correlation

(a) Onset: In toxic and inflammatory myelinopathies, the process of segmental demyelination occurs over a period of hours, days, or weeks.

(b) Initial changes may occur in the lower extremities, but not always distally: The diffuse process may occasionally become manifest in the short cranial nerves, but more commonly, the nerves to the lower extremities are initially involved. Presumably this occurs because the myelinated axons of the sciatic nerve are longest, contain the most myelin, and are statistically most likely to be involved in a random demyelinating process.

(c) Generalized weakness with mild sensory loss: The large-diameter, heavily myelinated motor axons and ventral roots are involved, resulting in diffuse symmetrical weakness or paralysis of the extremities and bulbar muscles. Relative sensory sparing may reflect in part the continued function of small-diameter myelinated and unmyelinated fibers. Sensory ataxia may occur from involvement of proprioceptive afferent fibers. The patterns of sensory and motor loss are illustrated in Figure 8.

(d) Absent tendon reflexes in all extremities: Both the afferent and efferent limbs of the monosynaptic stretch reflex are mediated by large-diameter myelinated fibers, especially vulnerable in the toxic and inflammatory myelinopathies. Generalized areflexia is a hallmark of these conditions.

(e) Marked slowing of nerve conduction: The widespread demyelination prolongs conduction and may give rise to conduction block. Conduction velocity in remyelinated fibers with thin myelin sheaths may be reduced.

(f) Elevated CSF protein: Inflammatory and toxic demyelination heavily involve the spinal roots, with leakage of protein into the surrounding subarchnoid space.

(g) Rapid recovery: Recovery is dependent on remyelination to restore impulse conduction. Effective remyelination of an internode may take only a few weeks and clinical recovery may be dramatic.

(h) No signs of CNS disease: Most toxic and inflammatory PNS myelinopathies spare the CNS for various reasons. One is that many myelinotoxic agents are unable to cross the blood-brain barrier; another is that many inflammatory conditions are immune-mediated and the response is directed at substances present in peripheral myelin.[6] Some hereditary metabolic diseases of myelin (leukodystrophies) have profound CNS involvement (see Chapter 9).

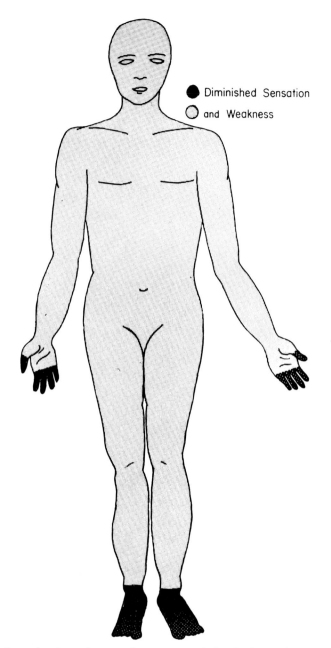

FIGURE 8. Pattern of motor and sensory loss in a severely involved case of the Guillain-Barré syndrome. There is diffuse weakness of limb, intercostal, and facial muscles. Sensory impairment is usually mild and involves only the distal portions of the limbs.

Neuronopathy

GENERAL. The term *neuronopathy* describes conditions in which the initial morphologic or biochemical changes occur in the neuron cell body.[1] Clinical manifestations of PNS neuronopathies are restricted to the segments innervated by the affected cell bodies. They are a heterogeneous, poorly understood group of conditions and, in the broadest sense, include many disorders of motor, sensory and autonomic neurons. They may commence prenatally or in infancy, adolescence, or adult life. Infectious neuronopathies include familiar conditions such as poliomyelitis and herpes zoster ganglionitis. The hereditary motor neuropathies (spinal muscle atrophies) and some hereditary sensory and autonomic neuropathies (e.g., familial dysautonomia) are generally conceptualized as PNS neuronopathies (see Chapter 10). Some toxic neuronopathies (e.g., mercury) also affect CNS neurons. Toxic PNS sensory neuronopathies have been produced in experimental animals by doxorubicin and pyridoxine megavitaminosis. Motor and sensory neuronopathy syndromes have been reported as remote complications of carcinoma.

HYPOTHETICAL MECHANISM. No single mechanism explains the pathophysiology of these heterogenous conditions. Indeed, even when the pathologic changes are obvious, as in some of the infectious or hereditary conditions, there is as yet no rationale for these events, e.g., the affinity of the virus of poliomyelitis for the anterior horn cell. Recent studies of experimental doxorubicin PNS sensory neuronopathy indicate that the pathogenesis and evolution of the changes is best understood as an initial disruption of metabolism of sensory nerve cells followed rapidly by degeneration throughout the length of their processes.[9] The dorsal root and Gasserian ganglion neurons are believed to be particularly vulnerable to some circulating toxins because of the special permeability of their blood vessels.

Cardinal Pathologic Features of Experimental Doxorubicin Toxic Sensory Neuronopathy (Figure 9)

(a) Circulating doxorubicin leaks through the normally fenestrated blood vessels in dorsal root and autonomic ganglia.
(b) Doxorubicin binds to nuclei of cells and disrupts protein synthesis.

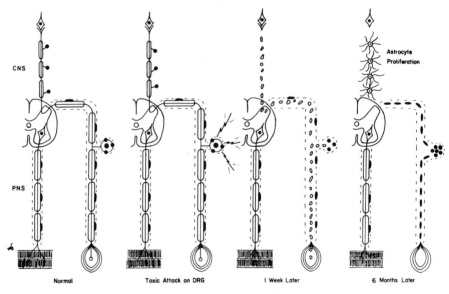

TOXIC SENSORY NEURONOPATHY

FIGURE 9. A diagram of the cardinal features of a rapidly involving toxic sensory neuronopathy. The jagged lines (lightning bolts) indicate that the toxin is directed at neurons in the dorsal root ganglion (DRG). Degeneration of these cells is accompanied by fragmentation and phagocytosis of their peripheral-central processes. The Schwann cells remain; there is no axonal regeneration.

(c) Pathologic changes appear in the neuronal perikaryon, soon followed by degeneration throughout the length of the axon.

(d) Motor cells are not affected and muscle undergoes no change.

(e) Regeneration cannot occur and sensory loss is therefore permanent.

Clinicopathologic Correlation in the Subacute Sensory Neuronopathy Syndrome

(a) Rapid or subacute onset: This reflects the latency before degeneration occurs in the sensory neurons.

(b) Initial sensory loss may occur anywhere: Characteristic of this disorder is the early appearance of numbness of the face *pari passu* with diffuse sensory loss in the extremities. Presumably this occurs because Gasserian ganglion neurons are affected at the same time as dorsal root ganglion neurons.

(c) Diffuse sensory loss and ataxia with preservation of strength: The loss of sensation and sensory ataxia reflect the disappearance of sensory neurons. In most subacute sensory neuronopathies, large-fiber modalities are heavily affected so that the proprioceptive deficit is greater than pain or thermal sense loss. Sparing of anterior horn cells accounts for preservation of strength. The pattern of sensory loss is depicted in Figure 10.

(d) Absent tendon reflexes: One of the hallmarks of this condition that reflects the large fiber sensory loss.

(e) Normal motor nerve conduction, slowed or absent sensory conduction: This mirrors the pattern of selective nerve cell loss.

(f) CSF protein variably elevated: This reflects the etiology of the neuronopathy. Inflammatory neuronopathies may be associated with elevated CSF protein.

(g) Variable recovery: This reflects the death of the nerve cell body and consequent permanent loss of axons. Some cells may be only slightly impaired and transiently function poorly, but are able to reconstitute themselves without losing their axons. This phenomenon, or collateral sprouting from surviving axons, may account for what variable recovery occurs in these conditions.

(h) Signs of CNS disease: The pure PNS sensory neuronopathy syndromes are not accompanied by CNS degeneration aside from fiber loss in the central projections of the sensory neurons (dorsal columns). However, some sensory neuronopathy syndromes (e.g., carcinomatous sensory neuronopathy, methyl mercury intoxication) accompany pathologic processes that involve the CNS as well (see Chapters 12 and 13).

FOCAL (MONONEUROPATHY) and MULTIFOCAL (MULTIPLE MONONEUROPATHY) NEUROPATHIES

Ischemia

GENERAL. The PNS, unlike the CNS, is usually minimally affected by large-vessel disorders. The principal reason for this resistance is the richly collateralized blood supply of peripheral nerve. In general, ischemia of peripheral nerve is synonymous with widespread small artery or arteriolar disease, and is most frequently associated with diabetes mellitus or the necrotizing vasculitides (see Chapter 15).

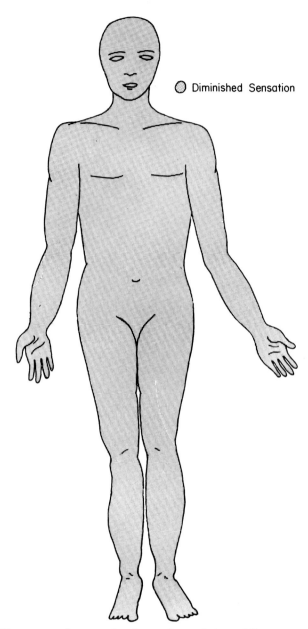

Diminished Sensation

FIGURE 10. The pattern of sensory loss in an advanced stage of the sensory neuronopathy syndrome. Sensation is diminished, often markedly, throughout. This distribution reflects diffuse destruction of sensory ganglion neurons.

PATHOGENETIC HYPOTHESIS. There is considerable controversy surrounding the nature and mechanism of vascular injury to peripheral nerve. It is generally held that in the vasculitides the nerve fiber damage results from local ischemia.[10]

Cardinal Pathological Features

(a) Compromise of several small arteries at one level in a nerve results in ischemia to an entire segment of nerve (mononeuropathy). Occasionally, multiple levels of *several* nerves may be simultaneously affected, resulting in a diffuse patchy neuropathy (multiple mononeuropathy). The lesions may summate to produce bilaterally symmetrical involvement.

(b) Axonal degeneration occurs in many fibers and Wallerian-like degeneration appears below the level of ischemia. Central fascicular degeneration is often pronounced.

(c) Infarct necrosis is rare and connective tissue elements usually are spared.

(d) Muscles undergo denervation atrophy.

(e) Collateral circulation begins.

(f) Regenerative potential is usually good (especially in diabetes mellitus) because of intact connective tissue. The vasculitides may have a poor prognosis because of continuing arteriolar necrosis and involvement of other organs.

Clinicopathologic Correlation in Diabetic Multiple Mononeuropathy Syndrome (see Chapter 4)

(a) Rapid onset is characteristic but not invariable, possibly reflecting occlusion of vessels. Pain frequently accompanies this neuropathy, often local and probably related to ischemia of the nervi nervorum.

(b) Initial findings are in the distribution of the ischemic nerves. The distribution of sensory loss in a typical case of multiple mononeuropathy is depicted in Figure 11.

(c) Weakness more striking than sensory loss: This may reflect the relative resistance of small myelinated and unmyelinated sensory axons to ischemia. Pain may persist for several weeks.

(d) Reflex loss in distribution of affected nerves: This probably reflects the vulnerability of large-diameter myelinated fibers to ischemia.

(e) Motor nerve conduction slightly reduced and may be accompanied by denervation atrophy. Sensory conduction may be near normal, as in (d), above.

(f) CSF protein: May be elevated in any diabetic patient and does not reflect ischemia to the distal nerves.

(g) Gradual recovery: Reflects the slow rate of axonal regeneration and will vary inversely with the locus of the ischemia, that is, the more distal lesion will recover sooner. Mild lesions, featured predominantly by segmental demyelination may recover rapidly, as in lesions of the third cranial nerve.

Infiltration

GENERAL. This heterogeneous group includes unusual tissue reactions that disrupt the continuity of nerve fibers and connective tissue and may eventually totally destroy the internal architecture of a nerve. Leprosy, amyloidosis, sarcoidosis, leukemic and lymphomatous infiltrates, perineurial xanthoma, Schwannoma, and sensory perineuritis are examples.

MECHANISM. Each condition produces secondary effects on nerve fibers. Most are subacute conditions and randomly destroy fibers. Some, especially the granulomas, give rise to an inflammatory response which, in concert with fibroblast proliferation, totally disrupt axons and Schwann cell tubes. Eventually, segments of nerve fascicles are converted into bundles of scar tissue through which regenerating fibers cannot pass.

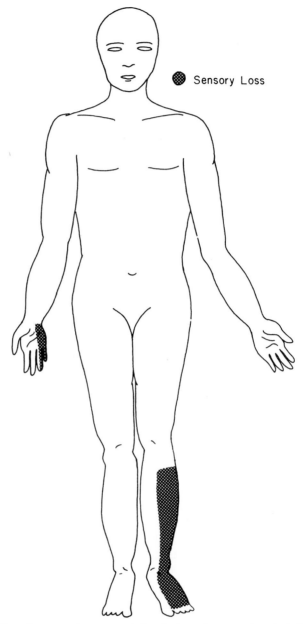

Sensory Loss

FIGURE 11. This illustrates the scattered distribution of sensory loss in ischemic multiple mononeuropathy, with involvement of contralateral ulnar and peroneal nerves.

Cardinal Pathologic Features of Lepromatous Leprosy (see Chapter 16)

(a) Formation of granulomas in vulnerable cutaneous nerves.

(b) Axons are disrupted and Schwann cell tubes disorganized at level of granuloma.

(c) Wallerian degeneration occurs distal to the level of granuloma, resulting in anesthetic skin.

(d) Reactive connective tissue proliferation prevents axonal regeneration.

Clinicopathologic Correlation in Lepromatous Leprosy (Chapter 16)

(a) Gradual onset: This reflects the indolent granulomatous response to the bacilli.

(b) Predominant involvement of superficial cutaneous nerves: The granulomas mainly develop in superficially situated nerves, as *M. leprae* bacilli proliferate more rapidly at lower temperatures. The manifestations are therefore predominantly sensory. Leprosy bacilli initially colonize Schwann cells, especially those associated with unmyelinated and small myelinated axons, resulting in selective pain and temperature sensory loss and anhidrosis.

(c) Permanent anesthesia: The granulomatous lesion totally destroys the architecture of the nerve.

(d) Nerve entrapment may occur because of the granulomatous enlargement of nerve trunks.

(e) CSF protein normal: The spinal roots are not involved in this disease of nerve.

Physical Injuries

GENERAL. Nerves are very susceptible to the effects of externally applied pressure. In general, damage to a nerve fiber appears to increase in proportion to the velocity, force, and duration of the traumatic agent, with the additional factors of traction and friction exaggerating the degree of injury.

There is widespread agreement about the basic three-stage classification of nerve injury, although the pathogeneses of these lesions, especially the mild lesions, remain controversial.[11,12,13] This section outlines and illustrates the salient stages of nerve response to injury. Chapters 17 and 18 discuss the features of acute and chronic nerve trauma.

CLASSIFICATION. This classification is based on three stages (Classes 1, 2 and 3) of seriate vulnerability of components of peripheral nerve to injury; thus, slight injury affects myelin, more severe injury, the axon, and the most severe disrupts connective tissue.

Class 1 (Neurapraxia). Conduction block is the hallmark of Class 1 compression injury and may be due either to transient ischemia or to paranodal demyelination. Ischemia results in a rapidly reversible loss of function associated with transient vascular blockade. Paranodal demyelination occurs with more severe compression and is a mild structural nerve injury. Dysfunction persists in the distribution of the affected nerve until paranodal remyelination occurs, usually after a few weeks (Figure 12).[14]

Class 2 (Axonotmesis). Axons are interrupted by a crush lesion, but the Schwann cell basal lamina and endoneurial tissue remain intact. Wallerian degeneration occurs below the site of injury. Axonal regeneration commences promptly after injury, and the growing axons reach proximal targets before distal sites of innervation (Figure 13).

Class 3 (Neurotmesis). The axon is severed and the connective tissue disrupted, ranging from endoneurial and Schwann cell tube transection to total nerve severence.[12] Wallerian degeneration is inevitable and axon regeneration is severely limited by distorted connective tissue. Neuroma formation and aberrant regeneration are common (Figure 14).

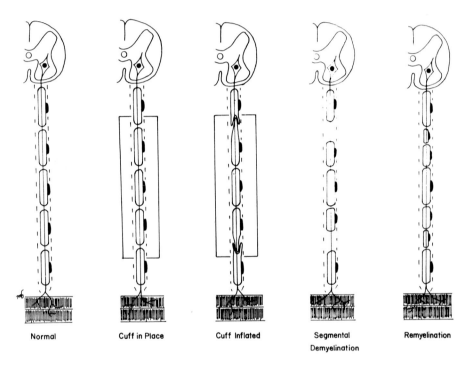

| Normal | Cuff in Place | Cuff Inflated | Segmental Demyelination | Remyelination |

CLASS I — ACUTE NERVE INJURY
(e.g. Compression)

FIGURE 12. Class 1 (neurapraxia) nerve injury associated with compression by a cuff. Axon movement at both edges of the cuff causes intussusception of the attached myelin across the node of Ranvier into the adjacent paranode. Affected paranodes demyelinate. Remyelination begins following cuff removal and conduction eventually resumes. Conduction is normal in the nerve above and below the cuff since the axon has not been damaged.

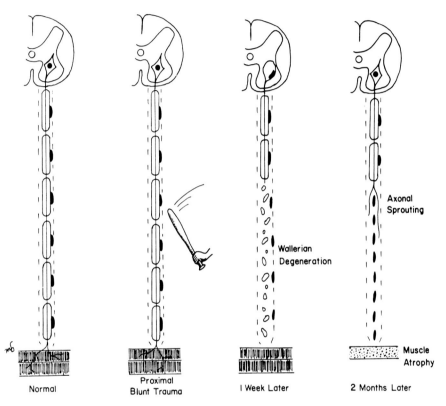

Normal   Proximal   I Week Later   2 Months Later
           Blunt Trauma

Axonal
Sprouting

Wallerian
Degeneration

Muscle
Atrophy

CLASS 2 NERVE INJURY

FIGURE 13. Class 2 nerve injury (axonotmesis) from a crush injury to a limb. Axonal disruption occurs at the site of injury. Wallerian degeneration takes place throughout the axon distal to the injury with loss of axon, myelin, and nerve conduction. Preservation of Schwann cell tubes and other endoneurial connective tissue ensures that regenerating axons have the opportunity to reach their previous terminals and, hopefully, re-establish functional connections.

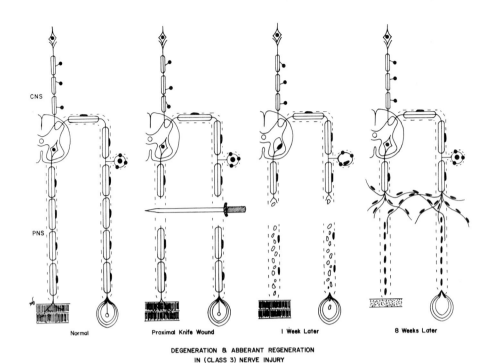

FIGURE 14. Class 3 nerve injury (neurotmesis) with severance of all neural and connective tissue elements. There is little hope of functional recovery without skilled surgery. Regenerating axons are entering inappropriate Schwann cell tubes (aberrant regeneration).

Clinicopathologic Correlation of Nerve Injuries (see Chapter 17 and 18)

Class 1. This lesion is commonly associated with moderate focal compression of nerve, for example, "Saturday night palsy." The motor deficit usually exceeds sympathetic and sensory loss. This reflects the low vulnerability of unmyelinated sympathetic and small myelinated sensory fibers, and the dependence of motor function upon larger myelinated axons which undergo focal demyelination. Nerve conduction remains preserved in the intact, still myelinated axons below the injury. The good prognosis and rapid recovery (usually weeks) from Class 1 lesions reflects both the preservation of axonal continuity and the ability of Schwann cells rapidly and effectively to remyelinate the demyelinated segments. Unlike axonal lesions, recovery occurs simultaneously throughout the distribution of the affected nerve.

Class 2. This lesion is commonly associated with severe closed-crush injuries to an extremity. Complete loss of sensory, sympathetic, and motor function may occur from interruption and unmyelinated and myelinated fibers. Nerve conduction fails below the lesion as the axons degenerate. Muscle atrophy may ensue. The prognosis is good (especially after distal lesions) since the axons can regenerate within their original Schwann cell tubes and the pattern of motor and sensory restoration will be appropriate. The course of recovery is slow (usually months) and proximal to distal, reflecting the rate and of course axonal regeneration.

DISORDERS OF PERIPHERAL NERVES

22

Class 3. These lesions are usually associated with severe traction injuries or open wounds. They have a poor prognosis because connective tissue disruption and proliferation interfere with axonal regeneration. Surgical repair with or without autotransplants is often required.

REFERENCES

1. SPENCER, PS AND SCHAUMBURG, HH: *Classification of neurotoxic disease: a morphological approach.* In SPENCER, PS AND SCHAUMBURG, HH (eds): Experimental and Clinical Neurotoxicology. Williams & Wilkins, Baltimore, 1980, p 92.
2. SCHAUMBURG, HH AND SPENCER, PS: *Clinical and experimental studies of distal axonopathy: a frequent form of nerve and brain damage produced by environmental chemical hazards.* Ann NY Acad Sci 329:14, 1979.
3. SPENCER, PS ET AL.: *Does a defect in energy metabolism in the nerve fiber underlie axon degeneration in polyneuropathies?* Ann Neurol 5:501, 1979.
4. SPENCER, PS AND SCHAUMBURG, HH: *Ultrastructural studies of the dying-back process. IV. Differential vulnerability of PNS and CNS fibers in experimental central-peripheral distal axonopathies.* J. Neuropathol Exp Neurol 36:300, 1977.
5. SPENCER, PS AND SCHAUMBURG, HH: *Ultrastructural studies of the dying-back process. III. The evolution of experimental peripheral giant axonal degeneration.* J Neuropathol Exp Neurol 36:276, 1977.
6. ASBURY, AK, ARNASON, BG AND ADAMS, RD: *The inflammatory lesion in idiopathic polyneuritis: Its role in pathogenesis.* Medicine 48:173, 1969.
7. WAKSMAN, BH AND ADAMS, RD: *Allergic neuritis: an experimental disease of rabbits induced by the injection of peripheral nervous tissue and adjuvants.* J Exp Med 102:213, 1955.
8. PLEASURE, DB, FELDMAN, B AND PROKOP, DJ: *Diphtheria toxin inhibits the synthesis of myelin proteolipid and basic proteins by peripheral nerve in vitro.* J Neurochem 20:81, 1973.
9. CHO, ES, SPENCER, PS AND JORTNER, BS: *Doxorubicin.* In SPENCER, PS AND SCHAUMBURG, HH (eds): Experimental and Clinical Neurotoxicology. Williams & Wilkins, Baltimore, 1980, p 430.
10. DYCK, PJ, CONN, DL AND OKAZAKI, H: *Necrotizing angiopathic neuropathy: three dimensional morphology of fiber degeneration related to sites of occluded vessels.* Mayo Clin Proc 47:461, 1972.
11. SEDDON, HJ: Surgical Disorders of the Peripheral Nerves. ed 2, Churchill Livingston, Edinburgh, 1975.
12. SUNDERLAND, S: Nerves and Nerve Injuries. ed 2, Churchill Livingston, Edinburgh, 1978.
13. THOMAS, PK: *Nerve injury.* In BELLAIRS, R AND GRAY, EG (eds). Essays on the Nervous System. Clarendon Press, Oxford, p 44.
14. OCHOA, J: *Nerve fiber pathology in acute and chronic compression.* In OMER, GE AND SPINNER, M (eds): Management of Peripheral Nerve Problems. WB Saunders, Philadelphia, 1980, p 487.

Chapter 3

THE INFLAMMATORY POLYNEUROPATHIES (GUILLAIN-BARRÉ SYNDROME AND RELATED DISORDERS)

THE GUILLAIN-BARRÉ SYNDROME (POST-INFECTIOUS POLYNEUROPATHY, ACUTE IDIOPATHIC INFLAMMATORY POLYNEUROPATHY).

Definition

The Guillain-Barré syndrome is a rapidly evolving, paralytic illness of unknown etiology. Its salient pathologic feature is widespread inflammatory PNS demyelination, presumably secondary to a hypersensitivity reaction.[1] Although the etiology is unknown, many cases follow nonspecific viral infections, and some are clearly associated with other events such as immunization, surgery, fever therapy.[2]

Pathology, Animal Models and Pathogenesis

PATHOLOGY. Endoneurial infiltration by mononuclear inflammatory cells is the hallmark of this condition. This is followed by widespread, multifocal segmental demyelination with relative sparing of axons (See Figure 7, Chapter 2). The endoneurial infiltrates are mostly lymphocytes and monocytes, with occasional plasma cells. They are frequently perivenous. Polymorphonuclear leukocytes are present only in the most fulminant cases. The blood vessels appear normal.

Both segmental demyelination and inflammation are usually most pronounced in the ventral roots, limb-girdle plexuses, and proximal nerve trunks; changes also occur in dorsal roots, autonomic ganglia, and distal peripheral nerves.[3] Axonal degeneration is an occasional finding, and is widely held to result from axonal interruption in zones of especially intense inflammation. Chromatolytic change may then occur in the anterior horn and dorsal root ganglion cells. Loss of these cells, or proximal axonal transection, probably accounts for poor clinical recovery in some cases. The primary lesions usually are confined to the PNS, and inflammatory change in the CNS is extremely rare.[1]

Within two weeks of the onset of acute demyelination, Schwann cell proliferation occurs—a prelude to remyelination of the denuded internodes. In later stages of the disease, remyelination is the predominant feature and the inflammation subsides. A few inflammatory cells may persist for years within the endoneurium of otherwise normal-appearing nerves, and possibly are significant in the pathogenesis of recurrent cases.[1]

The morphologic events of the acute demyelinating process have been extensively investigated[4,5] and, in combination with animal studies, have strongly contributed to an understanding of the pathogenesis of the Guillain-Barré syndrome. Ultrastructural study of the acute demyelination in this syndrome reveals phagocytes disrupting the Schwann cell, stripping away and phagocytizing the normal-appearing myelin. The axon usually is unaffected. This pattern of myelin loss does not occur in the other demyelinating neuropathies (diphtheria, etc.) and, among human disorders, appears unique to the Guillain-Barré syndrome and related conditions.

ANIMAL MODELS. PNS inflammatory demyelination also occurs in three animal diseases: experimental allergic neuritis,[6] coonhound paralysis[7] and Marek's disease.[8] Experimental allergic neuritis (EAN) is a disorder induced in any mammal by injection of peripheral nerve. EAN can also be produced by sensitization with galactocerebroside (discussed later in this chapter under Chronic Relapsing Polyneuropathy). Peripheral nerve-induced EAN is considered especially relevant to human Guillain-Barré syndrome since it mimics the clinical and pathologic features of the human illness.[6] Its salient features are: (1) generalized ascending paralysis beginning about two weeks after injection with mammalian peripheral myelin or myelin P_2 basic protein; (2) paralysis is accompanied by widespread PNS inflammatory demyelination and recovery follows disappearance of the inflammation and remyelination; (3) the disease can be transferred passively to another animal by lymphoid cells,[9] that is, this appears to be a disease of delayed hypersensitivity; (4) the disease can be prevented by immunosuppression of the animal.[2] Coonhound paralysis is an acute illness occurring in susceptible dogs after a raccoon bite[7] or injection with raccoon saliva,[10] and Marek's disease is a disorder of susceptible fowl associated with infection by an oncogenic group B herpes virus.[8] Neither of these naturally occurring conditions has been as well studied as EAN, and their relevance to the Guillain-Barré syndrome remains *sub judice.*

PATHOGENESIS. It is generally held that Guillain-Barré syndrome is an autoimmune disorder of delayed hypersensitivity[1,2] analogous to experimental allergic neuritis, although this is by no means fully established.[11,12] The demyelination in EAN allegedly is controlled by lymphocytes that have become transformed in response to the injected antigen (peripheral myelin or P_2 basic protein). The transformed lymphocytes attract macrophages to peripheral nerve and presumably direct an attack on myelin. The myelin sheath degenerates, impulse conduction is disrupted, and weakness ensues. Since the process is directed against peripheral myelin, all nerves and roots are potential targets, and the involvement is frequently diffuse, albeit with a proximal predilection. Recovery is associated with remyelination, which usually begins within a few weeks of the onset of the inflammatory event and may be rapid.[1,2]

Two cardinal problems remain if EAN is to be fully accepted as the model of the Guillain-Barré syndrome. First, in the Guillain-Barré syndrome the antigen is unknown; and second, the disease must somehow be related to the diverse conditions (Table 2) that precede it.[2] Also, it may develop in situations where cell-mediated immunity is depressed,[13] as in Hodgkin's disease. Theories abound, but none is wholly satisfactory.[14,15] It has been suggested that, in cases following viral infection, many of the implicated viruses incorporate host cell membrane in their coats, then become immunogenic.[2] Cases following immunization may result from injection of a substance antigenically similar to peripheral myelin, and the hypersensitivity reaction is subsequently misdirected. None explains the association with surgery, pregnancy, or neoplasm; however, it has been proposed that these conditions are associated with immunologic alterations, and this may culminate in an attack on peripheral myelin.[2] It is also possible that all antecedent events act simply to rekindle a latent hypersensitivity reaction in a susceptible individual.

It has also been suggested that circulating demyelinating antibodies may have a role in the pathogenesis of the disease.[14,15] Antimyelin antibodies have been found in the sera of most acute cases,[16] and the sera are capable of causing experimental demyelination. The source of these antibodies and their importance in the pathogenesis of the Guillain-Barré syndrome are currently under debate.[14,15,17,18,19]

Clinical Features

INCIDENCE. The Guillain-Barré syndrome is a world-wide illness. It is the most frequent cause of acute paralytic illness in young adults (9.5 cases per million in US). The age distribution is bimodal, the majority of cases occur among young adults, and there is second, lesser peak in the 45 to 64 age group. Males are slightly more susceptible. Cases occur throughout the year.[20]

PREDISPOSING FACTORS. Table 2 lists antecedent events that have been implicated in Guillain-Barré syndrome. Studies of HLA antigens among Guillain-Barré syndrome patients have revealed no consistent pattern that would indicate a predisposition.[21] Sixty percent of cases have an antecedent

TABLE 2. Antecedent Events For Guillain-Barré Syndrome

1. VIRAL INFECTIONS	2. OTHER INFECTIONS	6. MALIGNANCY
Measles	Mycoplasma pneumoniae	Hodgkins disease
Mumps	Salmonella typhosa	Carcinoma
Rubella	Listerosis	Lymphoma
Influenza A	Brucellosis	
Influenza B	Tularemia	7. PREGNANCY
Varicella-zoster	Ornithosis	
Cytomegalo virus		
Epstein-Barr virus	3. VACCINES	
Infectious mononucleosis	Rabies	
Vaccinia	Swine Flu	
Variola		
Infectious hepatitis	4. SURGERY	
Coxsackie		
ECHO	5. FEVER THERAPY	

upper respiratory or gastrointestinal illness within one month of onset. Immunization against rabies or with A/New Jersey influenza (Swine Flu) vaccine usually produces symptoms within 10 days to 3 weeks following the injection.[20] The pattern of illness is generally similar whatever the predisposing factor, although slight variations have been described; for example, an increase in sensory complaints and cranial nerve findings occurred in cases associated with the US Swine Flu immunization. Infectious mononucleosis may be accompanied by an inflammatory demyelinating polyneuropathy indistinguishable from the Guillain-Barré syndrome.[2] Usually a meningoencephalitic illness is associated with the neuropathy of infectious mononucleosis, and signs of central nervous system involvement may dominate the clinical picture.

SIGNS AND SYMPTOMS. There is now broad agreement on the semiology of the Guillain-Barré syndrome.[11,22,23] It may be most simply described as a rapidly progressive, largely reversible, motor neuropathy. Progressive and usually symmetrical weakness, combined with hyporeflexia, are the cardinal clinical features. Weakness usually begins in the distal lower limbs and may appear to spread upwards (ascending paralysis) over the entire body. This pattern is by no means inevitable; many cases may present with weakness in proximal lower limb muscles. Initial involvement may also occur in the upper limbs. The eventual degree of paralysis is variable, encompassing a broad spectrum that includes the occasional individual who never progresses beyond a mild foot-drop, to others with extreme weakness of all four extremities and facial muscles. Severe involvement may eventuate, with flaccid quadriplegia, inability to breathe, swallow, or speak. Limb weakness is generally symmetrical, and early muscle atrophy uncommon.

Facial weakness, present in many cases, is a striking feature of this illness, and helps to distinguish the Guillain-Barré syndrome from most other neuropathies, apart from those related to sarcoidosis. Facial diplegia and other lower cranial nerve palsies usually occur, together with weakness of the extremities. Extraocular muscle paralysis, present in about 10 percent of cases, may be the presenting sign and, rarely, the only muscles affected.

The tendon reflexes are usually absent, even in cases where weakness is confined to the distal extremities. On occasion, feeble tendon reflexes may be elicited in strong proximal muscle groups. Preservation of tendon reflexes in severely weakened muscles should seriously challenge the diagnosis.

Sensory symptoms, usually distal paresthesias, are present in most cases, rarely persist or progress (in contrast to the weakness), and generally are not accompanied by signs of a profound loss of sensation. Mild impairment of distal position and vibration sensation, and slight loss of pinprick over the toes, are commonly present. Marked sensory loss accompanied by pain or severe dyesthesias is very unusual.

Autonomic dysfunction occurs in many cases, probably reflecting involvement of the myelinated preganglionic fibers and the ganglia. Orthostatic hypotension and hypertension are frequent, may result from denervation supersensitivity, are very difficult to treat, and can seriously complicate the management of patients with respiratory compromise. In individuals who appear otherwise clinically stable, fatalities follow sudden, unexplained fluctuation in blood pressure or cardiac dysrhythmias. Tachycardia occurs in one-half of the cases, and transient bladder paralysis has been documented in several individuals. Persistent, severe bladder or bowel dysfunction has not been described.

Difficulty in walking is a common early complaint. It may take several forms, including bilateral foot-drop or a waddling, wide-based, unsteady gait. Rarely, limb ataxia, paralysis of eye movements, and diffuse hyporeflexia may be the sole manifestations (Miller Fisher syndrome).[24]

Central nervous system involvement is not part of this illness. Features such as a sharply defined abdominal sensory level, unequivocally extensor plantar responses, an internuclear ophthalmoplegia, or vertical nystagmus, render the diagnosis doubtful.[25]

Increased intracranial pressure and papilledema may occur rarely late in the illness. Raised intracranial pressure is often associated with an increase in the CSF protein level. This association has generated speculation that the elevated CSF protein is somehow responsible for the raised pressure, either by increasing the CSF viscosity or blocking the arachnoid villi. However, these hypotheses are no longer favored and the pathogenesis of the raised intracranial pressure remains obscure.

Most individuals do not appear systemically ill while becoming weak, and constitutional signs such as fever, chills, and weight loss are unusual.

COURSE. Rapid progression of weakness is characteristic of the Guillain-Barré syndrome; paralysis is maximal by one week in more than half, by three weeks in 80 percent, and one month in 90 percent. The remaining 10 percent will usually progress for variable intervals up to eight weeks. The Guillain-Barré syndrome should not be diagnosed with confidence in individuals who are either maximally weak within two days, or progress for more than two months.

Recovery usually begins within two to four weeks after progression ceases. The pattern of recovery is extremely variable, normally proceeds at a steady pace, and within six months 85 percent of cases are ambulatory. Occasional individuals experience a dramatic improvement and are able to return to work within two months following a quadriparetic episode. Rare cases show little or no improvement. Recurrences occur in approximately 3 percent of cases, and the clinical profile is an acute monophasic illness resembling the original episode. Recovery may be slow. Several recurrences may occur, and may be antedated by immunizations, surgery, or nondescript illnesses. The physiologic basis for rapid onset and recovery in the Guillain-Barré syndrome has been recently reviewed.[19]

PROGNOSIS. Although in time most individuals have an excellent functional recovery, this is not a benign illness. The overall mortality is 5 percent, and more than 50 percent of all individuals retain evidence of damage to the peripheral nervous system. Sixteen percent remain significantly handicapped by weakness. We have encountered several individuals with persistent dysesthesias in the feet in addition to weakness of dorsiflexion, and many instances of mild facial assymetry and hyporeflexia. There may be persistent abnormalities of nerve conduction.

Few features of the initial clinical illness are of help in predicting the eventual outcome. In general, individuals who experience only mild distal extremity weakness and subsequently improve within weeks of the first sign, have excellent recovery. Atrophy and denervation potentials in distal muscles indicate axonal transection or nerve cell death, and often are associated with incomplete or very prolonged recovery. Curiously, objective sensory loss, papilledema, and CSF pleocytosis are of no value as prognostic signs.

Laboratory Studies

ROUTINE CLINICAL LABORATORY. A moderate increase in circulating polymorphonuclear leukocytes is present early in the illness, and lymphocytosis occurs later. Serum immunoglobulins IgG, IgA and IgM may be elevated.

SPECIAL LABORATORY TESTS. Circulating, activated, protein-synthesizing lymphocytes are present in early cases, and their numbers allegedly correlate with the severity of the illness.[2] Complement-dependent antimyelin antibodies are present in the serum of many acute cases. Lymphocytes from acute Guillain-Barré syndrome patients may also be activated by exposure to peripheral nerve in tissue culture.[26] Serologic evidence of infection with either cytomegalovirus or Epstein-Barr virus is described in a substantial number of individuals with the Guillain-Barré syndrome.[27]

CEREBROSPINAL FLUID. The CSF protein is usually normal during the first three days of illness; it then steadily rises and may even reach extraordinarily high levels. A mid-zone colloid gold curve is often present in the early stage, reflecting an elevated IgA component. The CSF protein may remain elevated for several months, even after recovery is underway.[2]

Mononuclear cells, usually less than 10 per mm^3, are present in up to one-half of the cases. Exceptionally, they may number up to 50 cells per mm^3.

ELECTRODIAGNOSTIC STUDIES. Early in the illness, distal motor nerve conduction may be normal. Presumably, in such cases the disease process is confined to spinal roots and proximal nerves. Should the demyelination be present in distal nerves as well, then more profound slowing of motor conduction, characteristic of segmental demyelination, will occur. Analysis of the F response, a measurement of proximal motor conduction, may be of value in cases of suspected Guillain-Barré syndrome that display normal distal motor conduction.[28]

Sensory nerve conduction is often normal and electromyography usually does not reveal widespread denervation changes, unless axons have been damaged in the inflammatory process or nerves have become compressed in a chronically bedridden individual.

NERVE BIOPSY. Nerve biopsy is seldom indicated in the Guillain-Barré syndrome. The diagnosis can usually be established on clinical grounds with the aid of less invasive techniques. The distal cutaneous or subcutaneous nerves chosen for conventional biopsy are frequently not involved in the inflammatory demyelinating process and the specimen may be normal. Should occasional fibers display Wallerian degeneration, the biopsy results may be misleading.

TREATMENT. The patient suspected of having the Guillain-Barré syndrome must be admitted to the hospital even if the involvement is minimal, since the neuropathy often progresses rapidly and unpredictably. In general, such patients should be admitted directly to a respiratory care unit and remain until the condition has stabilized or is clearly improving. The tidal volume, oxygen saturation, vital capacity, blood pressure, and ability to cough and swallow should be closely monitored, as they can change without warning.

If mechanical ventilation is necessary (as determined by the degree of respiratory effort, the vital capacity, and the blood gases), it should be instituted early rather than waiting until the last moment.[29] Endotracheal intubation is usually performed initially, and replaced by a cuffed tracheostomy after five days if there is insufficient improvement. Postural drainage and chest percussion may be helpful in preventing atelectasis and pneumonia.

Loss of autonomic reflexes may eventuate, with peripheral pooling of blood, poor venous return, and low cardiac output. Positive-pressure respiration may further impede venous return and aggravate this situation. Rapid decrease in blood pressure may occur, and should be treated initially by fluid replacement. Pharmacologic manipulation of blood pressure in the Guillain-Barré syndrome patients is extremely perilous and should be avoided unless absolutely necessary. Attempts to prevent cardiac dysrthythmias by measures such as the combined administration of atropine and a beta adrenergic blocking drug have not yet been adequately evaluated.

Some patients will be unable to swallow or to gag. Feeding should be done through a small nasogastric tube. The patient should be sitting when food is given, and kept sitting for 30 to 60 minutes afterwards to minimize the risk of aspiration.

The patient may be unable to urinate because of abdominal muscle weakness or autonomic involvement. Abdominal compression may be helpful, and catheterization is occasionally necessary. Fecal impaction should be avoided by the use of stool softeners, laxatives, and enemas as required. The paralyzed patient must be turned frequently to avoid pressure sores. A sheepskin or water bed may be used. Low-dose subcutaneous heparin has been employed in an attempt to prevent deep venous thrombosis in the legs and lessen the consequent risk of pulmonary embolism. Passive movement of the limbs must be given, and a footboard should be used to prevent contracture of the calf muscles. If the eyes do not close completely, corneal damage must be prevented with protective solutions and the eyes taped shut at night; a temporary lateral tarsorrhaphy may be required.

The patient may be under severe psychologic stress because of paralysis and the intensive-care environment, and mild sedation occasionally may be necessary. He may be unable to communicate at all, but hospital personnel must not forget that he can see, hear, and understand. The Guillain-Barré syndrome is one cause of the 'locked in' syndrome.

If the patient with the Guillain-Barré syndrome can be carried through the acute stage of progressive paralysis (usually two or three weeks), strength will gradually return. Since most patients make a gratifying recovery after months of weakness, the importance of extremely fastidious supportive care in the acute stage cannot be overstressed.

Anti-inflammatory agents (especially glucocorticoids) have long been advocated in the acute Guillain-Barré syndrome, since it is known that immunosuppressive therapy can prevent EAN. A recent controlled clinical trial has demonstrated that prednisilone is of no benefit in the acute stage and may be detrimental. Its use is therefore contraindicated.[29] Plasmapheresis early in the course of the illness is currently under scrutiny because of promising results in some cases.

Differential Diagnosis

With the decline of poliomyelitis and diphtheria in Europe and North America, the Guillain-Barré syndrome is not usually a difficult diagnosis for a neurologist or experienced internist.

Hypokalemia and tick paralysis are misdiagnosed as the Guillain-Barré syndrome. In addition to being an embarrassing mistake, considerable risk may accrue to the patient with severe hypokalemia if not promptly treated. Therefore, serum electrolytes are immediately obtained on all cases of acute paralysis, and a careful search for a tick is undertaken if the patient comes from an appropriate region.

Acute myelitis or cervical spine fracture have, on occasion, been confused with the Guillain-Barré syndrome. A sharp sensory level and sphincter paralysis at the outset of the illness should raise the suspicion of spinal cord involvement.

Botulism may simulate the Guillain-Barré syndrome. Early prominence of extraocular muscle and lower cranial nerve muscle involvement, pupillary abnormalities, the absence of sensory complaints and normal CSF protein all may raise the possibility of botulism. On occasion, clinical distinction between these entities may be very vexing, especially if there is only mild pupillary involvement in the botulism cases.

Poliomyelitis is generally a febrile illness, frequently occurs in epidemics, is associated with nuchal rigidity and headache, results in assymetrical paralysis and usually is accompanied by an excess of 50 mononuclear cells per mm^3 in the CSF.

Other neuropathies

Porphyria may mimic the Guillain-Barré syndrome. The limb weakness is often proximal in both conditions, but greater involvement of the upper extremities is more characteristic of porphyria. Urine measurement of porphobilinogen and delta aminolevulinic acid should be performed in suspected cases of acute intermittent porphyria.

Toxic neuropathies. Dapsone, nitrofurantoin and thallium all produce neuropathies that may have a subacute onset, and are occasionally confused with the Guillain-Barré syndrome. Individuals, usually adolescent males, who abuse paint thinner or glue (sniffers, huffers), may have rapid onset of a predominantly motor neuropathy and respiratory paralysis. These individuals rarely have cranial nerve palsies, muscle atrophy is profound and, in general, sensory complaints are a persistent problem. A careful history that specifically inquires about medication or social habits will usually disclose those problems.

Case History and Comment

CASE HISTORY. A 35-year-old draftsman and talented amateur musician developed an upper respiratory infection with cough, fever, chills and myalgia, requiring a week of bed rest. He recovered, and 16 days later, noted a pins-and-needles sensation in his feet on awakening. While driving to work, he discovered that he could not manipulate the car's foot controls rapidly. By noon, he was walking with an unsteady gait. Later, he required assistance in climbing the stairs to his home. The next morning he noted an abnormal sensation in his fingers and had difficulty dialing the telephone for an ambulance.

On arrival at the hospital he was apprehensive and complained of weakness and unpleasant sensations in his feet and fingers. Vital signs were normal as was the remainder of the general physical examination. Neurologic examination revealed that he could not arise from a chair, stand, or walk unassisted, but could sit without support. Muscle strength in the lower extremities and distal upper extremities was ⅗ (MRC scale), and ⅘ in the proximal upper extremities. Cranial nerves were unremarkable and the vital capacity was in excess of 3 liters. The tendon reflexes were absent. There was a slight loss of touch, position, and vibration sense in the toes and ankles. Other sensory modalities were intact throughout. The CSF contained 3 mononuclear cells per mm^3 and the protein was 38 mg per dl. Peroneal motor nerve conduction velocities were 50 and 49 meters per second; median nerve motor conduction velocities were 53 and 56 meters per second.

The patient was admitted to the respiratory care unit and vital signs monitored every hour. On the second day, muscle strength in the legs was ⅖ and he could not sit unassisted. By the third day, he was found to have weakness in opening and closing his jaw and slight weakness of neck flexion. The upper extremity muscles were ⅖, the vital capacity was 2 liters and he could not turn in bed unassisted. By the fifth day, facial diplegia was present, and he could not dorsiflex his toes or feet. The vital capacity had declined to 1 liter, an endotracheal tube was inserted and ventilatory support was begun. Repeated lumbar puncture revealed no cells in the CSF and a protein of 280 mg per dl. By the eighth day, he was quadriplegic, had normal eye movements, and could only elevate his shoulders slightly and swallow weakly. He could make no unassisted respiratory effort. Left lower lobe pneumonia developed and was successfully treated with antibiotics. Total ventilatory support was necessary for two weeks. Movements of the face and proximal upper extremities then began to recover, and he began to make a slight voluntary respiratory effort. Within another ten days, ventilatory support was no longer needed. A peritracheal abscess was treated by incision and antibiotics. At this time he was able to sit without support and feed himself. One week later the tracheostomy was removed. He was transferred to the rehabilitation unit, and two months later had regained 80 percent of extremity strength. There was still mild left facial weakness, and tendon reflexes in the lower extremities were absent. Five months following the illness he returned to work, and has since been able to lead an active life. Five years later, the only residual functional deficit is an inability to play the piano with his former dexterity. On examination, the only abnormality is bilateral absence of the Achilles reflex.

COMMENT. Progression of weakness was rapid, requiring prompt hospitalization. The initial lumbar puncture, performed on the second day of illness, revealed a normal CSF protein value, as expected, and subsequently the protein rose to 280 mg per dl. The motor nerve conduction velocities obtained early in the illness were within normal limits, indicating that the bulk of the active demyelination was probably occurring in roots and proximal nerves. Prompt admission to the respiratory care unit enabled close monitoring, and eventual total support of respiratory function. The patient recovered without corticosteroid therapy and, in light of the pneumonia and tracheal infection that occurred, this decision appears sound. The pattern of illness was so typical of the Guillain-Barré syndrome that further studies, such as nerve biopsy, were not justified. The gratifying recovery, without major residual deficit, probably reflects the paucity of axonal degeneration in this case. The diminished pianistic skills may have resulted from asynchronous, slightly slowed conduction in remyelinated nerves and spinal roots.

CHRONIC RELAPSING INFLAMMATORY NEUROPATHY (CRIP) AND CHRONIC INFLAMMATORY POLYNEUROPATHY (CIP)

Definition

Affected individuals have an illness clinically similar to the Guillain-Barré syndrome, although usually with a more gradual onset, but subsequently undergo either a chronic relapsing (CRIP)[30,31] or a chronic progressive course (CIP).[32] The salient histologic features of both chronic forms are remarkably similar to those of the Guillain-Barré syndrome. It is generally held that CRIP and CIP represent clinical variants of the same condition, and may have a pathogenetic mechanism in common with the Guillain-Barré syndrome.[30]

Pathology and Pathogenesis

PATHOLOGY. Thinly myelinated or demyelinated axons, varying degrees of onion-bulb formation, and loss of myelinated fibers are the light microscope hallmarks of both conditions. Endoneurial edema and varying degrees of perivenular mononuclear cell infiltrates are occasionally present. It is alleged that onion-bulb formation is a more prominent feature of the recurrent cases, and lymphocytic infiltration more common in the chronic progressive forms. These changes are distributed throughout proximal nerves and spinal roots. Multifocal or localized pathology occurs but is rare, and may give rise to striking hypertrophy of proximal nerve trunks, for example the brachial plexus.

PATHOGENESIS. It is generally held that the pathogenesis of these disorders is similar to the Guillain-Barré syndrome, that is, they are autoimmune disorders of delayed hypersensitivity analogous to EAN. This notion has been reinforced by two factors: the continued presence of inflammatory cells in the nerves of individuals with the Guillain-Barré syndrome, long after clinical recovery from the monophasic illness and, more importantly, some animals with EAN (usually an acute monophasic illness) pursue a chronic progressive or relapsing course.

The variety of EAN induced in rabbits by sensitization with galactocerebroside may help to illuminate the pathogenesis of the chronic demyelinating neuropathies.[18] The galactocerebroside EAN animal displays a long latent period to disease, a subacute onset, and has a chronic course. In these respects, it more closely resembles CIP than does the usual monophasic illness characteristic of EAN produced by myelin injection. Another contrast between the two EAN models is that the immunologic process in the galactocerebroside-immunized animal appears not to be cell-mediated. Lymphocytes have not been observed during the demyelination, which is largely confined to the spinal roots of these animals.

Clinical Features

INCIDENCE. CIP and CRIP are rare. The peak incidence of CIP is in the fifth and sixth decades and males appear to be more frequently affected.

PREDISPOSING FACTORS. Occasional patients with CIP and CRIP have experienced an antecedent, nonspecific, upper respiratory infection. On the basis of HLA antigen testing, studies of CRIP have suggested that there may exist disease suseptibility genes for this disorder.[33]

SIGNS AND SYMPTOMS. As with the Guillain-Barré syndrome, the cardinal symptoms and signs reflect predominant motor involvement. Weakness of the extremities, intercostal muscles, and lower cranial nerves all occur in CIP and CRIP.[30,31,32]

Sensory complaints are almost as common as weakness, and objective signs of sensory loss are more frequent in the chronic disorders than in the Guillain-Barré syndrome. Hyporeflexia or areflexia have been observed in almost all individuals.

Papilledema was present in 7 percent of one series of patients with CIP, and 11 percent in this same series had nerves that were enlarged to palpation.[32]

COURSE AND PROGNOSIS. The development and course of illness are considered the salient features that distinguish between recurrent examples of the Guillain-Barré syndrome, CRIP, and CIP. Recurrent Guillain-Barré syndrome is characterized by an acute onset and a maximal neurologic deficit within 4 weeks of the initial complaint in each episode. CRIP and CIP generally have a more protracted onset and an indolent progression. The occurrence of subsequent relapsing episodes suggests CRIP,[30] and steady progression, CIP.[32] Clearly, there are many instances where these guidelines become blurred; for example, it may be impossible to distinguish between a fluctuation in the course of a progressing CIP and a relapse in the course of CRIP. This factor, in concert with the histopathologic similarities, leads the authors to believe that CIP and CRIP are variants of the same condition.

The course of CRIP displays considerable variation in the interval between relapses, the severity of an episode, and rate and degree of recovery. Subsequent attacks are generally similar to the initial episode and disability varies considerably. With treatment, improvement is generally good between episodes. Life-threatening episodes with respiratory insufficiency are more common early in the illness. Persistent disability following repeated attacks is variable, and in many instances the attacks cease after a few years.

The course of CIP is usually stepwise but may be gradual. If untreated, this condition may become disabling or fatal. The prognosis of CIP is uncertain since most clinical studies have not attempted to distinguish between this disorder and CRIP.

Laboratory Studies

ROUTINE CLINICAL LABORATORY. Mild elevations of plasma gamma globulin may occur in CIP.

CEREBROSPINAL FLUID. The CSF protein is elevated at some stage of the illness in almost every case of CIP or CRIP, but may fluctuate to normal levels in individuals with either condition.

Mononuclear cells, usually less than 10 per mm^3, are occasionally present in both disorders.

ELECTRODIAGNOSTIC STUDIES. Slowed conduction, sometimes profound, in both motor and sensory nerves, is characteristic of CIP and

CRIP, although not always present. Serial motor nerve conduction studies in CRIP reveal that during times of clinical improvement, conduction velocities may increase.

NERVE BIOPSY. Nerve biopsy may be extremely helpful in the diagnosis of these conditions if one is fortunate enough to select a diseased area. The histologic picture is characteristic for these disorders and consists of: (1) reduction in the number of myelinated fibers (2) axons with abnormally thin myelin, or demyelinated and (3) varying degrees of onion-bulb formation. Endoneural edema and scattered mononuclear cell infiltrates are present in some instances.

Treatment

CIP. It is generally held that corticosteroids are the treatment of choice for CIP. There is suggestive evidence from a controlled study that an alternate day, high-level prednisone regimen results in slight improvement.[32] Some patients continue to worsen despite high-dose corticosteroid and azathioprine treatment. There are few well documented, controlled therapeutic studies of this disorder, and it is possible that some of the therapeutic failures may represent cases of hereditary neuropathy misdiagnosed as CIP.

CRIP. It is generally held that ACTH or glucocorticoids are efficacious in this disorder and sometimes produce dramatic therapeutic responses. Unfortunately, most studies usually include cases of recurrent Guillain-Barré syndrome and have not distinguished them from individuals with CRIP. Thus, some cases of rapid improvement in CRIP following corticosteroid therapy may merely reflect the natural history of recurrent Guillain-Barré syndrome. The issue is further complicated by allegations that corticosteroids also induce remissions in relapsing Guillain-Barré syndrome.

Plasma exchange has recently been introduced as therapy for CRIP, and recent studies have described marked improvement in weakness following the exchange regimen.[34,35] This technique offers an effective alternative to individuals who cannot tolerate corticosteroid or other immunosuppressive therapy, or who have a severe acute relapse necessitating admission to an intensive care unit. However, such improvement is likely to be temporary. The success of this technique may also be evidence for a role of humoral components in the pathogenesis of CRIP.[18]

Hemodialysis has been unsuccessful in the treatment of CRIP.

Differential Diagnosis

CRIP. The differential diagnosis of CRIP is seldom a problem after several episodes have occurred. The characteristic combination of clinical remissions, elevated CSF protein, and profound slowing of motor nerve conduction usually suffice. On occasion, acute intermittent porphyria may mimic this disorder and the appropriate laboratory determinations should be done. Repeated exposure to exogenous toxins should also be ruled out by a careful occupational and environmental history. The differential diagnosis between CRIP and recurrent Guillain-Barré syndrome has been discussed elsewhere.

CIP. The differential diagnosis of CIP is sometimes very difficult. Unless the nerve biopsy displays unequivocal evidence of inflammatory cells and demyelinated fibers, this disorder may be indistinguishable from some hereditary neuropathies. These genetic disorders also are characterized by gradual progression, profound slowing of motor nerve conduction, and onion-bulb formation (see Chapter 16). A careful family history should always be obtained, especially if the illness begins in childhood or adolescence.

Case History of CRIP*

CASE HISTORY. A 65-year-old woman with a history of chronic bronchitis and pylelonephritis noticed pain and weakness in both hands. During the following month she developed progressive weakness of her legs which led to several falls. She also became aware of pain in both arms, tingling paresthesias in her fingers and toes, and some numbness of her fingers. She was admitted to hospital two months following the appearance of the initial symptoms. Examination on admission revealed obesity, hypertension (250/150), and basal crepitations in both lungs. She showed mild right facial weakness, but no other cranial nerve abnormality. She displayed a generalized weakness of her arms and legs affecting proximal and distal muscles, the arms being more affected than the legs. Her tendon reflexes were all absent and the plantar responses flexor. Apart from loss of vibration sense distally in the legs, no sensory abnormality was detected. A blood count was normal and ESR 27 mm at 1 hour. The total serum protein level was normal but electrophoresis showed a slight decrease in albumen and beta globulin. The fasting blood sugar level was normal. No evidence of active urinary infection was discovered and radiography of the chest was normal. The CSF contained 120 mg per dl of protein and 1 lymphocyte per mm^3 three weeks following admission. Motor nerve conduction velocity in the right ulnar nerve, recording from the abductor digiti minimi, was 30 m/s. Fifth finger-wrist sensory nerve action potentials were absent in the right hand.

The weakness in her limbs progressively increased following admission. Her hypertension was treated with bethanidine. Prednisone at a dosage of 30 mg daily was commenced after two weeks. However, this was discontinued after six days because of increasing hypertension and the development of edema. The weakness continued to advance to almost complete paralysis of all four limbs, and because of respiratory distress, she was transferred to the respiratory unit 20 days following admission, although assisted respiration did not become necessary. Over the following month there was some improvement with some return of power in the limbs. A repeat CSF examination, two months following admission, revealed a protein content of 380 mg per dl and 2 lymphocytes per mm^3. By the end of the third month, her condition was noted to have deteriorated again and she was started on 30 mg daily of prednisolone. A sural nerve biopsy revealed a substantial loss of myelin sheaths in transverse sections. Examination of isolated osmicated nerve fibers showed extensive segmental demyelination and remyelination. Her condition remained unaltered and, toward the end of the fourth month, she suddenly developed chest pain and died. The autopsy revealed a recent red infarct in the right lung and complete blockage of the right pulmonary artery with antemortem thrombus. Otherwise the examination showed bilateral chronic pyelonephritis and left ventricular hypertrophy. No carcinoma was detected.

*(Case 5. Thomas et al,[30] with permission)

Portions of cervical, thoracic, and lumbar spinal cord, together with dorsal and ventral spinal nerve roots and dorsal root ganglia from these three levels, were available from the autopsy. The dorsal and ventral spinal roots all showed a moderate loss of myelin sheaths in transverse section, especially in the cervical and lumbar regions. The ventral roots were affected to a greater extent than the dorsal. Little axonal loss was detectable. Single osmicated fibers from a lower lumbar ventral root were examined and showed profuse demyelination and remyelination, with very few normal surviving internodes. Perivenular collections of inflammatory cells, composed predominantly of lymphocytes, were seen at all three levels, most numerous in the ventral roots. The dorsal root ganglia appeared normal apart from some loss of ganglion cells with proliferation of satellite cells. No abnormalities were detected in the spinal cord.

REFERENCES

1. ASBURY, AK, ARNASON, BG AND ADAMS, RD: *The inflammatory lesion in idiopathic polyneuritis: its role in pathogenesis.* Medicine 48:173, 1969.
2. ARNASON, BG: *Inflammatory polyradiculopathies.* In DYCK, PJ, THOMAS, PK AND LAMBERT, EH (eds): Peripheral Neuropathy, Vol 2, WB Saunders, Philadelphia, 1975, p 1110.
3. PRINEAS, JB: *Pathology of the Guillain-Barré syndrome.* Ann Neurol 9 (suppl):6, 1981.
4. WIŚNIEWSKI, H, TERRY, RD, WHITAKER, RD, COOK, SD AND DOWLING, PC: *The Landry Guillain-Barré syndrome. A primary demyelinating disease.* Arch Neurol 21:269, 1969.
5. PRINEAS, JB: *Acute idiopathic polyneuritis. An electron microscope study.* Lab Invest 26:133, 1972.
6. WAXMAN, BH AND ADAMS, RD: *Allergic neuritis: an experimental disease of rabbits induced by the injection of peripheral nervous tissue and adjuvants.* J Exp Med 102:213, 1955.
7. CUMMINGS, JF AND DELAHUNTA, A: *Chronic relapsing polyradiculoneuritis in a dog. A clinical, light and electron-microscopic study.* Acta Neuropathol 28:191, 1974.
8. STEVENS, JG, PEPOSE, JS AND COOK, ML: *Marek's disease: A natural model for the Landry-Guillain-Barré syndrome.* Ann Neurol 9 (suppl):102, 1981.
9. ARNASON, BG AND CHELMICA-SZORC, E: *Passive transfer of experimental allergic neuritis in Lewis rats by direct injection of sensitized lymphocytes into sciatic nerve.* Acta Neuropath 22:1, 1972.
10. HOLMES, DF, ET AL.: *Experimental coonhound paralysis: animal model of Guillain-Barré syndrome.* Neurol 29:1186, 1979.
11. ASBURY, AK: *Diagnostic considerations in Guillain-Barré syndrome.* Ann Neurol 9 (suppl):1, 1981.
12. WHITAKER, JN: *The protein antigens of peripheral nerve myelin.* Ann Neurol 9 (suppl):56, 1981.
3. DRACHMAN, DA, ET AL: *Immunosuppression and the Guillain-Barré syndrome.* Arch Neurol 23:385, 1970.
14. IQBAL, A, OGER, J-F AND ARNASON, BGW: *Cell mediated immunity in idiopathic polyneuritis.* Ann Neurol 9 (suppl):65, 1981.
15. COOK, SD AND DOWLING, PC: *The role of autoantibody and immune complexes in the pathogenesis of Guillain-Barré syndrome.* Ann Neurol 9 (suppl):70, 1981.
16. COOK, SD, ET AL: *Circulating demyelinating factors in acute idiopathic polyneuropathy.* Arch Neurol 24:136, 1971.
17. NYLAND, H, MATRE, R AND MRK, S: *Immunologic characterization of sural nerve biopsies from patients with Guillain-Barré syndrome.* Ann Neurol 9 (suppl):80, 1981.
18. SAIDA, T, SAIDA, K, SILBERBERG, DH AND BROWN, MJ: *Experimental allergic neuritis induced by galactocerebroside.* Ann Neurol 9 (suppl):87, 1981.
19. SUMNER, A: *The physiological basis for symptoms in Guillain-Barré syndrome.* Ann Neurol 9 (suppl):28, 1981.
20. SCHOENBERGER, LB, ET AL: *Guillain-Barré syndrome: Its epidemiology and associations with influenza vaccination.* Ann Neurol 9 (suppl):31, 1981.
21. STEWART, GJ, ET AL: *HLA antigens in the Landry-Guillain-Barré syndrome and chronic relapsing polyneuritis.* Ann Neurol 4:285, 1978.

22. McLEOD, JG, ET AL: *Acute idiopathic polyneuritis: a clinical and electrophysiological follow up study.* J Neurol Sci 27:145, 1976.

23. SOFFER, D, FELDMAN, S AND ALTER, M: *Clinical features of the Guillain-Barré syndrome.* J Neurol Sci 37:135, 1978.

24. FISHER, M: *An unusual variant of acute idiopathic polyneuritis (syndrome of ophthalmoplegia, ataxia and areflexia).* N Eng J Med 255:57, 1956.

25. ASBURY, AK, ET AL: *Criteria for diagnosis of Guillain-Barré syndrome.* Ann Neurol 3:565, 1978.

26. COOK, SD, DOWLING, PC AND WHITAKER, JN: *The Guillain-Barré syndrome: relationship of circulating immunocytes to disease activity.* Arch Neurol 22:470, 1970.

27. DOWLING, PC AND COOK, SD: *Role of infection in Guillain-Barré syndrome: laboratory confirmation in 41 cases.* Ann Neurol 9 (suppl):44, 1981.

28. McLEOD, JG: *Electrophysiological studies in the Guillain-Barré syndrome.* Ann Neurol 9 (suppl):20, 1981.

29. HUGHES, RAC, KADLUBOWSKI, M AND HUFSCHMIDT, A: *Treatment of acute inflammatory polyneuropathy.* Ann Neurol 9 (suppl):125, 1981.

30. THOMAS, PK, ET AL: *Recurrent and chronic relapsing Guillain-Barré polyneuritis.* Brain 92:589, 1969.

31. PRINEAS, JB AND McLEOD, JG: *Chronic relapsing polyneuritis.* J Neurol Sci 27:427, 1970.

32. DYCK, PJ, ET AL: *Chronic inflammatory polyradiculoneuropathy.* Mayo Clin Proc 50:621, 1975.

33. ADAMS, D, ET AL: *HLA antigens in chronic relapsing idiopathic inflammatory polyneuropathy.* J Neurol Neurosurg Psychiat 42:184, 1979.

34. SERVER, A, ET AL: *Treatment of chronic relapsing inflammatory polyradiculoneuropathy by plasma exchange.* Ann Neurol 6:258, 1979.

35. GROSS, MLP AND THOMAS, PK: *The treatment of chronic relapsing and chronic progressive idiopathic inflammatory polyneuropathy by plasma exchange.* J Neurol Sci 52:69, 1981.

Chapter 4

METABOLIC NEUROPATHY: DIABETES

DEFINITION AND CLASSIFICATION

A wide range of peripheral nerve disorders may occur in diabetes mellitus. The varied clinical manifestations of peripheral neuropathy in diabetics probably reflect the multiple causes of nerve degeneration in this disorder. In general, diabetic neuropathies may be classified into two types: the symmetrical polyneuropathies and the isolated nerve lesions (mononeuropathies).[1]

> **Symmetrical polyneuropathy syndromes:**
> Rapidly reversible neuropathy
> Distal, primarily sensory neuropathy
> Autonomic neuropathy
>
> **Mononeuropathy and multiple mononeuropathy syndromes:**
> Cranial nerve lesions
> Focal peripheral nerve lesions
> Proximal, lower-extremity neuropathy (diabetic amyotrophy)

It should be emphasized that mixed syndromes are common, with isolated mononeuropathies, for example, occurring on a background of symmetrical sensory polyneuropathy. For this reason, some authorities have argued that no rational classification is possible.[2] Yet, as will be discussed, the classification outlined here is explicable in terms of the likely underlying pathology.

Pathology, Pathogenesis and Animal Models

Pathology

SYMMETRICAL POLYNEUROPATHIES. Although it is widely assumed that diabetic symmetrical neuropathies have a metabolic basis, pathologic studies have not demonstrated a consistent pattern or distribution of lesions, and they have been of little assistance in elucidating the pathogenesis.[3] Furthermore, these lesions have usually been advanced, nonspecific, and described in individuals with chronic neuropathy. Identification of the early structural lesions in human diabetic neuropathy might provide clues about an underlying metabolic disorder. Nerves obtained at autopsy or biopsy display a mixture of axonal loss and segmental demyelination. Axonal loss is the predominant change in these chronic cases, clearly restricting potential recovery in such individuals. It is claimed that there is selective vulnerability of certain fiber types in diabetic sensory neuropathy, and that this correlates with the clinical syndrome. This idea receives support from one study which demonstrates predominantly small-fiber abnormalities in individuals with pain and autonomic symptoms as major complaints.[4]

Electron microscopy so far has added little. Lipid bodies within Schwann cells may be more numerous than in other neuropathies, and thickening of the basal lamina of Schwann cells and perineurium[5] has been described.

Skeletal muscles may show grouped muscle fiber atrophy typical of denervation. Histochemical fiber-type grouping, indicative of collateral sprouting by surviving axons followed by reinnervation, is prominent. Abnormalities are also detectable in terminal axons at motor endplates, and the basal lamina surrounding muscle fibers may be thickened.

Abnormalities of the vasa nervorum are more common in diabetics than in the general population and were, in the past, considered significant in the pathogenesis of symmetrical neuropathies. Thickening of the walls of endoneurial capillaries by layers of reduplicated basal lamina is prominent.[6] It is now generally conceded that such changes are present to an equal degree in diabetics without evidence of chronic neuropathy, and this etiologic explanation can no longer be upheld.

There are few studies on the autonomic nervous system in patients with diabetic autonomic neuropathy. Enlargement and degeneration of sympathetic chain ganglion cells has been described, together with a reduced density of myelinated fibers and segmental demyelination in the greater splanchnic nerve, and a reduced innervation of lower-limb arterioles.[7]

MONONEUROPATHY. It is widely held that isolated peripheral nerve lesions in diabetics have a vascular basis. Three clinical facts support this notion: they are most common in the elderly, in whom vascular disease is likely to be frequent, may have an abrupt onset, and often improve spontaneously.[1,6]

Two autopsy studies of diabetics who died shortly following the onset of oculomotor palsy describe focal lesions in the intracavernous portion of the corresponding third nerve.[8,9] Destruction of myelin and, to a lesser extent, of axons, is prominent in the central portion of these nerves. No vascular occlusion was demonstrated, but there was pronounced narrowing and hyalinization of adjacent arterioles in one case.[9]

Pathogenesis

SYMMETRICAL POLYNEUROPATHIES. The clinical features of symmetrical polyneuropathies, which often selectively involve particular fiber types, favors a metabolic basis. Elevated levels of neurotoxic ketones have been sought but not found.[10] Distal axonopathy may be one of the mechanisms operating in individuals with the common progressive distal symmetrical sensory neuropathy. No valid animal models are currently available to test this hypothesis; however, there are claims of distal axonopathy in experimental diabetes.[11] Further confounding a metabolic explanation is the inconsistent relationship of severity of neuropathy to control of blood glucose. There are many instances of "well-controlled" patients who develop severe sensorimotor neuropathy, and others with "poor control" who have no evidence of neuropathy. Although it is generally conceded that neuropathy is most likely to develop in poorly controlled cases, and recovery less likely to occur in such individuals, observed variation in individual susceptibility suggests that multiple factors may be involved in the pathogenesis of diabetic neuropathy, of which hyperglycemia is but one.[1]

Among the proposed biochemical mechanisms underlying diabetic neuropathy, accumulation of nerve sorbitol[12] and depletion of nerve myoinositol[13] have received most attention. Sorbitol accumulates in the lens of the eye, alters the state of hydration and may, by this mechanism, lead to cataract formation. Sorbitol also accumulates in nerve, but not in sufficient quantities to lead to osmotic damage unless it is confined to a particular cell compartment.

Myoinositol is a cyclic hexitol normally present in nerve, and is a precursor of polyphosphoinositides which are present in membranes where they may regulate the patencies of ion channels. Nerve myoinositol concentration is reduced both in human and in experimental diabetes.[13] It has been claimed that the addition of small quantities of myoinositol to the diet of animals prevents reduction in nerve conduction velocity in experimental diabetes.[14] The administration of dietary inositol to humans with diabetic neuropathy appears to have little beneficial effect.[15]

MONONEUROPATHY. In contrast to the symmetrical neuropathies, vascular factors probably have a significant role in the pathogenesis of focal diabetic peripheral nerve lesions.[6] The clinical pattern—abrupt onset of painful, focal nerve lesions—is strikingly analogous to the pattern of neuropathy encountered in other vascular neuropathies (see Chapter 15). Vascular occlusions have not been adequately documented in humans with mononeuropathy, and further investigation of this condition is required to support this attractive, but still unproven, assumption.[6,8,9,16,17]

ANIMAL MODELS. There is no satisfactory animal model of human diabetic neuropathy. Studies of peripheral nerves from rats with experimentally induced diabetes frequently yield contradictory results. Nerve conduction velocity is reduced in both alloxan- and streptozotocin-induced diabetes in the rat in comparison with age-matched controls.[18,19] This reduction in nerve conduction velocity is readily abolished by insulin treatment,[20] and may result from impaired growth produced by the diabetic state.[21] The significance of morphologic studies of such animals is also currently debated. Degenerative changes in distal hind limb nerves have been described, but it is uncertain whether these represent a distal axonopathy due to diabetes or to an abnormal susceptibility of diabetic nerve to pressure.[11] A true but mild distal axonopathy probably develops, but changes in nerve trunks comparable to those of human diabetic neuropathy have not been demonstrated.

CLINICAL FEATURES
OF SYMMETRICAL POLYNEUROPATHY
AND MONONEUROPATHY SYNDROMES

INCIDENCE. Diabetic neuropathy occurs throughout the world equally among men and women. Although it is a common condition, estimates of prevalence vary widely, and most series are confounded by imprecise definition of what constitutes neuropathy. Many agree that there is a prevalence of about 50 percent for individuals with diabetes of 25 years' duration.[2] Neuropathy is present in less than 10 percent of individuals at the time of the initial diagnosis of diabetes, and is uncommon in diabetic children.

PREDISPOSING FACTORS. Neuropathy develops more readily and recovery is less likely in individuals with poorly controlled blood sugar levels,[2] and conduction slowing may correlate with degree of hyperglycemia.[22] However, there is considerable variation in individual susceptibility, and there are many instances of severe neuropathy in well-controlled diabetic subjects. Genetic factors may be important.

Symptoms and Signs

Symmetrical Polyneuropathy Syndromes

RAPIDLY REVERSIBLE NEUROPATHIES. Newly diagnosed, untreated diabetics may display reduced nerve conduction velocity on electrodiagnostic testing, without clinical signs or symptoms of peripheral nerve involvement. This reduced conduction velocity is rapidly reversed by lowering blood sugar concentration to near normal levels. Occasional untreated diabetics likewise manifest distal, painful paresthesias that respond promptly to control of the diabetic state. It seems unlikely that these rapidly reversible phenomena are associated with structural breakdown in peripheral nerve fibers. As yet, it is not clear whether the occurrence of these rapidly reversible changes correlates with the later development of persistent neuropathy. A recent study suggests that nerve conduction in insulin-requiring diabetics is not improved following rigid control of blood sugar for short intervals.[23]

DISTAL (PRIMARILY) SENSORY NEUROPATHY. Distal sensory polyneuropathy is the commonest type of diabetic peripheral nerve disorder.[2] It may be asymptomatic, with abnormal signs first detectable on routine neurologic examination, or it may present with a variety of symptoms. These occasionally indicate a predominant involvement of either larger or smaller diameter nerve fibers; in severe instances, fibers of all diameters are affected. The onset of symptoms may be insidious in individuals with longstanding diabetes mellitus, or it may lead to discovery of the condition in maturity-onset cases where undetected diabetes has been present for a considerable time. Symptoms may also arise in a more precipitate manner, sometimes following an episode of severe ketosis, or after initiation of treatment.

Three consistent patterns are present either singly or in combination in most diabetics with distal sensory neuropathies.

(1) The most common is a proposed "large-fiber" pattern, in which symptoms present as paresthesias in the feet and lower legs.[2] Prominent signs are absent ankle jerks, impaired appreciation of light touch in a stocking distribution, and reduction or loss of vibration sense in the feet. In more severe cases, joint position sense is impaired, the hands are involved, and slight distal weakness appears. Morphologic confirmation of this large fiber hypothesis has yet to be obtained.

(2) Less frequent is a proposed "small-fiber" pattern, which usually presents with pain.[4] Dull aching may be experienced in the feet or deep pain, sometimes described as "in the bones" in the legs. Burning sensa-

tions in the soles are common, and are especially troublesome at night. Prominent signs include impairment of cutaneous pain and temperature and similar impairment of deep pain sensation in the legs. Autonomic nervous system involvement may be associated with this variety. Strength, tendon reflexes, and the sensations of light touch, vibration and position, are relatively spared. Electrophysiologic and pathologic studies on nerves from these patients have supported the notion of predominant "small-fiber" involvement, and the sum of evidence suggests an axonal disorder.

(3) Most rare, fortunately, is a "pseudotabetic" pattern, featured in the lower limbs. Romberg's sign is present and tendon reflexes are absent in the legs. Ulceration of the feet and joint deformation *(neuropathic arthropathy)* are hallmarks of this condition, developing in individuals with long-standing diabetes mellitus associated with profound sensory loss. Ulcers are most often situated on the ball of the foot over the heads of the medial metatarsal bones, but may occur at other pressure sites, such as on the toes or heel. Diabetic neuropathic arthropathy generally involves the distal joints, in contrast to the *Charcot joint* of tabes dorsalis, which commonly affects the knees, hips, and ankles. Autonomic disorders associated with this variety, especially impotence, bladder atony, and pupillary abnormalities, enhance the analogy to tabes dorsalis.

AUTONOMIC NEUROPATHY. Diabetic autonomic neuropathy generally is associated with symmetrical sensory neuropathy, although there are instances where impairment of autonomic function constitutes the major neurologic disturbance. It is probably widely underdiagnosed, since the signs are often subtle and best detected by special tests not routinely employed in clinical practice. Autonomic involvement may be asymptomatic or cause incapacitating disability.[2]

Three types of autonomic dysfunction are prominent in diabetics: gastrointestinal, cardiovascular, and genitourinary.

Gastrointestinal. Asymptomatic disturbances of esophageal motility are sometimes demonstrable by cineradiography, and may be associated with gastroparesis and delayed emptying of the stomach. Vomiting from this condition is rare. Episodic nocturnal diarrhea is the best known diabetic alimentary disturbance; the feces are watery and the patient may experience urgency and incontinence. Colonic dilatation in diabetics sometimes occurs, and is usually attributed to autonomic neuropathy.

Cardiovascular. Impairment of vasomotor reflexes is present in many patients with evidence of sensory neuropathy, even in mildly affected cases.[2] Postural hypotension is rare, but when present, can be extremely disabling. It is aggravated by the administration of insulin, tricyclic antidepressants, diuretics, and phenothiazines. Cardiac denervation, either vagal alone or a combination of vagal and sympathetic denervation, is well described. Vagal denervation is featured by a high resting heart rate and loss of the sinus arrythmia that occurs with respiration. Some instances of sudden death in young diabetics may be attributable to cardiac arrythmia.

Genitourinary. Bladder dysfunction usually has an insidious onset.[24] It commonly begins with increasing intervals between voiding, followed by difficulty in the initiation of micturition, an intermittent weak stream, and postmicturition dribbling. A large residual urinary volume is present, and there is poor sensation of filling until bladder capacity is reached. Some cases develop urinary retention and overflow. Retrograde ejaculation secondary to poor closure of the denervated internal bladder sphincter, resulting in passage of seminal fluid into the bladder rather than along the urethra, may also occur.[25] Impotence is sometimes the initial manifestation of autonomic neuropathy; it usually steadily worsens and rarely, if ever, is improved by control of hyperglycemia.

Other prominent autonomic features are various abnormalities of pupillary function and sweating. Gustatory sweating may be an especially troublesome complication, with profuse facial sweating usually beginning shortly after eating and extending to the scalp and shoulders symmetrically. Nocturnal total body sweating, not related to hypoglycemia, also occurs. Diminished sweating of the distal extremities may lead to hot, dry skin that fissures easily.

Mononeuropathy Syndromes

CRANIAL NERVE LESIONS. Isolated or multiple palsies of the nerves to the extraocular muscles are particularly found in older diabetics.[2,8,9] Frequently, there is no other evidence of neuropathy and, on occasion, this may be the first indication of diabetes in an otherwise asymptomatic adult. The third nerve is most commonly affected, the sixth less frequently. Fourth nerve lesions are rare. Involvement may be unilateral or bilateral. The onset is usually abrupt and associated with an intense, retro-orbital aching sensation. Occasionally, paralysis evolves in a subacute, painless manner. Sparing of the pupillomotor fibers is frequent, with diabetic third nerve palsy and, when present, helps differentiate clinically lesions that compress the nerve, such as an aneurysm of the internal carotid artery. The probable explanation is that the pupilloconstrictor fibers, situated around the periphery of the nerve, are not affected by ischemic demyelination that disrupts the central part of the nerve.[8] Satisfactory recovery of nerve function is usual, occurring within several weeks in most cases.

Isolated lesions of other cranial nerves, especially the seventh, probably occur more frequently in diabetics than in the general population.

ISOLATED PERIPHERAL NERVE LESIONS. Almost every major peripheral nerve can be affected by diabetic mononeuropathy. Lesions of the ulnar, median, radial, lateral cutaneous nerve of the thigh, sciatic and peroneal nerves, have been described. It is alleged that diabetic nerves are especially vulnerable to compression, and mononeuropathies frequently appear at common sites of entrapment and external compression.[26] As with the cranial neuropathies, the onset of symptoms is usually abrupt and frequently painful. Recovery may be satisfactory if the lesion is sited distally. Proximal lesions may be associated with prolonged deficits, presumably because of the greater distance required for axonal regeneration. It is widely held that rapid recovery of a peripheral mononeuropathy indicates a demyelinative lesion.

Proximal Lower Extremity Motor Neuropathy (Diabetic Amyotrophy)

The syndrome of proximal, asymmetrical weakness of the lower extremities has been recognized as a type of diabetic neuropathy for nearly a century. The term *diabetic amyotrophy* is now generally employed to describe the condition.[27]

This syndrome usually appears in middle aged or elderly individuals. Cardinal manifestations include progressive, painful, asymmetrical proximal weakness of anterior thigh muscles (iliopsoas, quadriceps, adductors), loss of knee jerks, few sensory findings, and spontaneous recovery. There is considerable variation in onset, progression, and symmetry, and not all cases recover satisfactorily. Some cases also display distal atrophy and weakness. For these reasons, it has been proposed that diabetic amyotrophy constitutes a clinical spectrum characterized at one end by a rapid-onset, asymmetrical type, likely due to ischemia, and at the other, by a chronic, slow-onset, symmetrical type of probable metabolic origin.[17] Despite this variation, diabetic amyotrophy represents an easily recognizable clinical syndrome. For the present, it is probably best classified as a multiple mononeuropathy because of the usual absence of the appropriate sensory loss of the widespread *proximal* and asymmetrical muscle involvement. It is not simply a femoral neuropathy since, in nearly all cases, there is weakness of muscles innervated by other nerves such as the obturator or sciatic. Many cases appear to display unilateral lumbar plexus involvement. Elevation of the CSF protein is a feature of most cases, and may indicate spinal root involvement.

Course and Prognosis

Symmetrical Polyneuropathy Syndromes

RAPIDLY REVERSIBLE NEUROPATHIES. The course of these conditions is usually brief, and prognosis for recovery is excellent once the diabetic state is controlled with hypoglycemic agents.

DISTAL, PRIMARILY SENSORY NEUROPATHY. There are few studies that address the prognosis of this common condition.[2,27] Some individuals with the large fiber variety of sensory neuropathy display a steady, insidiously progressive neurologic deficit. A few will fluctuate, improve transiently, and then slip back. Most will plateau and experience moderately annoying sensory symptoms and mild distal lower-extremity weakness. Severe disability and limitation of activities are the exception, unless an associated autonomic or mononeuropathy syndrome also develops. The painful small fiber type is often self-limited, but the pseudotabetic variety generally progresses relentlessly, and is much more disabling. This is partly due to the associated joint deformities and foot ulceration.

AUTONOMIC NEUROPATHY. The course of autonomic neuropathy varies from an imperceptible progression to the relentless development of an incapacitating disability.[2] Nocturnal diarrhea may occur in brief episodes, with long asymptomatic intervals. The other prominent autonomic phenomena do not improve, and the prognosis for autonomic disability is among the worst for all the neuropathies of diabetes mellitus. Psychologic disability is especially common in males who develop genitourinary dysfunction and impotence.

Mononeuropathy and Multiple Mononeuropathy Syndromes

CRANIAL NEUROPATHIES. The course of these disorders is characterized by rapid development of severe dysfunction of involved nerves, followed by a satisfactory recovery. Other cranial nerves may subsequently be involved. Repeated palsies of the same cranial nerve are rare.

ISOLATED PERIPHERAL NERVE LESIONS. The prognosis of mononeuropathies involving limb nerves is better in cases with an acute onset.[2] In general, the more distal the lesion, the more rapid and complete the recovery. An exception to this rule is the median nerve lesion that occurs at the wrist, reinforcing the notion that superimposed trauma worsens the prognosis in diabetic mononeuropathies.[27]

PROXIMAL LOWER-EXTREMITY NEUROPATHY. The prognosis is generally good if the onset is abrupt and maximum disability occurs asymmetrically over a brief interval.[28] Such lesions appear analogous to other, presumably ischemic, mononeuropathies of diabetes, except that here multiple proximal nerves are involved.[16] Those individuals who experience an insidious onset of symmetrical proximal weakness often experience less satisfactory recovery, and may remain permanently disabled.

Laboratory Studies

GENERAL. Determination of blood glucose and the response to glucose ingestion are crucial in establishing a diagnosis of diabetes mellitus. Neuropathy rarely, if ever, antedates detectable abnormalities of carbohydrate metabolism.

The CSF protein is moderately elevated in most varieties of diabetic neuropathy. Levels as high as 500 mg per dl may rarely occur. For undetermined reasons, many diabetic subjects with no evidence of neuropathy have elevated CSF protein levels.

In individuals with autonomic dysfunction, it is often useful to determine early in the course of illness the state of the appropriate cardiovascular, gastrointestinal, and genitourinary reflexes.

Electrodiagnostic Studies

SUBCLINICAL NEUROPATHY. Quantitative analysis of vibration and tactile sensation in asymptomatic diabetics commonly reveals diminished sensory perception.[29] The most useful routine electrodiagnostic test in subclinical neuropathy is assessment of sensory nerve conduction. The sensory action potential displays temporal dispersion and reduced amplitude and velocity.[30] Motor conduction may also be reduced in patients without manifestations of neuropathy, but the degree of slowing is much greater in overt neuropathy and correlates well with severity.

Newly diagnosed diabetics may display reduced nerve conduction velocity without clinical evidence of neuropathy (*vide supra*). This is rapidly corrected by treatment of the diabetic state.[31,32]

SYMMETRICAL, PRIMARILY SENSORY NEUROPATHIES. In patients with any of the three types of sensory neuropathy outlined above, changes in sensory conduction are the most consistent abnormality.[2,30] Reduction in motor conduction velocity may be striking in cases with sensorimotor deficit. Electromyography reveals signs of denervation if distal muscles are clinically affected, and fibrillation potentials may be detectable in distal muscles even in the absence of definite weakness or wasting.

MONONEUROPATHY SYNDROMES. Electrodiagnostic abnormalities tend to be confined to affected limb nerves or their innervated muscles.[2] Cranial nerves, except for the seventh, are rarely subjected to electrodiagnostic investigation in diabetic cranial neuropathies. Slowed conduction in the femoral nerve is usually present in diabetic amyotrophy, as are signs of denervation in anterior thigh muscles. In patients with no clinical evidence of focal lesions, localized slowing may be detected at common sites of nerve entrapment, such as the ulnar nerve in the cubital tunnel at the elbow or the median nerve in the carpal tunnel.

TOLERANCE TO ISCHEMIA. Diabetic nerve displays an unexplained increased tolerance to ischemia, whether or not there is clinical or electrophysiologic evidence of neuropathy. The usual conduction block that develops in nerve fibers with ischemia is delayed, so that diabetics retain sensory and motor function for longer periods during ischemia produced by application of a pressure cuff.[33]

Nerve Biopsy

Nerve biopsy is seldom helpful in establishing a diagnosis of diabetic neuropathy, since there are no characteristic morphologic changes.[2] In general, its use is discouraged except for individuals investigating the pathophysiology of diabetic nerve disorders. In exceptional instances, where diabetes mellitus is present as an incidental finding in an individual with neuropathy from another cause, nerve biopsy may establish the correct diagnosis. Examples are a diabetic patient with autonomic neuropathy secondary to amyloidosis, an individual with mononeuropathy due to polyarteritis nodosa, or leprous neuropathy in a patient from an endemic area.

Treatment

GENERAL. Diabetic neuropathies of all types are more likely to develop, and to recover less well, if the metabolic state is poorly supervised. Strict control of blood sugar concentration is therefore mandatory whether or not neuropathy is present. When neuropathy has developed, there is no clear evidence that any particular means of achieving control is preferable. The recently introduced continuous administration of insulin to regulate blood glucose levels may ameliorate neuropathy. Patients in whom neuropathy appears shortly after the initiation of treatment usually recover completely after several months of insulin therapy or treatment with hypoglycemic drugs.

Treatment with myoinositol has proven unrewarding, and the common practice of administering vitamins of the B group does not alter the neuropathy. Aldose reductase inhibitors, gangliosides, and the French drug, Isaxonine®, also are under evaluation as therapeutic agents.

SYMPTOMATIC. Sensory neuropathy is frequently accompanied by persistent, severe pain which, on occasion, can be incapacitating. Simple analgesics rarely help and the chronicity of the problem contraindicates the use of opiates. Various regimens are suggested by diabetologists. Trials of diphenylhydantoin, carbamazepine and phenothiazines (in that order) are advocated by most. Depression occurs in most prolonged painful conditions, and is especially frequent in the middle-aged diabetic patient with painful neuropathy. In our experience, physician reassurance and the collaborative atmosphere present in most diabetes clinics is often of more benefit than antidepressant pharmacotherapy.

Trophic ulcers of the feet ("diabetic foot") result from several factors, of which sensory loss is the most important. They may respond to a reduction in weight bearing, enlargment of shoe size, local debridement, and appropriate antibiotics. Impaired healing may be due to coexistent ischemic vascular disease, and osteomyelitis may accompany an infected ulcer.[2]

Autonomic neuropathy furnishes a host of difficult therapeutic problems. Diabetic diarrhea may be helped by codeine phosphate or diphenoxylate, but not all cases respond favorably. A single 250 mg dose of tetracycline sometimes aborts the attack if given at the outset. Its mechanism of action is uncertain. In mild cases of postural hypotension, simple measures such as the use of elastic support stockings may be helpful. In more severe cases, sodium-retaining steroids, such as fluorocortisone, may be effective, but edema can become a troublesome side effect. In patients with bladder atony, regular voiding according to a time schedule is advisable, with micturition assisted by suprapubic pressure. Urinary infections require prompt treatment. Resection of the bladder neck is sometimes helpful where there is severe difficulty in voiding,[34] but dribbling incontinence can follow. Impotence related to autonomic neuropathy, once established, does not recover. Testosterone is contraindicated since it does not remove the impotence, and merely aggravates the situation by increasing libido. Penile prostheses[35] or implants are only occasionally successful.

Mononeuropathies frequently yield severe motor deficits. The cranial mononeuropathies that commonly affect extraocular muscles may be accompanied by severe pain. Since they are self-limited conditions, opiates may be judiciously used with little risk of addiction. Facial palsy with paralysis of the orbicularis oculi may lead to exposure keratitis and require tarsorrhaphy.

The limb mononeuropathies frequently require repetitive physical therapy.[2] Anterior tibial weakness from a common peroneal palsy may require foot support, and persistent wristdrop from a radial nerve palsy may necessitate tendon-transfer surgery.

Diabetic amyotrophy syndromes frequently require major analgesic therapy,[36] which can usually be given without fear of addiction in these self-limiting conditions. Physical therapy of the adductor, quadriceps, and hip flexor muscles is very important. These individuals may eventually require orthopedic appliances (leg braces) and assistance with walking.

Differential Diagnosis

Diabetes mellitus is a common condition and other causes for neuropathy may be coincidental.

PARANEOPLASTIC SENSORY NEUROPATHY. This purely sensory condition usually has a subacute onset, involves the lower extremities, affects all modalities, and may be associated with signs of CNS dysfunction. In these aspects, it differs from most cases of diabetic sensory or sensorimotor neuropathy and, when present, such findings should initiate a search for an occult carcinoma or lymphoma.

COMBINED SYSTEM DISEASE (B$_{12}$ DEFICIENCY). This condition shares many features with diabetic sensory neuropathy: *viz.* gradual onset in later life, abnormal sensations in the lower limbs, "large-fiber" pattern of sensory loss and absent ankle jerks. Hyperreflexic knee jerks, positive Babinski responses, psychiatric disturbance, and anemia may suggest this condition, and a low serum B$_{12}$ level establishes the diagnosis.

POLYARTERITIS NODOSA. Mononeuropathy from this condition differs in few clinical respects from that due to diabetes mellitus. Polyarteritis should be suspected if the individual is youthful and has evidence of systemic illness (fever, elevated ESR, elevated blood urea nitrogen). Nerve biopsy is often diagnostic.

LEPROSY. Thickening of nerve trunks, the distribution of sensory loss (ears, malar eminences, forearms, and lateral legs) and the coexistence of cutaneous lesions in advanced cases of leprosy should suggest this diagnosis, especially in individuals from endemic areas. Detection of early cases, in which one nerve is prominently involved, may require nerve biopsy.

ANEURYSM OF INTERNAL CAROTID OR POSTERIOR COMMUNICATING ARTERY WITHOUT SUBARACHNOID HEMORRHAGE. Like diabetic oculomotor neuropathy, this aneurysm occurs with abrupt onset and orbital pain. Sparing of the pupillomotor fibers strongly suggests a diabetic basis, and such patients should not undergo neuroradiologic procedures. Pupillary dilatation is often sufficient indication for carotid angiography.

Patients in whom the presence of mild diabetes is overlooked may be subjected to extensive and discomforting investigation, or misdirected therapy. Three prominent examples of this phenomenon are:

(1) Myelography in cases of distal sensory neuropathy, genitourinary autonomic neuropathy, and diabetic amyotrophy.
(2) Evaluation for occult carcinoma in individuals with symmetrical sensory neuropathy, or for lumbar plexus neoplasm in cases of asymmetric diabetic amyotrophy.
(3) Unwarranted psychotherapy or androgen therapy in males with impotence secondary to autonomic neuropathy.

Case Histories and Comment

Symmetrical, Primarily Sensory Neuropathy with Subsequent Cranial Mononeuropathy

CASE HISTORY. A 32-year-old female was discovered to have diabetes mellitus at a pre-employment physical examination. Treatment with diet and tolbutamide adequately controlled hyperglycemia until age 45, when she additionally required 10 units of NPH insulin twice a day. At age 47, unpleasant, burning pain appeared over the soles of both feet. This steadily worsened until age 50 and began to disturb sleep. Wearing shoes produced great discomfort and she preferred to walk about the house barefoot. Outpatient evaluation at that time revealed no abnormalities other than symmetrical, lower-extremity sensory and reflex changes. Strength and sweating were normal. Knee jerks were normal; ankle jerks were absent. Vibratory stimuli (128 cps) were not felt at toes or ankles but were appreciated normally at the knees. Position sense was moderately diminished at the toes. Pin-prick and light touch sensation were slightly diminished over both feet and lower legs to a level just two inches below the knee, and both stimuli elicited an abnormal "burning" sensation. Electromyography of the leg muscles was normal, as was motor conduction in the peroneal nerves. Sensory conduction in the peroneal nerves was profoundly slowed to 20 m per sec (normal 40–60), and sensory conduction in the median nerves was at the lower limit of the normal range (50 m per sec). Treatment with diphenylhydantoin failed to alleviate the pain, and she declined further medication. During the following 10 years, she scrupulously maintained dietary and insulin control of hyperglycemia. In that time, there was gradual progression of sensory loss in the legs and occasional numb sensations of the fingers. The spontaneous burning pain did not worsen and did not limit her activities.

At age 61, while on vacation, she awakened one morning with severe throbbing pain in the right eye and vomited repeatedly. Double vision appeared by noon, and the right lid was half closed. The following day, she was admitted to the hospital with continued orbital pain and vomiting. On examination there was complete ptosis of the right lid and paralysis of all extraocular muscles innervated by the oculomotor nerve. The pupils were equal, and reacted normally to light, and to accommodation-convergence. Vision was 20/30 in both eyes. Facial sensation was normal as was other cranial nerve function. In the upper extremities, there was no perception of vibration over the fingers or wrists, and pin prick was poorly perceived over the finger tips. Other sensory modalities were intact, and no dysesthesias were reported. Tendon reflexes were normal in the arms. In the lower extremities, vibration sensation was absent except at the iliac crests. Pin and touch sense were severely diminished up to the mid-shin, and were perceived better on moving up the proximal limb, becoming normal at mid-thigh. In the feet, the skin was cool and moist, sweating appeared normal and pedal pulses were present. Joint position sense was poor at the toes, normal at ankles. Rubbing her soles elicited only mild discomfort. There was slight (4/5) weakness of dorsifexion of ankles and toes. Gait was slow, deliberate, narrow-based, and required no support. Romberg's sign was not present. Toe walking was performed well, but she could not walk on her heels. Tendon jerks were absent in the lower limbs.

The orbital pain was relieved by large doses of codeine and subsided on the third hospital day. The CSF was clear, contained no cells, and showed a protein level of 130 mg per dl. CT scan was unremarkable. She refused electrodiagnostic studies and was discharged after one week. After two months, strength returned to the right eyelid and, in the subsequent month, extraocular muscles regained a full range of motion.

COMMENT. This case demonstrates that several types of neuropathy may occur in the same diabetic individual. Despite excellent control of hyperglycemia, a primarily large-fiber type, dysesthetic symmetrical sensory neuropathy occurred. Initially, it was featured by distal loss of vibration sense and tendon reflexes. Typically, progression of neuropathy was slow, and the patient was still functional after ten years without therapy. The abnormal sensations either subsided or she accomodated to them. Definite weakness was present in the legs after 10 years, but was not apparent to the patient. Autonomic dysfunction was not symptomatic or detected by bedside maneuvers, indicating that unmyelinated fibers were relatively spared. A painful cranial mononeuropathy, typically involving the third nerve, developed in old age and had a benign course. Sparing of the pupillomotor fibers strongly argued against an aneurysm compressing the third nerve and, together with the negative CT scan, obviated the need for carotid angiography.

Proximal Lower Limb Neuropathy (Diabetic Amyotrophy): Two Examples

CASE HISTORY. A 54-year-old female was diagnosed as diabetic and treated by diet alone. She did well for five years, and then began to lose weight in the sixth year, losing nearly 40 lbs in a nine-month period. The weight loss was accompanied by pain in the legs and steadily increasing leg weakness over a five-month period. She required assistance in walking on admission to hospital. There was severe muscle wasting in the lower limbs, more marked in proximal than distal muscles, and more on the right side than the left. Tendon reflexes were absent in the legs, depressed in the arms, and a right Babinski response was present. Sensation was preserved throughout. The CSF protein was 240 mg per dl. Rigorous control of hyperglycemia was attained by insulin administration. The wasted muscles improved dramatically within 20 months and, after three years, there was only minimal weakness in the lower limbs.

CASE HISTORY. A 65-year-old male, diabetic for 10 years and well controlled by diet and tolbutamide, suddenly developed deep pain in the left anterior thigh. Weakness of the proximal left lower limb developed within the day; the pain progressed for one week and then subsided, leaving a slight burning sensation above the knee. On examination, there was 2/5 weakness on the left iliopsoas, quadriceps femoris and adductor muscles, the left knee jerk was absent and there was a poorly defined area of diminished pinprick appreciation over the mid anterior thigh. Cerebrospinal fluid protein was 100 mg per dl. Eight weeks later, there was moderate atrophy of the left thigh, strength was unchanged, and electromyographic signs of denervation were present in the above-named muscles. Motor conduction in the peroneal and median nerves was within normal limits. Six months following the original episode, he had recovered 4/5 strength in the proximal muscles, sensory loss was not detected, and he was able to walk unaided. The left patellar reflex remained absent.

One year following the original episode, persistent dull pain developed in the right buttock. Two weeks later, incapacitating (2/5) weakness appeared in most muscles of the right lower limb. The gluteus maximus, hamstrings, gastrocnemius, anterior tibial, peroneal muscles, quadriceps femoris and ileopsoas, were involved. Tendon reflexes were absent in the right leg. Pain persisted for one month, occasionally requiring opiates for relief. No sensory loss was detected. Four months later there was atrophy and no improvement in strength; the other muscles remained at 2/5. Two years later, he remains unchanged and walks with a frame and a right short leg brace.

COMMENT. Both patients displayed evidence of lesions that could be localized to multiple levels of lower limb nerves and were accompanied by pain. The two cases differed strikingly in rate of progression and symmetry, and constitute good examples of the clinical extremes and pathogenetic dilemmas surrounding diabetic amyotrophy. The first case, featured by the gradual onset of a relatively symmetrical pure motor syndrome with good recovery, suggests a metabolic axonopathy (see Chapter 2), save for the predominantly proximal distribution and absence of sensory findings. The second case initially was featured by abrupt onset of asymmetrical combined femoral and obturator nerve deficits. Later, a similar affliction additionally involved the contralateral sciatic nerve. This clinical profile strongly suggests a vascular multiple mononeuropathy syndrome.

REFERENCES

1. THOMAS, PK AND ELIASSON, SG: *Diabetic neuropathy*. In DYCK, PJ, THOMAS, PK AND LAMBERT, EH (EDS): Peripheral Neuropathy, Vol 2, WB Saunders, Philadelphia, 1975, p 956.

2. PIRART, J: *Diabetic neuropathy: a metabolic or a vascular disease*. Diabetes, 14:1, 1965.

3. THOMAS, PK AND LASCELLES, RG: *The pathology of diabetic neuropathy*. Q J Med 35:489, 1966.

4. BROWN, MJ, MARTIN, JR AND ASBURY, AK: *Painful diabetic neuropathy: a morphometric study*. Arch Neurol 33:164, 1976.

5. JOHNSON, PC, BRENDEL, K AND MEEZAN, G: *Human diabetic perineurial cell basement membrane thickening*. Lab Invest 44:265, 1981.

6. ASBURY, AK AND JOHNSON, PC: *Pathology of peripheral nerves*. WB Saunders, Philadelphia, 1978.

7. APPENZELLER, O AND RICHARDSON, EP: *The sympathetic chain in patients with diabetic and alcoholic polyneuropathy*. Neurology (Minneap) 16:1205, 1966.

8. DREYFUS, PM, HAKIM, S AND ADAMS, RD: *Diabetic ophthalmoplegia: report of a case, with postmortem study and comments on vascular supply of human oculomotor nerve*. AMA Arch Neurol Psychiat 77:337, 1957.

9. ASBURY, AK, ET AL: *Oculomotor palsy in diabetes mellitus: A clinicopathological study*. Brain 93:555, 1970.

10. ZLATKIS, A, ET AL: *Volitale metabolites in serum of normal and diabetic patients*. J Chromatogr 182:137, 1980.

11. BROWN, M., ET AL: *Distal neuropathy in experimental diabetes mellitus*. Ann Neurol 8:168, 1980.

12. GABBAY, KH: *The sorbitol pathway and the complications of diabetes*. N Engl J Med 288:831, 1973.

13. WINEGRAD, AI AND GREENE, DA: *Diabetic polyneuropathy: the importance of insulin deficiency, hyperglycemia and alterations in myoinositol metabolism in its pathogenesis*. N Engl J Med 295:1416, 1976.

14. JEFFERYS, JGR, ET AL: *Influence of dietary myoinositol on nerve conduction and inositol phospholipids in normal and diabetic rats*. J Neurol Neurosurg Psychiat 41:333, 1978.

15. GREGERSEN, G, ET AL: *Myoinositol and function of peripheral nerves in human diabetes*. Acta Neurol Scand 58:241, 1978.

16. RAFF, MC AND ASBURY, AK: *Ischemic mononeuropathy and mononeuropathy multiplex in diabetes mellitus*. N Engl J Med 279:17, 1968.

17. ASBURY, AK: *Proximal diabetic neuropathy*. Ann Neurol 2:179, 1977.

18. ELIASSON, SG: *Nerve conduction changes in experimental diabetes*. J Clin Invest 43:2353, 1964.

19. SHARMA, AK AND THOMAS, PK: *Peripheral nerve structure and function in experimental diabetes*. J Neurol Sci 23:1, 1974.

20. JAKOBSEN, J: *Early and preventable changes of peripheral nerve structure and function in insulin-deficient diabetic rats*. J Neurol Neurosurg Psychiatry 42:509, 1979.

21. SHARMA, AK, BAJADA, S AND THOMAS, PK: *Influence of streptozotocin-induced diabetes on myelinated nerve fiber maturation and on body growth of the rat*. Acta Neuropathol 53:257, 1981.

22. GRAF, RJ, ET AL: *Nerve conduction abnormalities in untreated maturity-onset diabetes: relation to levels of fasting plasma glucose and glycosylated hemoglobin*. Ann Int Med 90:298, 1979.

23. SERVICE, JF, ET AL: *Effect of artificial pancreas treatment on peripheral nerve function in diabetes*. Neurology 31:1375, 1981.

24. ELLENBERG, M: *Diabetic neurogenic vesical dysfunction*. Arch Int Med 117:348, 1966.

25. ELLENBERG, M AND WEBER, H: *Retrograde ejaculation in diabetic neuropathy*. Ann Int Med 65:1237, 1966.

26. MULDER, DW, ET AL: *The neuropathies associated with diabetes mellitus: a clinical and electromyographic study of 103 unselected diabetic patients.* Neurology (Minneap) 11:275, 1961.

27. GILLIATT, RW: *Clinical aspects of diabetic neuropathy.* In Cumings, JN AND KREMER, M (EDS): *Biochemical Aspects of Neurological Disorders.* Blackwell Scientific Publications, Oxford, 1965, p 117.

28. GARLAND, HT: *Diabetic amyotrophy.* Br Med J 2:1287, 1955.

29. CONOMY, JP, BARNES, KL AND CONOMY, JM: *Cutaneous sensory function in diabetes mellitus.* J Neurol Neurosurg Psychiatry 42:656, 1969.

30. LAMONTAGNE, A AND BUCHTHAL, F: *Electrophysiological studies in diabetic neuropathy.* J Neurol Neurosurg Psychiatry 33:442, 1970.

31. GREGERSON, G: *Variations in motor conduction velocity produced by acute changes of the metabolic state in diabetic patients.* Diabetologia 4:273, 1978.

32. WARD, JD, BARNES, CG AND FISHER, DJ: *Improvement in nerve conduction following treatment in newly diagnosed diabetics.* Lancet 1:428, 1971.

33. HOROWITZ, SH AND GINSBERG-FELLNER, F: *Peripheral nerve responses during ischemia in the evaluation of diabetic neuropathy.* Muscle and Nerve 1:388, 1978.

34. BALFOUR, J AND ANKENMAN, GJ: *Atonic neurogenic bladder as a manifestation of diabetic neuropathy.* J Urol 76:746, 1956.

35. MASSEY, EW AND PLEET, AB: *Penile prosthesis for impotence in multiple sclerosis.* Ann Neurol 6:451, 1979.

36. CHOKROVERTY, S, ET AL: *The syndrome of diabetic amyotropy.* Ann Neurol 2:181, 1977.

Chapter 5

ALCOHOLISM, NUTRITIONAL DEFICIENCIES AND MALABSORPTION

Nutritional neuropathy in North America and Europe is almost synonymous with the thiamine/combined-B-vitamin-deficiency polyneuropathy associated with alcoholism. The selective vitamin B_{12} and pyridoxine (B_6) deficiency polyneuropathies have become rare, as has peripheral nerve damage secondary to malabsorption syndromes. While it is acknowledged that polyneuropathy occurs with selective deficiencies of many B vitamins and nicotinic acid, disorders such as beriberi and pellagra are now medical curiosities in Western medical practice.

Most deficiency syndromes affecting the nervous system are now held to result from lack of multiple vitamins, frequently combined with other dietary imbalance. Rarely can an instance of polyneuropathy be defined in terms of a single vitamin deficiency.[1]

ALCOHOL-NUTRITIONAL DEFICIENCY POLYNEUROPATHY SYNDROME

Definition and Etiology

This disorder is most simply defined as the polyneuropathy associated with chronic abuse of alcohol. In North America, it usually occurs in association with nutritional deprivation.[2]

The precise dietary imbalance in most cases of alcohol-nutritional deficiency polyneuropathy is usually not identified. Thiamine deficiency frequently has a dominant role, but other vitamins and nutrients may also be lacking.[3] In addition, alcohol itself might also be neurotoxic. Thus, while most cases of alcoholic neuropathy in North America are associated with excessive intake of carbohydrate relative to thiamine and other vitamins, neuropathy also is reported to occur occasionally in well nourished alcoholics.[4]

Pathology and Pathogenesis

PATHOLOGY. Postmortem examination of the nervous system from cases of beriberi and alcohol-nutritional deficiency neuropathy consistently reveals severe degenerative changes in distal limb peripheral nerves and in the cervical portion of the gracile fasciculi. Degeneration of the distal vagus and recurrent laryngeal nerves, and "axonal reaction" of anterior horn and dorsal root ganglion cells are present in advanced cases.[1]

Several studies of nerve biopsies from human alcohol-nutritional deficiency neuropathy strongly indicate that initial axonal changes are followed by alterations in myelin.[4,5] These findings, taken in concert with the distal distribution of changes, are evidence that this condition is a distal axonopathy. Confirmation of this notion awaits definitive experimental animal studies. Unfortunately, there is neither satisfactory experimental mammalian model for many nutritional deficiency neuropathies, nor firm evidence that ingested ethyl alcohol results in PNS degeneration.

PATHOGENESIS. The pathogenesis of the presumed alcohol-nutritional deficiency distal axonopathy is widely held to be similar to that of other metabolic axonopathies (see Chapter 2). Supposedly, lack of thiamine and other vitamins—cofactors for several key biochemical reactions—disrupts both axonal and nerve cell body metabolism, triggering the eventual breakdown of distal axonal integrity.[6] It is possible that alcohol itself has some role in this process.

In vitamin-deficient alcoholics, at least four additional factors have been proposed in the pathogenesis of polyneuropathy: one is decreased intake of vitamins as the alcoholic loses interest in nourishment,[2] second is malabsorption associated with alcohol-induced pancreatic damage,[7] third is an increased metabolic need for thiamine as alcohol and carbohydrates (pretzels, spaghetti, etc.) become the major foods,[1] and fourth is that alcohol, whether in the blood or the intestinal lumen, interferes with absorption of thiamine.[8]

When well nourished alcoholics develop polyneuropathy it is often presumed that alcohol itself somehow produces axonal damage.[4] Elucidation of this controversial idea awaits further studies; it is also possible that other undiscovered causes for neuropathy are present in these individuals.

Clinical Features

INCIDENCE. Alcohol-nutritional deficiency polyneuropathy is unusual in North American general practice, but is common in some municipal institutions. In the Boston City Hospital Series, 9 percent of all alcoholics had evidence of polyneuropathy.[1] The disorder is more frequent in women.

SYMPTOMS AND SIGNS. Clinical evidence of malnutrition, usually weight loss, is present in one half of alcoholics with polyneuropathy; a history of prolonged alcohol abuse, combined with a diet high in carbohydrates, can sometimes be elicited. In approximately one half of cases, symptoms consist only of mild aching in the calf muscles and discomfort over the soles. Examination of such individuals usually reveals depression or loss of Achilles reflexes, with impairment of pin and touch sensation over the feet and thinned legs.[9]

Symptoms in more severely involved cases usually consist of distal lower-limb paresthesias, pain, and weakness. The legs are always affected before the arms, and often are involved exclusively.[3] Mixed sensorimotor neuropathy is the rule. In the early stages, only sensory symptoms and signs may be present, but eventually weakness appears. Pure motor neuropathy is not described. Distressing symptoms of pain and paresthesias of the feet occur in about one quarter of cases, and some develop the full-blown "burning feet" syndrome. This condition, also associated with some toxic (e.g., thallium) and non-alcohol-related malnutrition states, evolves subacutely over weeks or months. The soles are initially affected with aching pain that may become pricking, electric, or stabbing, sometimes evolving into an intense burning sensation.[9] The entire plantar surfaces become exquisitely sensitive to touch, and the pressure of shoes and stockings cannot be tolerated. These sensations spread to the dorsum of the feet, eventually may cover the entire leg, and usually are accompanied by excessive perspiration.[1]

Weakness is initially distal. Foot and wrist drop may occur, and, when accompanied by atrophy, evolve into disabling contractures. Prominent weakness of the thigh muscles can be evident. Symptoms of lower cranial nerve involvement may appear in advanced cases, and include difficult swallowing, hoarseness, and impaired phonation. Postural hypotension occasionally occurs, while other symptoms of autonomic involvement are extremely rare.[1]

Clear signs of PNS impairment are present in cases with only minimal symptoms.[10] The Achilles reflexes are diminished or absent in individuals with any degree of weakness. Tenderness upon squeezing the calf muscles is characteristic. Sensory impairment generally involves all modalities, and a symmetrical glove-and-stocking pattern is the rule. Motor and sensory loss in extreme cases may extend to the proximal limbs. Severe dysesthesias of the soles are always accompanied by sensory loss.[1]

Signs of nutritionally-induced CNS impairment may accompany the polyneuropathy. Gait and lower limb ataxia, formerly attributed exclusively to PNS involvement, probably primarily reflect degeneration in the anterior cerebellar vermis. Some evidence of Wernicke's disease (nystagmus, oculomotor palsy, confusion, Korsakoff's psychosis), is occasionally detectable.[3]

Laboratory Studies

CLINICAL LABORATORY. Abnormal values of routine clinical laboratory tests are common and usually reflect nutritional anemia or alcohol-induced liver disease. Special laboratory tests have been advocated as helpful in establishing the presence of vitamin deficiencies. Blood pyruvate and thiamine levels are less reliable. The best index of thiamine deficiency is low serum or erythrocyte transketolase activity, and the restoration of normal activity response during treatment with vitamin B_1.[11,12]

CEREBROSPINAL FLUID. The CSF is acellular and the protein usually normal. A modest elevation in protein may be present in advanced cases.

ELECTRODIAGNOSTIC STUDIES. Electromyographic abnormalities are present even in the earliest (asymptomatic) stages, and increase *pari passu* with the degree of clinical impairment. Electromyographic signs of denervation in distal leg muscles are detectable in cases with only mild sensory impairment and no weakness. Motor and sensory nerve conduction velocity is usually normal in early or moderately severe cases. Sensory amplitudes may be diminished early in distal segments of limb nerves. Taken together, these electromyographic and nerve conduction abnormalities are typical of axonal degeneration, and support the notion that alcohol-nutritional deficiency neuropathy represents a distal axonopathy.[4,5,13]

COURSE PROGNOSIS AND TREATMENT. The prognosis of untreated alcoholic-nutritional deficiency neuropathy is poor. Axonal degeneration continues and leg weakness becomes extreme. Weakness in the upper extremities is not as profound, and proximal strength and tendon reflexes remain relatively spared. Signs of Wernicke's encephalopathy or delerium tremens may overshadow the polyneuropathy, and can constitute a life-threatening situation.[3]

With treatment, the prognosis is excellent if the polyneuropathy is still in an early stage. Treatment begun in the later stages of neuropathy may rapidly alleviate paresthesias, but objective improvement in strength may not appear until much later. Proximal muscles usually regain bulk and strength within several months. A year may elapse before foot-drop lessens. Rarely, distal atrophy, contractures, and sensory loss are permanent.

Treatment includes abstinence from alcohol, a high calorie, protein-rich diet, and multiple vitamin supplements.[1] Thiamine initially should be administered by intramuscular injection of 50 mg daily for a week.[7] Multiple vitamin therapy should also be given. Physical therapy should stress range-of-motion exercises, and splints may be necessary to avoid contractures in severe cases.

Differential Diagnosis

The diagnosis of alcohol-nutritional deficiency neuropathy is straightforward in an individual with evidence of liver disorder, malnutrition, and a history of alcoholism. Paraneoplastic neuropathies (see Chapter 13) may share common clinical and neurologic features (e.g., weight loss, paresthesias) and should be considered in cases refractory to nutritional therapy and abstinence from alcohol.

Alcoholism is a common condition, and its associated polyneuropathy is clinically indistinguishable from many other distal axonopathies. Therefore, the diagnosis of alcoholic polyneuropathy should be entertained with caution in individuals with coexistent metabolic disorders, or in those who also may be exposed to neurotoxic agents (see Chapters 11 and 12).

Case History and Comment

CASE HISTORY. A 41-year-old bachelor and construction worker had consumed a pint of whiskey, but otherwise a balanced diet, almost daily for ten years, without apparent ill effect. He sustained a fractured humerus in early June and was unable to work. His daily whiskey consumption increased to a quart, and he gradually lost interest in preparing meals or shopping. In addition to alcohol, his diet consisted mainly of spaghetti, pretzels, potato chips, and pizza. By Christmas, he appeared tremulous and seemed unsteady. In April, he fell down the stairs, was knocked unconscious and was admitted to hospital. General physical examination disclosed no evidence of weight loss, but an enlarged liver and rhinophyma were present. He was alert, cooperative, and oriented. Memory was intact. Cranial nerves and upper limb strength and sensation were normal. The gait was broad-based and he lost balance frequently. Coordination of the arms was normal, the heel-knee-shin maneuver was irregular, and toe-tapping was jerky. Tendon reflexes were absent throughout, save for weak biceps and triceps jerks. Strength was normal proximally in the legs. The dorsiflexors of ankles and toes could be overcome with ease, and he was unable to stand on toes or heels. Gentle pressure upon the calf muscles elicited severe pain, as did squeezing the anterior thighs. Pin and touch sensation were markedly impaired over the feet, and gradually shaded into normal appreciation at knee level. Both pin and touch elicited an unpleasant "stabbing" sensation over the soles. Vibration sense was diminished over the toes and ankles, while position sense was intact. Routine laboratory tests disclosed a mild hypochromic microcytic anemia. Liver function tests were unremarkable.

The day following admission he became tremulous and, in the ensuing three days, developed visual hallucinations and florid delerium tremens. He was hospitalized for three weeks and given a high protein diet with vitamin supplements. He refused electrodiagnostic studies or lumbar puncture, and was discharged to live with a sister. She supervised his diet and general well being, but could not limit his alcohol consumption. Six months later, gait was still broad-based and tendon reflexes were unchanged. Strength was nearly normal, and there was no muscle tenderness or dysesthetic response in the legs. Sensation to pin and touch was still impaired over the feet and ankles.

COMMENT. This case demonstrates many of the salient clinical features of alcoholic-nutritional deficiency neuropathy. It also illustrates the role of increased carbohydrate consumption in its genesis, and the ability of therapy rapidly to reverse some of the changes. Evidence of cerebellar dysfunction is also present, and may never recover.

SPECIFIC VITAMIN DEFICIENCY POLYNEUROPATHY SYNDROMES

Thiamine (B$_1$)

GENERAL. Although thiamine-deficiency polyneuropathy in North America is generally associated with alcoholism, in other areas of the world a thiamine-poor diet alone causes nervous system damage; for example, polyneuropathy ('dry' beriberi) resulting from a diet exclusively of polished rice. Recurrent vomiting, independent of alcoholism, is a well-documented gastrointestinal cause of Wernicke's encephalopathy (cerebral beriberi). One of Wernicke's original cases was a young woman with an esophageal stricture.[14] Cardiac failure with peripheral edema ('wet' beriberi) is a further consequence of deficiency of this vitamin.

STRUCTURE, SOURCE, REQUIREMENT, ABSORPTION. Thiamine is a water-soluble vitamin, formed by a pyrimidine ring and a thiazole moiety linked by a methylene bridge. It is synthesized by many plants and bacteria, and is present in most vegetable and nonfatty animal tissues. Most of the thiamine in cereal grains is in the outer layers, hence the occurrence of beriberi in individuals eating only milled rice. The minimal daily requirement for an adult is 0.7 to 0.9 mg. Daily gastrointestinal absorption capacity is limited to 5 to 10 mg. Only approximately 25 mg is stored in the body—excessively administered oral thiamine being excreted in the feces. These two factors emphasize the need for daily parenteral treatment of the thiamine-deficiency neurologic syndromes, and may explain the rapidity with which symptoms develop.[3] Certain bacteria and raw fish contain thiaminases, and a diet containing raw carp may contribute to the development of beriberi. Thiamine-deficiency neurologic syndromes are generally associated with diminished intake rather than malabsorption although, as noted above, recurrent vomiting may precipitate Wernicke's disease.

MECHANISM OF ACTION. Thiamine diphosphate is a coenzyme for several important biochemical reactions, including the oxidative decarboxylation of pyruvate and ketoglutarate and the transketolase reaction of the pentose phosphate pathway.[3] It is also alleged that thiamine has a specific role in nerve conduction, independent of its coenzyme function in general metabolism.[15]

PATHOLOGY AND PATHOGENESIS. The pathology and pathogenesis of thiamine-deficiency polyneuropathy are widely held to be identical to those described in the preceding section. There is no satisfactory mammalian experimental model of thiamine-deficiency neuropathy.[16] Degeneration of long and large myelinated nerve fibers is a consistent feature in pigeons made thiamine deficient.[17] Unfortunately, this avian model has not been studied with modern morphologic or electrophysiologic techniques.

GENERAL CLINICAL FEATURES OF THIAMINE DEFICIENCY. The most devastating neurologic effects of thiamine deficiency are Wernicke's disease, and its associated syndrome, Korsakoff's psychosis. Cerebellar degeneration and polyneuropathy often accompany Wernicke's disease.[3] The signs, symptoms, course and prognosis of thiamine-deficiency polyneuropathy ('dry' beriberi) are indistinguishible from those described for alcohol-nutritional deficiency. Cardiac failure ('wet' beriberi) may be associated with neuropathy.

DIAGNOSIS AND TREATMENT. The most reliable biochemical test of thiamine deficiency is the measurement of whole-blood or erythrocyte transketolase activity before, and following, the addition of thiamine diphosphate *in vitro*. An increase in enzyme activity following treatment further supports this diagnosis.[11,12]

Treatment consists of intramuscular injection of 50 mg thiamine daily for two weeks, followed by 5 mg per day orally. Since these individuals often suffer multiple vitamin deficiencies, other water-soluble vitamins should also be given.[1] In individuals suspected to have Wernicke's disease, treatment is urgently indicated and may dramatically reverse extraocular dysfunction.[3]

Riboflavin (B₂)

GENERAL. Riboflavin deficiency almost invariably occurs in combination with other vitamin deficiencies. It is usually secondary to a riboflavin-deficient diet, but has also been described following gastrectomy and attributed to malabsorption. Riboflavin deficiency is alleged to be one of the factors responsible for the "burning feet" syndrome seen in certain malabsorptive and undernutrition states, but the administration of riboflavin alone does not relieve the neurologic symptoms.[1]

Niacin (Nicotinic Acid, B₃)

GENERAL. Deficiency of niacin or its amino acid precursor, tryptophan, precipitates pellagra. Pellagra may result from a diet poor in these substances (primary pellagra) or from gastrointestinal malabsorption (secondary pellagra). Degeneration of CNS neurons and coexistent dementia are well documented in pellagrins, and clearly are secondary to niacin-tryptophan depletion. Claims of a niacin-induced peripheral neuropathy are viewed with skepticism, and this entity remains *sub judice.* It is generally held that the peripheral neurologic manifestations of pellegra can be attributed to coexisting deficiencies of other vitamins.[7]

Pyridoxine (B₆)

GENERAL. Naturally occurring, selective pyridoxine deficiency is extremely rare, largely because this vitamin is present in many foods; the condition may be induced both because it is destroyed during food processing and because certain drugs act as pyridoxine antagonists. Isoniazid antituberculolosis therapy accounts for almost all instances of human pyridoxine-deficiency polyneuropathy. Isoniazid toxicity and its pathogenesis are described in Chapter 11.

Paradoxically, the daily administration of excessive amounts of pyridoxine to experimental animals results in degeneration of dorsal root ganglion cells and the appearance of a permanently disabling toxic sensory neuronopathy syndrome.*[18]

STRUCTURE, SOURCE, REQUIREMENT, ABSORPTION. Three closely related compounds—pyridoxine, pyridoxal and pyridoxamine—are designated as vitamin B₆. The coenzyme form is pyridoxal-5-phosphate and the three compounds owe their enzymatic activity to tissue conversion to this moiety. The vitamin is widely and uniformly distributed in all foods. The minimal daily requirement for an adult is 0.6 to 1.3 mg. Ingested ethyl alcohol interferes with the metabolism of pyridoxal phosphate, possibly providing an additional factor in the alcoholic-nutritional deficiency neuropathy syndrome. Gastrointestinal absorption is rapid, occurs by passive diffusion and, despite extensive postsurgical loss of small intestine, pyridoxine-deficiency neurologic syndromes rarely result from malabsorption.[7]

MECHANISM OF ACTION. Pyridoxal phosphate acts as a cofactor for many enzymes in amino acid metabolism (transaminases, synthetases, hydroxylases), and is especially important in the metabolism of tryptophan, glycine, serine and glutamate. Pyridoxine has a vital, poorly understood role in neuronal excitability, possibly related to gamma-aminobutyric acid metabolism.

PATHOLOGY AND PATHOGENESIS. See *Isoniazid Toxicity* in Chapter 11.

GENERAL CLINICAL FEATURES OF PYRIDOXINE DEFICIENCY. Pyridoxine-deficiency neurotoxicity produced in human volunteers by administering desoxypyridoxine, a pyridoxine antagonist, includes generalized

*A comparable syndrome recently has been recognized in humans daily consuming in excess of 2g of pyridoxine. (Ann Neurol, 12:107, 1982.)

seizures as well as peripheral neuropathy of the type seen in isoniazid toxicity.[19] Some genetic conditions characterized by abnormalities in B_6 metabolism are featured by generalized seizures and CNS damage, unless large amounts of pyridoxine are given.[20]

DIAGNOSIS AND TREATMENT. The most common diagnostic index is the measurement of tryptophan metabolites, particularly xanthurenic acid, following tryptophan loading.[21] Also useful is the *in vitro* assessment of erythrocyte glutamic pyruvate transaminase in the presence and absence of pyridoxine.[7]

Oral treatment with 30 mg of pyridoxine is advocated for prophylaxis in pregnancy, and for individuals taking isoniazid.

Pantothenic Acid

GENERAL. Selective pantothenic acid deficiency is extremely rare because of the ubiquitous occurrence of this vitamin. Since pantothenic acid is not stored in the body to any great extent, severely malnourished individuals rapidly deplete their reserve of this and other vitamins. Pantothenic acid-deficiency syndromes secondary to malabsorption are not known.

Experimental human pantothenic acid deficiency is alleged to result in the "burning feet" syndrome, and one report describes relief of this condition in malnourished individuals by the administration of pathothenic acid.[22] These observations were not confirmed by a subsequent investigation of human pathothenic acid deficiency.[1] The existence of a polyneuropathy caused by selective pantothenic acid deficiency appears moot.

Vitamin B_{12}

GENERAL. Vitamin B_{12} deficiency is generally related to malabsorption. Dietary inadequacy of B_{12} is rare and encountered solely in strict vegetarians. Malabsorption usually results from either inadequate gastric production of intrinsic factor (pernicious anemia, gastrectomy) or from disorders of the terminal ileum (celiac disorders, intestinal resection). The prominent clinical features common to all conditions from which B_{12} deficiency may develop are hematologic, gastrointestinal, and neurologic (both CNS and PNS).[7] There exists an enormous clinical and experimental knowledge of the hematologic and CNS[23] effects of B_{12} deficiency that is beyond the scope of this review. In contrast, remarkably little is known about the peripheral neuropathy.

STRUCTURE, SOURCE, REQUIREMENT, ABSORPTION. Vitamin B_{12} is a complex organometallic compound characterized by a cobalt atom sited within a corrin ring. It cannot be synthesized in the human body, but can be formed by some bacteria normally present in the intestine. The principal dietary source of vitamin B_{12} is meat and dairy products. The minimum adult daily requirement is 3 μg. Dietary vitamin B_{12} combines with a glycoprotein intrinsic factor (IF) that is produced by the parietal cells of the stomach. The B_{12}-IF complex travels to the distal ileum where B_{12} is absorbed into the blood. Thus, disorders of the stomach or lower intestine may result in B_{12} deficiency. Normally, about 4 mg of B_{12} are stored in the body. In view of the extremely low minimal daily requirement, it takes 3 to 4 years of malabsorption to produce a human deficiency state.[7] This may explain the repeated failures of earlier investigators to produce nervous system degeneration in short-term animal experiments.

MECHANISM OF ACTION. Methylcobalamin is necessary for the demethylation of methyltetrahydrofolate (TFH). This involves the methylation of homocysteine to methionine. TFH is required for the production of the active folate coenzymes that are necessary for DNA synthesis. Nitrous oxide is known to inactivate methylcobalamin, but not adenoslycobalamin, and gives rise to megaloblastic changes in bone marrow. One report suggests that prolonged exposure of monkeys to N_2O gives rise to a myelopathy with combined posterior and lateral column degeneration, possibly similar to human combined-system disease.[24]

PATHOLOGY AND PATHOGENESIS. Little is known about either the pathology or pathogenesis of the PNS lesions of human B_{12} deficiency.[1,25] This contrasts strikingly with the extensive studies of the human CNS lesions,[23] and the findings of a recent ultrastructural investigation of similar CNS lesions appearing in primates following prolonged, carefully controlled B_{12} deficiency.[25,26] Human and primate CNS lesions are confined to the white matter, are prominent in the dorsal and lateral funiculi of the spinal cord and peripheral visual pathways, and are scattered in the cerebrum. Vacuolation of myelin with relative sparing of axons appears to be the initial change while, at later stages, there is loss of axons and gliosis.

The PNS lesions have not been extensively studied morphologically. Most reports are limited to descriptions of nerve biopsies processed by conventional histologic methods.[27,28] Degeneration of both myelin and axons are described, but it is difficult to determine whether the polyneuropathy is axonal or demyelinative. There is a manifest lack of detailed study of the extent of the human PNS lesions utilizing modern histologic techniques, and no suitable animal model of the PNS lesion of B_{12} deficiency. Curiously, the B_{12}-deficient primate, which displays profound CNS demyelinative lesions closely mimicking those of humans, does not become anemic or develop peripheral neuropathy.[25,26]

Theories concerning the biochemical basis underlying the nervous system lesions that accompany B_{12} deficiency have included occult cyanide poisoning and lipid metabolic abnormalities resulting from impairment of the methylmalonyl CoA mutase reactions. These theories have been thoroughly reviewed elsewhere.[26] More recently, methyl group deficiency has been considered.[24]

GENERAL CLINICAL FEATURES OF B_{12} DEFICIENCY POLYNEUROPATHY. The frequency of peripheral neuropathy among the neurologic complications of vitamin B_{12} deficiency is controversial. Two scholarly reviews of this issue yield the following diametrically opposing statements: "In our opinion peripheral neuropathy is probably the commonest neurological complication of vitamin B_{12} deficiency,"[1] and "One may conclude that the neurologic manifestations of pernicious anemia are due primarily to the spinal cord lesions. In the course of the myelopathy the peripheral nerves may also be involved, but the latter affection is less frequent than the former and of less clinical significance."[7]

Taken together, there is overwhelming evidence that PNS changes occur in individuals with severe B_{12} deficiency. Clinical evidence of neuropathy initially appears in the legs and consists of early absent or diminished Achilles reflexes, distal leg sensory deficits for multiple modalities and occasionally, distal leg weakness that exceeds the accompanying pyramidal signs. Since myelopathy accompanies the PNS degeneration, in most cases it is extraordinarily difficult to determine whether the paresthesias in the feet are secondary to changes in the dorsal columns or in the peripheral nerves.[1] Signs of pyramidal tract involvement (Babinski sign) usually appear early, and often accompany the diminished or absent Achilles reflexes. Electrophysiologic investigations have generally supported the existence of lower limb peripheral nerve involvement, but have not helped in elucidating its nature.[29]

DIAGNOSIS AND TREATMENT. Specific assays for serum B_{12} are now generally available in developed countries. The normal range of vitamin B_{12} in serum is 200 to 900 pg per ml; values less than 100 pg per ml indicate clinically significant deficiency.

Treatment consists of 100 ug of vitamin B_{12}, (as hydroxocobalamin) intramuscularly on alternate days for a week, then weekly for 3 months. Since the defect is almost always one of absorption, replacement is given parenterally and must be maintained for life, usually at a level of 1000 ug every 3 months.

Malabsorption Neuropathies: Postgastrectomy and Sprue-Related Disorders

POSTGASTRECTOMY NEUROPATHY. Total gastrectomy abolishes the absorption of vitamin B_{12} due to lack of intrinsic factor and, if untreated, a fully developed vitamin B_{12}-deficiency neurologic syndrome (optic neuropathy, myelopathy, peripheral neuropathy) would seem likely. Myelopathy has been demonstrated in such individuals and paresthesias occur, but there are few reports of polyneuropathy.

Partial gastrectomy is clearly associated with peripheral neuropathy or myelopathy, or both, usually long (10 to 20 years) after surgery. Although it is widely held that malabsorption of vitamin B_{12} underlies these disorders, serum B_{12} levels are sometimes normal, and replacement therapy elicits a variable response. It appears likely that some cases of postgastrectomy neuropathy are unrelated to vitamin B_{12} deficiency.

SPRUE-RELATED DISORDERS (TROPICAL SPRUE, GLUTEN-INDUCED ENTEROPATHY, CELIAC DISEASE AND OTHER MALABSORPTION-ASSOCIATED ENTEROPATHIES). These disorders, of varied etiology and pathogenesis, result in impairment of the absorptive function of the small intestine.[30] They are characterized by varying degrees of fatty diarrhea (steatorrhea), weight loss, disturbance of calcium and protein metabolism, and anemia. The neurologic syndromes associated with these disorders allegedly include, in varying degrees, peripheral neuropathy, myelopathy, encephalopathy, and myopathy. Peripheral neuropathy and myelopathy are most frequently observed, but are poorly documented by modern histologic or electrophysiologic techniques. It is often stated that these neurologic disorders, like those following gastrectomy, are somehow related to selective malabsorption of vitamin B_{12}. Analysis of the few well studied cases of sprue-related neuropathy or myelopathy, or both, does not strongly support this assumption.[7] Treatment with vitamin B_{12} has not always ameliorated the symptoms, and individuals have recovered without such therapy. It has been suggested that the malabsorptive neurologic disorders possibly result from multiple nutritional deficiencies. Vitamin E deficiency has been advanced as a possible cause in some instances.[31]

REFERENCES

1. VICTOR, M: *Polyneuropathy due to nutritional deficiency and alcoholism.* In DYCK, PJ, THOMAS, PK AND LAMBERT, EH Peripheral Neuropathies, Vol 2, WB Saunders, Philadelphia, 1975, p 1030.

2. VICTOR, M AND ADAMS, RD: *On the etiology of the alcoholic neurologic diseases. With special references to the role of nutrition.* Am J Clin Nutr 9:379, 1961.

3. VICTOR, M, ADAMS, RD AND COLLINS, GH: The Wernicke-Korsakoff Syndrome. FA Davis, Philadelphia, 1971.

4. BEHSE, F AND BUCHTHAL, F: *Alcoholic neuropathy: clinical, electrophysiological and biopsy findings.* Ann Neurol 2:95, 1977.

5. WALSH, JC AND MCLEOD, JG: *Alcoholic neuropathy: an electrophysiological and histological study.* J Neurol Sci 10:457, 1970.

6. SPENCER, PS, ET AL: *Does a defect in energy metabolism in the nerve fiber underlie axon degeneration in polyneuropathies?* Ann Neurol 5:501, 1979.

7. PALLIS, CA AND LEWIS, PD: *The Neurology of Gastrointestinal Disease.* WB Saunders, Philadelphia, 1974.

8. HALSTED, CH, ROBLES, EA AND MAZEY, E: *Decreased jejunal uptake of labeled folic acid (^{3}H-PGA) in alcoholic patients: roles of alcohol and nutrition.* N Engl J Med 285:701, 1971.

9. BISCHOFF, A: *Die alkoholische Polyneuropathie: klinische, ultrastructurelle und pathogenetische Aspekte.* Dtsch Med Wochenschr 96:317, 1971.

10. CÖERS, C AND HILDEBRAND, J: *Latant neuropathy in diabetes and alcoholism.* Neurology (Minneap) 15:19, 1965.

11. WARNOCK, LG: *Transketolase activity of blood hemolysate, a useful index for diagnosing thiamine deficiency.* Clin Chem 21:432, 1975.

12. DREYFUS, PM: *Clinical application of blood transketolase determinations.* N Engl J Med 267:596, 1962.

13. CASEY, EB AND LEQUESNE, PM: *Electrophysiological evidence for a distal lesion in alcoholic neuropathy.* J Neurol Neurosurg Psychiatry 35:624, 1972.

14. WERNICKE, C: *Lehrbuch der Gehirnkrankenheiten fur Aerzte und Studirende,* Vol 2, T Fischer, Kassel, 1881, p 229.

15. ITOKAWA, Y AND COOPER, JR: *Ion movements and thiamine. II. The release of the vitamin from membrane fragments.* Biochem Biophys Acta 196:274, 1970.

16. PRINEAS, J: *Peripheral nerve changes in thiamine-deficient rats.* Arch Neurol 23:541, 1970.

17. SWANK, RL: *Avian thiamine deficiency.* J Exp Med 71:683, 1940.

18. KRINKE, G, ET AL: *Pyridoxine megavitaminosis produces degeneration of peripheral sensory neurons (sensory neuronopathy) in the dog.* Neurotoxicology 2:13, 1981.

19. VILTER, RW, ET AL: *The effect of vitamin B_6 deficiency induced by desoxypyridoxine in human beings.* J Lab Clin Med 42:335, 1953.

20. HUNT, AD, ET AL: *Pyridoxine dependency: A report of a case of intractable convulsions in an infant controlled by pyridoxine.* Pediat 13:104, 1954.

21. HANSSON, O: *Tryptophan loading and pyridoxine treatment in children with epilepsy.* Ann NY Acad Sci 166:306, 1969.

22. GOPALAN, C: *The "burning-feet" syndrome.* Indian Medical Gazette 81:22, 1946.

23. PANT, SS, ASBURY, AK AND RICHARDSON, EP: *The myelopathy of pernicious anemia. A neuropathological reappraisal.* Acta Neurol Scand 44(suppl 35):1, 1968.

24. DINN, JJ, ET AL: *Animal model for subacute combined degeneration.* Lancet 11:1154, 1978.

25. AGAMANOLIS, DP, ET AL: *Neuropathology of experimental vitamin B_{12} deficiency in monkeys.* Neurology (Minneap) 26:905, 1976.

26. AGAMANOLIS, DP, ET AL: *An ultrastructural study of subacute combined degeneration of the spinal cord in vitamin B_{12} deficient rhesus monkeys.* J Neuropathol Exp Neurol 37:273, 1978.

27. GREENFIELD, JG AND CARMICHAEL, EA: *The peripheral nerves in cases of subacute combined degeneration of the cord.* Brain 58:483, 1935.

28. CÖERS, C AND WOOLF, AL: The Innervation of Muscle. Blackwell Scientific Publications, Oxford, 1959.

29. MAYER, RF: *Peripheral nerve function in vitamin-B_{12} deficiency.* Arch Neurol 13:335, 1965.

30. COOKE, WT AND SMITH, WT: *Neurological disorders associated with adult coeliac disease.* Brain 88:683, 1966.

31. NELSON, JS, ET AL: *Progressive neuropathologic lesions in vitamin E-deficient rhesus monkeys.* J Neuropathol Exp Neurol 40:166, 1981.

ALCOHOLISM,
NUTRITIONAL
DEFICIENCIES AND
MALABSORPTION

67

Chapter 6

METABOLIC NEUROPATHY: UREMIA

DEFINITION AND ETIOLOGY

DEFINITION. Uremic neuropathy is best defined as the distal symmetrical sensorimotor polyneuropathy associated with chronic renal insufficiency. The nature of the underlying renal disease appears immaterial, since virtually all types of kidney disorders that can lead to uremia have now been associated with this neuropathy.[1]

ETIOLOGY. The etiology is elusive. It is widely held that uremic neuropathy is secondary to retained, dialyzable toxins or metabolites normally excreted by the kidneys. Two features support this notion: one is the close clinicopathologic resemblence of uremic and the toxic neuropathies,[2] the other is improvement following dialysis and, more dramatically, after renal transplantation.[3,4] The responsible agent clearly has a molecular weight exceeding that of urea or creatinine.[5] Elevation of myoinositol, parathyroid hormone, or magnesium, and the presence of vitamin deficiencies or transketolase inhibition, have been proposed as candidates, but none has been established as being responsible.[6-11]

Pathology and Pathogenesis

PATHOLOGY. Axonal degeneration is characteristic of this disorder, and it can be classified as a distal axonopathy. This conclusion is strongly supported both by comprehensive postmortem examination of the peripheral nervous system from several advanced cases, and by detailed ultrastructural study of nerve biopsy material from early and advanced cases.

Postmortem studies indicate the following common *distribution* of changes in all cases: striking loss of nerve fibers in distal nerve trunks of the legs, intense fiber breakdown in distal nerves with less active changes proximally, normal spinal roots and degeneration in the cervical portion of the gracile fasiculi. Anterior horn cells remain intact but show chromatolysis.[12,13] Nerve biopsy study of early and advanced cases indicates the *nature* of the PNS change to be nonspecific axonal shrinkage, secondary myelin breakdown, and eventually, fiber loss. Large myelinated fibers appear initially affected. In advanced cases, both small myelinated and unmyelinated axons degenerate. Blood vessels and connective tissue elements display only mild secondary reactions.[14,15]

PATHOGENESIS. The distribution and nature of the pathologic changes, taken in concert with clinical findings, constitute overwhelming evidence that uremic polyneuropathy is a distal axonopathy. Presumably, its pathogenesis is similar to that proposed for other metabolic or toxic axonopathies (see Chapter 2), and its elucidation awaits identification of the underlying metabolic disturbance. There is no animal model of uremic neuropathy.

Clinical Features

INCIDENCE. Evidence of uremic neuropathy is present in approximately half of all patients in hemodialysis programs, and the disorder is more common in males.[11] Since the recent proliferation of hemodialysis and renal transplant centers, advanced, disabled cases of neuropathy are less frequent. Many mild or subclinical cases probably are undetected. This notion is supported by the observation of nerve conduction abnormalities in individuals with chronic renal insufficiency and no clinical evidence of PNS dysfunction.[16,17]

Symptoms, Signs, Course

The cardinal clinical features of fully developed uremic neuropathy are similar to those described for most distal axonopathies and include distal to proximal progression of signs, legs affected more than arms, symmetrical loss of both motor and sensory function and slow recovery.[11,14]

SYMPTOMS. Initially, sensory symptoms often predominate, and tingling paresthesias of the legs are especially frequent. Occasionally, the "burning-feet" syndrome, similar in every respect to that encountered in nutritional deficiency, occurs. Weakness of foot dorsiflexion is the usual first motor complaint.

The "restless legs" syndrome commonly accompanies sensory symptoms in the early stages, and has statistical association with uremic neuropathy. Leg movements are especially frequent at night. Occasionally, this syndrome appears to herald the development of neuropathy.[18] Muscle cramps in distal extremities are common.

SIGNS. Loss of the Achilles reflex is usually an early sign in uremic neuropathy, often accompanied by diminished vibration sense in the toes. Advanced cases almost always display distal diminution of vibration, touch, and position sense. Pain and temperature senses are less frequently involved. Weakness and atrophy of distal muscles are also common in advanced uremic neuropathy. Although the overwhelming majority of cases develop a mixed sensorimotor neuropathy, rare instances of pure motor and pure sensory patterns are well documented. Autonomic dysfunction is uncommon, except in the more severe cases; prominent features include postural hypotension, impaired sweating, and abnormal Valsalva maneuver. Abnormalities of eighth nerve function, both auditory and vestibular, may be present;[20] their pathogenesis is obscure and may reflect, in part, CNS dysfunction or the effects of ototoxic antibiotics.

Isolated mononeuropathy syndromes may rarely occur in individuals with chronic renal failure, and are generally attributed to an abnormal susceptibility to pressure palsies.[17]

COURSE. Gradual onset of a progressively disabling sensorimotor neuropathy is usual. Most progress over several months to reach a plateau despite worsening of the renal state. However, there may be considerable variation in tempo, and cases with a near-apoplectic development of an advanced neuropathy occur.[12]

The advent of long-term hemodialysis and aggressive renal transplant services have significantly altered the natural history of uremic neuropathy,[17] and are discussed in the following section.

Laboratory Studies

CLINICAL LABORATORY. Abnormal values of routine clinical laboratory tests are common, and reflect the effects of chronic renal dysfunction such as anemia and electrolyte abnormalities.

CEREBROSPINAL FLUID. The CSF is acellular. Protein may be moderately elevated, perhaps reflecting coexistent uremic encephalopathy in these cases.[11]

ELECTRODIAGNOSTIC STUDIES. Abnormalities of motor nerve conduction may be present in the legs of asymptomatic individuals with chronic renal disease, and may reflect subclinical neuropathy.[16,17] In more advanced cases, nerve conduction velocity and muscle and nerve action potential amplitude generally parallel the degree of clinical and pathologic impairment, and probably reflect changes in large, rapidly conducting myelinated axons.[14] Following successful renal transplantation, nerve conduction gradually returns to normal levels, *pari passu* with clinical improvement.[4] Hemodialysis has much less effect on nerve conduction.

Electromyographic signs of denervation in distal leg muscles are a consistent early feature of uremic polyneuropathy, and frequently disappear following renal transplantation.

Prognosis and Treatment

PROGNOSIS. The prognosis of untreated uremic neuropathy is usually poor, and in the past it was among the disabling complications of chronic renal failure.[12]

TREATMENT. Successful renal transplantation is unquestionably effective in the prevention and reversal of uremic neuropathy. Mild cases display prompt relief of paresthesias and a steady return of strength and sensibility. Recovery is more prolonged in advanced cases and not always complete.[3,4,11]

Repeated hemodialysis is considerably less effective in ameliorating neuropathy. While it is generally held that some patients improve or become stable following repeated hemodialysis,[21,22] its effectiveness in treating uremic neuropathy is still debated.[23] Paresthesias frequently disappear soon after beginning dialysis.[17] Features of uremic neuropathy most resistant to dialysis are sensory loss for vibration, touch and position. The "restless legs" syndrome also responds poorly (if at all) to dialysis.[17,19]

It has been proposed that close monitoring of peripheral nerve function (electrophysiology, quantitative sensory testing) in individuals with chronic renal disease might prove helpful in indicating the need for dialysis. One clinical study, using quantitative tests of sensation, sensitive electrophysiologic techniques, and the services of an active nephrology unit, challenges this assumption and indicates a limited role for the neurologist in the decisions that dictate the need for dialysis.[23]

Differential Diagnosis

The diagnosis of uremic neuropathy is not difficult in an individual with *chronic* renal disease who develops signs of a progressive, distal, symmetrical sensorimotor polyneuropathy.

Uremia is a common condition, and its associated polyneuropathy is clinically indistinguishible from many other distal axonopathies. Therefore, the diagnosis of uremic polyneuropathy should be entertained with caution in individuals with coexistent metabolic disorders, or in those who may also be exposed to neurotoxic agents. This is an especially common dilemma in uremic patients who may be taking neurotoxic antibiotics such as nitrofurantoin.

Case History and Comment*

CASE HISTORY. A 38-year-old printer was admitted in February, 1967. He had been admitted to another hospital in 1966 because of headaches and occasional vomiting which had been present for three years. These symptoms became worse one week before admission. He was found to have malignant hypertension (220/150) and chronic pyelonephritis with bilateral contracted kidneys.

Hgb was 8.4 g per dl; plasma sodium 137 mEq per liter, potassium 5.3 mEq per liter; blood urea 330 mg per dl. His urine showed proteinuria with a few granular casts and polymorphonuclearleukocytes and an IVP bilateral small contracted kidneys.

While in hospital he developed weakness of both legs. He was treated initially by a 20-g protein, low-salt diet, and peritoneal dialysis with no improvement in his neuropathy and was therefore transferred to the Royal Free Hospital, London, for hemodialysis.

On admission to the Royal Free Hospital, no cranial nerve abnormality or abnormalities in the upper limbs were found. In the legs, there was bilateral wasting of the anterior tibial and small foot muscles, and weakness of all muscle groups below the knees, particularly dorsiflexion and eversion at the ankles and of extension of the toes. Knee jerks were present and symmetrical, but neither ankle jerk was obtainable. Plantar responses were flexor. No sensory loss was detectable.

Following hemodialysis, his neuropathy deteriorated, with increased weakness in his legs and the development of numbness and tingling paresthesias in his legs and hands. He became unable to walk. Examination showed mild weakness and wasting of the small hand muscles and more severe weakness distally in his legs, loss of both knee and ankle jerks, mild distal sensory impairment for all modalities in the legs, and slight cuta-

*(Case 4. Thomas, PK, et al, 1974, with permission)

neous sensory loss over the hands. A sural nerve biopsy was performed on August 6, 1967.

Slow recovery occurred, but the patient remained confined to a wheelchair for six months. Nine months after starting hemodialysis, he was able to walk and climb stairs. When examined in July 1970, he was still aware of some persisting weakness and numbness of his feet and had "restless legs" in bed at night. There was moderate distal weakness in his legs, mainly for dorsiflexion and eversion at the ankles. The knee jerks had returned, but the ankle jerks remained absent. Sensory testing still revealed distal impairment for all modalities in the legs. Successful renal transplantation was performed in November 1970, following which he was maintained on prednisolone and azathioprine. The sensory symptoms from his neuropathy improved substantially after the operation, although the weakness in his legs improved only slightly. When last reviewed in April 1971, he still showed distal weakness in his legs and his ankle jerks remained absent. The impairment of cutaneous and vibration sensibility was less extensive and joint position sense in his toes was no longer inaccurate.

Motor nerve conduction velocity in the median nerve shortly after his transfer to the Royal Free Hospital was slightly reduced (47 m per sec). A median sensory nerve action potential of reduced amplitude (4 μV), but with a normal velocity (55 m per sec) was obtained. Following the deterioration after the commencement of hemodialysis, motor nerve conduction velocity in the median nerve was 45 m per sec, but could not be estimated in the peroneal nerve as both extensor digitorum brevis muscles became completely denervated and had not become reinnervated at the time of his examination in July 1970. Motor-nerve conduction velocity in the median nerve was then 50 m per sec, and a median-sensory nerve action potential 6 μV in amplitude with a velocity of 56 m per sec was obtained. In April 1971, five months after renal transplantation, motor nerve conduction velocity in the median nerve was 55 m per sec. A median sensory nerve action potential 12 μV in amplitude was recorded with a velocity of 59 m per sec. The extensor digitorum brevis muscles had become reinnervated, and a motor conduction velocity of 27 m per sec was obtained in the common peroneal nerve.

COMMENT. This case displays many of the cardinal features of uremic neuropathy. PNS dysfunction appeared years following symptoms related to renal failure, and although initially motor signs predominated, an eventual sensorimotor neuropathy developed. Hemodialysis was associated with some improvement of neurologic dysfunction, but did not prevent the appearance of the "restless legs" syndrome. Renal transplantation was eventually necessary and resulted in substantial relief from sensory symptoms.

REFERENCES

1. ASBURY, AK AND JOHNSON, PC: *Pathology of Peripheral Nerve*. WB Saunders, Philadelphia, 1978, p 80.
2. SCHAUMBURG, HH AND SPENCER, PS: *The toxic neuropathies—a review*. Neurology (Minneap) 29:429, 1979.
3. BOLTON, CF, BALTZAN, MA, BALTAAN, RB: *Effects of renal transplantation on uremic neuropathy. A clinical and electrophysiologic study*. N Engl J Med 284:1170, 1971.
4. OH, SJ, ET AL: *Rapid improvement in nerve conduction velocity following renal transplantation*. Ann Neurol 4:369, 1978.

5.   TENCKHOFF, HA, ET AL: *Polyneuropathy in chronic renal insufficiency.* JAMA 192:1121, 1965.

6.   DEJESUS, PB, CLEMENTS, RS AND WINEGRAD, AI: *Hypermyoinositolemic polyneuropathy in rats. A possible mechanism for uremic polyneuropathy.* J Neurol Sci 21:237, 1974.

7.   REZNEK, RH, SALWAY, JG AND THOMAS, PK: *Plasma myoinositol levels in uremic neuropathy.* Lancet 1:675, 1977.

8.   AVRAM, MM, FEINFELD, DA, HUATUCO, AH: *Search for the uremic toxin: decreased motor nerve conduction velocity and elevated parathyroid hormone in uremia.* N Engl J Med 298:1000, 1978.

9.   EGAN, JD AND WELLS, IC: *Transketolase inhibition and uremic peripheral sensory neuropathy.* J Neurol Sci 41:379, 1979.

10. HOLLINRAKE, K, ET AL: *Observations on plasma magnesium levels in patients with uremic neuropathy under treatment by periodic hemodyialysis.* Neurology (Minneap) 20:939, 1970.

11. ASBURY, AK: *Uremic neuropathy.* In DYCK, PJ, THOMAS, PK AND LAMBERT, EH (EDS): *Peripheral Neuropathy,* Vol II, WB Saunders, Philadelphia, 1975, p 982.

12. ASBURY, AK, VICTOR M AND ADAMS, RD: *Uremic polyneuropathy.* Arch Neurol 8:413, 1963.

13. FORNO, L AND ALSTON, W: *Uremic polyneuropathy.* Acta Neurol Scand 43:640, 1967.

14. THOMAS, PK, ET AL: *The polyneuropathy of chronic renal failure.* Brain 94:761, 1971.

15. DYCK, PJ, ET AL: *Segmental demyelination secondary to axonal degeneration in uremic neuropathy.* Mayo Clin Proc 46:400, 1971.

16. PRESWICK, G AND JEREMY, D: *Subclinical polyneuropathy in chronic renal failure.* Lancet 2:731, 1964.

17. THOMAS, PK: *Screening for peripheral neuropathy in patients treated by chronic hemodialysis.* Muscle and Nerve 1:396, 1979.

18. CALLAGHAN, N: *Restless legs syndrome in uremic neuropathy.* Neurology (Minneap) 16:359, 1966.

19. NIELSEN, VK: *The peripheral nerve function in chronic renal failure.* Lancet 2:731, 1964.

20. WIGAND, ME, ET AL: *Kochleovestibulare Storung bei Uramie in Beziehung zum Elektrolytstoffwechsel und Glomerulumfiltrat.* Schweiz Med Wochenschr 102:477, 1972.

21. JEBSEN, RH, TENCKHOFF, H AND HONET, JC: *Natural history of uremic polyneuropathy and effects of dialysis.* N Engl J Med 277:327, 1967.

22. KONOTEY-AHULU, FID, ET AL: *Effect of periodic dialysis on the peripheral neuropathy of end stage renal failure.* Brit Med J 2:1212, 1965.

23. DYCK, PJ ET AL: *Comparison of symptoms, chemistry, and nerve function to assess adequacy of hemodialysis.* Neurology (Minneap) 29:1361, 1979.

Chapter 7

METABOLIC NEUROPATHY: THE PORPHYRIAS

DEFINITION AND ETIOLOGY

DEFINITION. The prophyrias are a group of six rare hereditary disorders characterized by disturbances in heme biosynthesis.[1] Three are associated with peripheral neuropathy and mental disturbance: variegate porphyria (VP), acute intermittent porphyria (AIP), and hereditary coproporphyria (HCP).[2] Porphyric neuropathy is a serious, life-threatening illness and occurs in acute episodes, often induced by drugs.[3] (Table 3).

ETIOLOGY. Each of the porphyrias is characterized by a unique pattern of overproduction, accumulation, and excretion of intermediates of heme biosynthesis. They reflect genetically determined deficiencies of specific enzymes in the heme synthetic pathway (Fig. 15). The primary enzymatic defects in two of the porphyrias associated with neuropathy are known: uroporphyrinogen-1 synthetase deficiency in AIP and coproporphyrian oxidase deficiency in HCP.[1]

Pathology and Pathogenesis

PATHOLOGY. Detailed postmortem studies of the PNS in AIP suggest that distal axonopathy is the pathologic pattern in this neuropathy. Curiously,

TABLE 3. Drugs That Induce Porphyric Attacks

Barbiturates	Chlorpropamide
Chlordiazepoxide	Phenytoin
Meprobamate	Glutethimide
Sulfonamides	Griseofulvin
Estrogens	Rifampicin
Oral contraceptives	

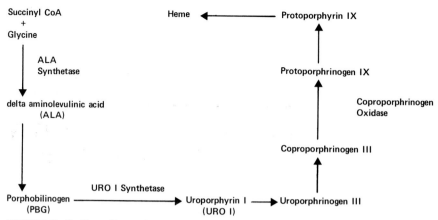

FIGURE 15. Outline of heme biosynthesis.

these studies suggest that in some cases, *short* motor axons appear preferentially affected, in striking contrast to the early changes in *long* axons which characterize most metabolic distal axonopathies.[4,5] Early weakness is a prominent clinical phenomenon in AIP; frequently it is proximal or assymetric, and may in part reflect selective involvement of short motor fibers. One study also demonstrates involvement of large-diameter axons supplying muscle spindles.[4] Selective involvement of short motor axons is not an inevitable finding, and there are also well documented instances of predominantly affected long motor and sensory fibers. This variability remains unexplained. Severe cases may exhibit axonal degeneration in the ventral roots, and fiber loss in the gracile columns occasionally occurs.[6] Nerve biopsies from cases of porphyric neuropathy display paranodal demyelination, probably secondary to axonal alterations.[7] The nature of the axonal change has not been studied by modern morphologic techniques, and despite considerable effort, there is no satisfactory animal model of human porphyric neuropathy. In sum, the mechanisms underlying this unusual distal axonopathy have not been elucidated by pathologic studies.

There are no characteristic postmortem CNS changes that can account for the prominent psychiatric phenomena in the porphyrias. Scattered areas of ischemic necrosis, present in some cases,[6] are scarcely an adequate substrate for the major behavioral aberrations characteristic of these conditions.

PATHOGENESIS. The pathogenetic link between peripheral neuropathy and biochemical abnormalities in heme synthesis is unknown.[1] AIP is the most studied of the three porphyrias, and several hypotheses have been proposed to explain both its neurologic and psychiatric manifestations. None is firmly supported by experimental evidence. Three suggestions are currently considered: (1) uroporphinogen-1 synthetase is deficient in neurons, leading to local cytotoxic accumulations of PBG or ALA;[2,8] (2) excess circulating ALA or PBG formed in the liver gains access to the nervous system and is toxic (an attractive notion since there exists a rough correlation between plasma levels of ALA, PBG, and neuropsychiatric symptoms);[1,9] (3) another hereditary metabolic defect, not directly related to heme synthesis, is present in the nervous system.[1,10]

Additionally, there is no satisfactory explanation for the precipitation of acute clinical attacks by such unrelated events as fasting, fever, drugs, toxins, and hormones.[1] The mechanism of drug idiosyncrasy is especially clinically relevant, since certain drugs (see Table 3) appear to be precipitating factors in most attacks in asymptomatic individuals with the genetic trait. It is suggested that these drugs induce hepatic cytochrome P450 which create an increased demand for hepatic heme-induced ALA synthetase.[1]

CLINICAL FEATURES
OF ACUTE INTERMITTENT PORPHYRIA

GENERAL. The neurologic manifestations of AIP, HCP and VP are identical, and presumably have a common pathogenesis.[1,2] These three conditions are distinguished principally by their different enzymatic defects, variations in urinary and fecal excretion of heme precursors, and the occurrence of photocutaneous lesions in VP. In other respects they are similar, and discussion of minor clinical variations is beyond the scope of this volume. Since AIP is the most commonly encountered and thoroughly delineated of the three conditions, this section is confined to its description.

INCIDENCE. AIP is rare, occurs world-wide and its incidence range is between 1:5000 and 1.5:100,000. In Lapland, the incidence is 1:1000, largely because of one kindred of 137 in this sparsely populated region. Diagnostic screening of psychiatric patients yields, not surprisingly, a higher incidence than in the general population.[1]

HEREDITY. AIP is autosomal dominant. It seems likely that homozygosity for this hereditary defect is not compatible with life. These conclusions are based on recent studies using erythrocyte urobilinogen 1-synthetase activity as the genetic marker, which has yielded more consistant data than the techniques employed in previous studies of carrier detection.[11]

Signs and Symptoms

SYMPTOMS AND SIGNS OF GENERAL DISEASE. This condition is often clinically latent; affected individuals may be asymptomatic or only manifest vague feelings of anxiety, malaise, and so forth. Latency is the rule in childhood, and attacks before puberty are extremely rare. Variability in phenotypic expression is common in autosomal dominant disorders; in AIP this genetic variability appears further compounded by the exquisite sensitivity of the disorder to environmental factors (drugs, fever, fasting).[1]

An acute attack of colicky abdominal pain, often combined with constipation, vomiting, fever, and leukocytosis is frequently the initial presentation.[12] The duration is variable (days to months), and intermittency is the rule. Exploratory laparotomy is frequent in unsuspected cases. The pathogenesis of the abdominal crises is obscure. Possibly they are related to autonomic neuropathy that results in gastrointestinal dysfunction with alternate periods of spasm and hypomotility.[12] Mental disturbance may accompany or occasionally precede abdominal attacks. Many patients have long histories of emotional instability, agitation, and occasionally, sociopathic behavior. Severe psychiatric episodes are frequently drug provoked, follow abdominal crises, and may be characterized by psychotic behavior, visual hallucinations and delirium.[13]

PNS SYMPTOMS. Symptoms of PNS dysfunction are rarely present in individuals without previous abdominal or mental disturbance. Most commonly, the peripheral neuropathy develops acutely or subacutely following the general manifestations of AIP. Indeed, the sequence of consultation may (in retrospect) be diagnostic: surgeon, psychiatrist, neurologist.[1]

Weakness is the cardinal symptom in the neuropathy of AIP. Pain in affected limbs or back may precede or be coincident.[2] Weakness may either begin in proximal or distal portions of any extremity, and both symmetrical and asymmetrical patterns occur. Sudden onset of asymmetrical, painful, shoulder-girdle weakness may initially suggest an erroneous diagnosis of brachial neuritis. Sensory symptoms occasionally are prominent and may herald neuropathy. Paresthesias, often distressingly severe, may occur in proximal or distal extremities, and in the face and neck.[3]

PNS SIGNS. Motor signs are predominant.[2] The pattern of weakness in early stages is extremely variable, upper limbs are usually most affected and proximal muscles may be weakest.[14] This contrasts strikingly with the pattern in other metabolic distal axonopathies, and correlates well with predominance of distal axonal degeneration in short nerves found at postmortem.[4] Some cases present with distal weakness of upper and lower extremities, and rare individuals display a monoplegic or hemiplegic pattern of flaccid paralysis. Most eventuate with severe, flaccid weakness of all extremities that also involves respiratory muscles. Muscle tenderness and cramps usually are present, and eventually profound wasting may occur.

Weakness of muscles innervated by cranial nerves, especially the facial and vagus, is frequent at later stages. Extraocular muscle palsy, ptosis and anisocoria are also described.[2]

Tendon reflexes are unpredictable. Usually they are absent or diminished; however, profound weakness may occur with relative preservation of tendon jerks, especially the Achilles reflex.

Sensory loss parallels the distribution of weakness. Diminished pain, thermal and touch sensation is usual, vibration is less frequently affected and joint position sense is often normal.

Autonomic dysfunction is common. Persistent tachycardia is present in almost every case, and is widely held to be characteristic of porphyric neuropathy. Other signs attributed to autonomic neuropathy are fluctuations in blood pressure, urinary and anal sphincter dysfunction, and fever. Many of the prominent gastrointestinal features of AIP may reflect autonomic involvement *(vide supra)*.

Laboratory Studies

CLINICAL LABORATORY. Abnormal values for routine clinical laboratory tests are common and usually reflect associated metabolic problems: inappropriate secretion of antidiuretic hormone, salt-losing renal lesions, and mild hepatic dysfunction. The urine may be brown if porphobilinogen is present in high concentrations. During attacks, urine porphobilinogen and ALA are usually readily detected in the urine; however, they may be absent between attacks and are variably present in asymptomatic carriers. Assay of erythrocyte urobilinogen 1-synthetase is widely regarded as the most accurate means of detecting AIP.[1]

CEREBROSPINAL FLUID. The cerebrospinal fluid is usually acellular and the protein content modestly elevated, rarely exceeding 100 mg per dl.

ELECTRODIAGNOSTIC STUDIES. Electromyographic signs of denervation appear in most involved muscles. Motor-nerve conduction velocities are generally normal or slightly decreased. There are no reports of sensory conduction in AIP neuropathy.[2]

NERVE BIOPSY. One report describes paranodal demyelination with slight segmental loss of myelin, and attributes this to a primary axonal alteration.[7]

Course, Treatment and Prognosis

COURSE. The progression of limb weakness or sensory signs is usually continuous and, in most cases, the neurologic deficit peaks within six weeks.[2] Variation exists, and stepwise progression, plateaus, mild fluctuations and prolonged courses are all documented.[3] It should be emphasized that *continuous* progression does not always mean *contiguous* progression in AIP. Proximal weakness in the arm may be followed by distal weakness in the same extremity, or by symmetrical weakness of the feet. Ascending paralysis or sensory loss is unusual in this disorder. Most attacks eventuate in weakness and sensory loss in all extremities, trunk and cranial nerves. Many patients are desperately ill, require both ventilatory and alimentary support, and can die from either respiratory or cardiac (sympathetic) complications. In the past, death was not unusual in severe cases. One study documented ten deaths in 29 attacks of neuropathy that occurred in 25 individuals—seven died during the first attack and three in subsequent episodes.[3]

Recovery usually commences within two months of the peak of neurologic disability. Reinnervation of proximal muscles and dermatomes occurs initially, and eventually strength and sensation are restored in the distal extremities. Thus, the pattern of recovery further supports the notion of distal axonopathy in this condition. Complete or near-complete recovery is the rule, although it may take years to restore function to distal extremities.[2]

Repeated attacks of AIP at widely ranging intervals may be accompanied by neuropathy, and are documented to occur within weeks or decades.[2]

TREATMENT. The most important measure in the management of AIP is prevention of acute attacks by instructing carriers about the provocative factors shown in Table 3. A dedicated search for carriers and genetic counseling are crucial in AIP.

Hematin and glucose both prevent induction of ALA synthetase in experimental animals and appear to reverse the human biochemical abnormalities in AIP, usually resulting in clinical improvement of abdominal and psychiatric signs within 48 hours. Glucose should be administered intravenously at a rate of 10 to 20 g every hour; if there is no improvement within 48 hours, intravenous hematin, 4 mg per kg, should be infused every 12 hours.[9]

Hyponatremia, hypomagnesemia, and azotemia require skilled manipulation of fluid and electrolyte therapy. Agitation, combativeness, and delirium usually respond well to phenothiazines.

Severe autonomic and somatic complications of AIP neuropathy frequently occur rapidly, may be life-threatening, and require sophisticated management. These patients, like individuals with the Guillain-Barré syndrome, are best treated in respiratory care facilities. Tachycardia and hypertension usually respond to beta-adrenergic blocking drugs. Respiratory failure is frequent in severe cases, and usually requires tracheostomy and ventilatory assistance.[2]

PROGNOSIS. Although AIP remains a serious illness, its prognosis has improved considerably in recent years, and fatalities are now rare. Most individuals recover from acute episodes and gradually regain strength and sensation.

Differential Diagnosis

The diagnosis of porphyric neuropathy is not difficult in an individual known to carry the genetic trait. Unsuspected AIP can constitute a formidable diagnostic problem for the surgeon and psychiatrist, since its clinical manifestations are protean. Differential diagnosis for the neurologist usually involves two conditions, the Guillain-Barré syndrome and toxic neuropathy.

(1) The Guillain-Barré syndrome may be readily misdiagnosed as AIP neuropathy since both may be asymmetrical, proximal, subacute, dominated by motor signs, accompanied by tachycardia and respiratory failure, and involve cranial nerves. The Guillain-Barré syndrome is not accompanied by abdominal crises or mental disturbances, and the urine does not contain porphobilinogen or ALA.

(2) Toxic neuropathies with a subacute onset may be caused by thallium, organophosphate, dapsone, nitrofurantoin, and lead. While the pharmaceutical agents usually are readily ruled out by history, lead presents a more difficult diagnostic problem. Plumbism may be accompanied by major gastrointestinal symptoms, porphyrin metabolism is deranged, and weakness often dominates the neurologic syndrome. There is a clear biochemical distinction between the two disorders: urine lead levels are not elevated in AIP, and erythrocyte urobilinogen 1-synthetase is normal in lead neuropathy.

Case History and Comment

CASE HISTORY. A 20-year-old male experienced intermittent abdominal cramping. Radiographic studies of the abdomen were negative. Two months later he noticed weakness and numbness in his fingers, which progressively involved hands, arms, and distal lower extremities. Within six days he was unable to walk, had difficulty swallowing, and was admitted to the hospital. General physical examination was unremarkable. Mental state appeared normal except for an inappropriate affect. There was severe proximal weakness and slight distal weakness of the arms, mild diffuse weakness of the legs, and bilateral facial weakness. Tendon reflexes were absent, except for brisk Achilles reflexes. Sensation was normal. Routine clinical laboratory tests were normal, as was examination of the CSF. Electromyography revealed denervation potentials in most muscles tested, and motor nerve conduction velocites were normal in arms and legs. He began to improve one week following admission, and was ambulatory at discharge five weeks later. Within three months there were no detectable neurologic signs, and he was told that he had recovered from an "atypical Guillain-Barré syndrome."

Two months later he developed fever, sore throat and cramping abdominal pains. He was given erythromycin and aspirin and soon afterwards he was admitted to the hospital. Examination revealed a temperature of 34°C, purulent exudate over the tonsils and, despite severe abdominal pain, a soft abdomen. Neurologic examination was unremarkable. He was treated with intravenous fluids and erythromycin. On the ninth hospital day his urine was noted to become red upon standing exposed to room air. A Watson-Schwartz test was positive, and subsequently elevated urine levels of ALA and PBG were obtained. He gradually improved and was discharged without signs or symptoms of neuropathy. He denied any family history of a similar condition.

COMMENT. This case demonstrates many of the cardinal findings of AIP neuropathy—rapid onset, proximal weakness and diffuse motor involvement—yet the diagnosis was only established following the serendipitous observation of red discoloration of the urine during a subsequent hospitalization. It seems likely that the febrile illness triggered the abdominal pain of the latter admission, and it is fortunate that he was not given a drug that might have precipitated another episode of neuropathy.

REFERENCES

1. MEYER, UA AND SCHMID, R: *The Porphyrias.* In STANBURY, JB, WYNGAARDEN, JB AND FREDRICKSON, DS (EDS): *The Metabolic Basis of Inherited Disease,* ed 4, McGraw-Hill, New York, 1978, p 1166.
2. RIDLEY, A: *Porphyric Neuropathy.* In DYCK, PJ, THOMAS, PK AND LAMBERT, EH (EDS): *Peripheral Neuropathy,* Vol. II, WB Saunders, Philadelphia, 1975, p 942.
3. RIDLEY, A: *The neuropathy of acute intermittent porphyrias.* Q J Med 38:307, 1969.
4. CAVANAGH, JB AND MELLICK, RS: *On the nature of the peripheral nerve lesions associated with acute intermittent porphyria.* J Neurol Neurosurg Psychiatry 28:320, 1965.
5. SWEENEY, VP, PATHAK, MH AND ASBURY, AK: *Acute intermittent porphyria. Increased ALA-synthetase activity during an acute attack.* Brain 93:369, 1970.
6. HIERONS, R: *Changes in the nervous system in acute porphyria.* Brain 80:176, 1957.
7. ASBURY, AK, SIDMAN, RL AND WOLF, MK: *Drug induced porphyrin accumulation in the nervous system.* Neurology (Minneap) 16:320, 1966.
8. DHAR, GJ, ET AL: *Effects of hematin in hepatic porphyria: Further studies.* Ann Int Med 83:20, 1975.
9. LABBE, RF: *Metabolic abnormalities in porphyria. The result of impaired biologic oxidation.* Lancet 1:1361, 1967.
10. SASSA, S, ET AL: *Studies in porphyria. IV. Expression of the gene defect of acute intermittent porphyria in cultured human skin fibroblasts and amniotic cells. Prenatal diagnosis of the porphyria trait.* J Exp Med 142:722, 1975.
11. GOLDBERG, A: *Acute intermittent porphyria. A study of 50 cases.* Q J Med 28:183, 1959.
12. GOLDBERG, A: *Diagnosis and treatment of the porphyrias.* Proc R Soc Med 61:193, 1968.
13. GARCIN, R AND LAPRESLE, J: *Manifestations nerveuses des porphyries.* Sem Hôp Paris 26:3404, 1950.
14. RIDLEY, A, HIERONS, R AND CAVANAGH, JB: *Tachycardia and the neuropathy of porphyria.* Lancet 2:708, 1968.

Chapter 8

METABOLIC NEUROPATHY: ENDOCRINE OTHER THAN DIABETES

HYPOTHYROIDISM

Definition and Classification

Two types of peripheral nerve disorders occur in hypothyroidism: symmetrical polyneuropathy,[1-8] and mononeuropathy.[8-10] The latter usually consists of the carpal tunnel syndrome. Sensorineural hearing loss is also associated with myxedema, but its etiology is obscure and it may not reflect primary alterations in the PNS.[4-11]

Pathology

MONONEUROPATHY. The carpal tunnel syndrome in hypothyroidism is probably secondary to compression of the median nerve by swollen tendons, synovial membranes, and other engorged connective tissues.[9] It seems unlikely that myxedemotous deposits occur within the perineurium and compress nerve fibers.[8] There are no contemporary morphologic studies of this entity; presumably the pathologic changes are similar to those described in entrapment neuropathy from other causes (see Chapter 18).

SYMMETRICAL POLYNEUROPATHY. There are no credible postmortem descriptions of the PNS changes in hypothyroid neuropathy. Contemporary studies, utilizing sural nerve biopsy specimens, indicate both axonal loss and segmental demyelination.[7,8] This conclusion is based both on teased fiber and ultrastructural examination. It appears likely that axonal change is primary, but this notion remains unproven. Neither deposits of foreign material nor excessive thickening of intraneural connective tissues are described. One study documents Schwann cells with excessive deposition of glycogen and nonspecific mitochondrial changes.[6]

Pathogenesis

MONONEUROPATHY. As already noted, the pathogenesis of the carpal tunnel syndrome is best understood as chronic compression of the median nerve by swollen connective tissue (see Chapter 18). Its severity does not correlate with that of the metabolic defect.

SYMMETRICAL POLYNEUROPATHY. It appears that metabolic derangement secondary to thyroid hypofunction may be responsible for the symmetrical polyneuropathy, giving rise to axonal degeneration with secondary or concomitant Schwann cell dysfunction. The nature of the metabolic disturbance is unknown.

Clinical Features

INCIDENCE. There are no reliable estimates for the incidence of either a symmetrical polyneuropathy or mononeuropathy.[8] Paresthesias of the fingertips (acroparesthesias) are common and usually reflect the carpal tunnel syndrome, the commonest peripheral nerve disturbance in hypothyroidism. Symmetrical polyneuropathy is rare.[6,7]

Symptoms and Signs

MONONEUROPATHY. Intermittent paresthesias in the hands, especially at night, are the main feature of the carpal tunnel syndrome.[9] The clinical manifestation of the hypothyroidism-associated type are identical to those usually found in this disorder, and are described in Chapter 18. Other entrapment neuropathies may occur, for example, meralgia paresthetica.

Symmetrical Polyneuropathy

SYMPTOMS. Distal-extremity paresthesias and muscle cramps are frequent in hypothyroidism,[2] and it has been suggested that they reflect subclinical polyneuropathy.[8] This notion is debated as these symptoms are not always accompanied by signs of PNS dysfunction, but there may be electrophysiologic abnormalities in such individuals.[12] Most patients with hypothyroid neuropathy initially complain of numbness in the feet. Within a few months, the hands are also affected. Leg weakness, accompanied by an unsteady gait, develops subsequently.

Symptoms of polyneuropathy are often accompanied or obscured by other manifestations of hypothyroidism such as constipation, scaly skin, fatigue, cold intolerance, hearing loss, and hoarseness.[8]

SIGNS. Touch, vibration, and position sense are decreased in the distal extremities in all instances; diminished pain or thermal sense is rare.[6] Tendon reflexes are usually absent in legs and depressed in the arms. Mild distal weakness of the legs is frequent, atrophy and fasciculations are rare. Proximal limb weakness, if present, is usually due to coexisting hypothyroid myopathy. Clumsiness and limb ataxia occasionally occur and are commonly attributed to cerebellar degeneration.[5] Prolonged relaxation of the tendon reflexes is characteristic of hypothyroidism, and does not reflect peripheral neuropathy.

Laboratory Studies

CLINICAL LABORATORY. Values of most routine laboratory tests are normal, but the serum cholesterol and creatine kinase concentrations may be elevated. Serum thyroxine levels are decreased in all varieties of hypothyroidism. Serum triiodothyronine levels and radioactive iodine uptake values are less predictable.

CEREBROSPINAL FLUID. The CSF protein is frequently mildly elevated in severe hypothyroidism, independent of malfunction of the peripheral nervous system.

Electrodiagnostic Studies

MONONEUROPATHY. Electrodiagnostic studies of individuals with the carpal tunnel syndrome are valuable, both in establishing the site of the lesion and in excluding a more diffuse neuropathy. Prolonged latency of motor and sensory impulses at the wrist and diminished amplitude of sensory action potentials are usually present. Electromyography of the thenar muscles reveals denervation changes in advanced cases (see Chapter 18).

SYMMETRICAL POLYNEUROPATHY. Motor nerve conduction velocity in the lower limbs is usually moderately slowed.[6] Electromyography occasionally reveals signs of denervation in distal muscles.[7] Coexistent carpal tunnel syndrome may complicate interpretation of upper-limb electrodiagnostic studies in individuals with symmetrical neuropathy.

Course, Treatment and Prognosis

MONONEUROPATHY. The severity of the carpal tunnel syndrome correlates poorly either with the degree or the duration of hypothyroidism. In general, the untreated course is a gradual increase in paresthesias, followed by sensorimotor loss in the distribution of the distal median nerve. Most cases improve following hormone replacement therapy; surgical section of the transverse carpal ligament usually is unnecessary.[8,10]

SYMMETRICAL POLYNEUROPATHY. The untreated course is relentless progression from initially mild sensory impairment to a severe distal symmetrical sensorimotor neuropathy. The natural history of untreated neuropathy is unknown since published reports all deal with treated cases. Symmetrical polyneuropathy responds well to hormone replacement therapy; usually there is dramatic improvement in signs, symptoms, and electrophysiologic function within six months.[6,7,8]

Differential Diagnosis

MONONEUROPATHY. The diagnosis of hypothyroidism should be entertained in individuals with the carpal tunnel syndrome, even if they appear euthyroid and the condition is unilateral. In blatantly hypothyroid patients with the carpal tunnel syndrome, it is unlikely that other factors are operant, but it is prudent to rule out chronic arthritic compression of the median nerves.

SYMMETRICAL POLYNEUROPATHY. It is not difficult to identify hypothyroid neuropathy when accompanied by florid myxedema, but the clinical features are nonspecific and the condition cannot be distinguished from many other symmetrical polyneuropathies. Fortunately, symptoms and signs of clinical hypothyroidism are clearly apparent in most cases and recovery after hormonal replacement therapy will confirm the diagnosis.

ACROMEGALY

Definition and Etiology.

Acromegaly is usually caused by growth hormone-secreting tumors develop in the pituitary gland. Two types of PNS involvement may develop: an entrapment mononeuropathy, usually the carpal tunnel syndrome,[13,14] and a distal symmetrical polyneuropathy.[15,16] Proximal muscle weakness (acromegalic myopathy) occurs independently of PNS changes, and may confuse the clinical profile.[13]

Pathology and Pathogenesis

MONONEUROPATHY. There is no contemporary description of morphologic changes in the acromegalic carpal tunnel syndrome. Presumably compression results from combined acral soft-tissue hyperplasia, synovial edema, bony overgrowth, and osteoarthritis.[13,14,17,18] The pathology and pathogenesis of this condition are discussed in Chapter 18.

SYMMETRICAL POLYNEUROPATHY. There are widely differing descriptions of the peripheral nerves in acromegaly. Earlier reports of a hypertrophic neuropathy in acromegaly[19,20] are not substantiated by a recent study which utilizes modern histopathologic techniques.[16] It is also possible that some early reports describe diabetic changes in peripheral nerve, since diabetes is a well known complication of acromegaly. The recent study examines sural nerve biopsies from four nondiabetic acromegalic subjects and describes a reduction in the number of myelinated and unmyelinated fibers, segmental demyelination, and occasional onion-bulb formations. It is not clear whether segmental demyelination in this condition is a primary change or secondary to axonal degeneration.[16]

The pathogenesis of acromegalic neuropathy is obscure. It is suggested that excessive growth hormone is responsible, but there is no clear relationship between symmetrical polyneuropathy and plasma levels of growth hormone.[13]

Clinical Features

INCIDENCE. The carpal tunnel syndrome is a well-known complication of acromegaly and can be detected in more than one third of cases.[13] Estimates of the incidence of symmetrical polyneuropathy vary; it is probably uncommon.

Symptoms and Signs

MONONEUROPATHY. The manifestations of the carpal tunnel syndrome in acromegaly do not differ from those usually encountered in this condition (see Chapter 10). It seems likely that acroparesthesias of the fingers, which occur in one third of all acromegalics, arise from this cause.

SYMMETRICAL POLYNEUROPATHY. Symptoms of polyneuropathy may develop at any time in the course of acromegaly, but mostly appear late in the illness.[13,16] Initial symptoms are paresthesias in the feet and hands, followed by the insidious development of weakness.

SIGNS. Decreased touch, vibration, and position sense in the lower extremities is characteristic. Tendon reflexes are usually absent in the legs and depressed in the arms. Mild distal weakness of the legs is frequent, and atrophy and fasciculations are rare. Thickening of peripheral nerve trunks has been described, but is an inconsistent finding.[20]

Laboratory Studies

CLINICAL LABORATORY. Values of most routine laboratory tests are normal, although the plasma glucose may be elevated. Serum growth hormone is usually elevated, and its level is not suppressed following glucose ingestion.

CEREBROSPINAL FLUID. The CSF is usually normal.

Electrodiagnostic Studies

MONONEUROPATHY. Nerve conduction studies of individuals with the carpal tunnel syndrome are diagnostically helpful, both in establishing the site of damage and in excluding more widespread nerve dysfunction (see Chapter 18).

SYMMETRICAL POLYNEUROPATHY. Motor and sensory nerve conduction in limb nerves is abnormal, with moderately reduced motor conduction velocity and depressed or absent sensory action potentials.[16]

Course, Treatment and Prognosis

MONONEUROPATHY. The untreated course is a gradual increase in paresthesias, followed by sensorimotor loss in the distribution of the distal median nerve. Most cases improve following removal of the pituitary adenoma, and surgery of the transverse carpal ligament usually is unnecessary.[13]

SYMMETRICAL POLYNEUROPATHY. The course is gradual worsening of distal motor and sensory manifestations. There are no studies of the effect of removal of pituitary adenoma on the course of the neuropathy.[13,16]

Differential Diagnosis

There is usually little difficulty establishing the diagnosis, since mononeuropathy or symmetrical polyneuropathy usually occur after the somatic manifestations of acromegaly have become obvious. This is not always true for the carpal tunnel syndrome, as the acromegalic changes develop insidiously and may at first be overlooked.

REFERENCES

1. NICKEL, SN AND FRAME B: *Neurologic manifestations of myxedema.* Neurology (Minneap) 8:511, 1958.

2. CREVASSE, LE AND LOGUE, RR: *Peripheral neuropathy in myxedema.* Ann Int Med 50:1433, 1959.

3. NICKLE, SN ET AL: *Myxedema neuropathy and myopathy. A clinical and pathologic study.* Neurology (Minneap) 11:125, 1961.

4. SANDERS, V: *Neurologic manifestations of myxedema.* N Eng J Med 266:547, 599, 1962.

5. CREMER, GM, GOLDSTEIN, NP AND PARIS, J: *Myxedema and ataxia.* Neurology (Minneap) 19:37, 1969.

6. DYCK, PJ AND LAMBERT, EH: *Polyneuropathy associated with hypothyroidism.* J Neuropathol Exp Neurol 29:631, 1970.

7. SHIRABE, T, ET AL: *Myxoedematous polyneuropathy: a light and electron microscopic study of the peripheral nerve and muscle.* J Neurol Neurosurg Psychiatry 38:241, 1975.

8. BASTRON, JA: *Neuropathy in Diseases of the Thyroid.* In DYCK, PJ, THOMAS, PK AND LAMBERT, EH (EDS): *Peripheral Neuropathy,* Vol. II, WB Saunders, Philadelphia, 1975, p 999.

9. MURRAY, IPC AND SIMPSON, JA: *Acroparaesthesia in myxoedema. A clinical and electromyographic study.* Lancet 1:1360, 1958.

10. Purnel, DC, Daly, DD and Lipscomb, PR: *Carpal-tunnel syndrome associated with myxedema.* Arch Int Med 108:751, 1961.

11. GREENE, R: *The thyroid gland: its relationship to neurology.* In VINKEN, PJ AND BRUYN, GE (eds): *Handbook of Clinical Neurology,* Vol 27, Metabolic and Deficiency Diseases of the Nervous System, Part I, Elsevier North Holland, New York, 1976, p 255.

12. FINCHAM, RW AND CAPE, CA: *Neuropathy in myxedema: a study of sensory nerve conduction in the upper extremities.* Arch Neurol 19:464, 1968.

13. PICKETT, JBE, ET AL: *Neuromuscular complications of acromegaly.* Neurology (Minneap) 25:638, 1975.

14. O'DUFFY, JD, RANDALL, RV, MACCARTY, CS: *Median neuropathy (carpal tunnel syndrome) in acromegaly. A sign of endocrine overactivity.* Ann Int Med 78:379, 1973.

15. DINN, JJ: *Schwann cell dysfunction in acromegaly.* J Clin Endocrinol Metab 31:140, 1970.

16. Low, PA, ET AL: *Peripheral neuropathy in acromegaly.* Brain 97:139, 1974.

17. SCHILLER, F, AND KOLB, FO: *Carpal tunnel syndrome in acromegaly.* Neurology (Minneap) 4:271, 1954.

18. BIGLIERI, EG, WALTINGTON, CO AND FORSHAM, PH: *Sodium retention with human growth hormone and its subfractions.* J Clin Endocrinol Metab 21:361, 1961.

19. WOLTMAN, HW: *Neuritis associated with acromegaly.* Arch Neurol Psychiatry 45:680, 1941.

20. STEWART, BM: *The hypertrophic neuropathy of acromegaly.* Arch Neurol 14:107, 1966.

Chapter 9

METABOLIC NEUROPATHY: HEREDITARY DISORDERS OF LIPID METABOLISM

This is a heterogeneous group of disorders characterized by accumulation of lipids in tissues, but with widely different clinical and morphologic manifestations. These are rare disorders, and in most, peripheral neuropathy is not the predominant feature.

SULFATIDE LIPIDOSIS (METACHROMATIC LEUKODYSTROPHY)

Biochemical Abnormality

Accumulation of galactosyl-3-sulfate and lipids containing the galactosyl-3-sulfate moiety characterizes this disorder. The enzyme arylsulfatase A is deficient in the more common forms, and its assay in blood leukocytes and cultured skin fibroblasts is used both as a standard diagnostic test and a means of heterozygote detection.[1]

General Features

Sulfatide lipidosis includes several autosomal recessive conditions. The three most common types, all associated with arylsulfatase A deficiency, are the late infantile, juvenile, and adult forms.[1] The late infantile form is by far the most common and its clinical features develop in four stages. Stage 1 manifests in the second year by weakness and hypotonia; a spastic gait occasionally appears in this stage. Stage 2 follows within 18 months, the child is unable to stand, speech is slurred, and intellect dulled. Stage 3 follows within 6 months, featured by quadriparesis, abnormal posture, and further deterioration in speech and intellect. In the final stage, patients are blind, unable to move, and fed by nasogastric tube. Lifespan is usually 5 to 6 years after the first signs. The juvenile form is clinically similar to the infantile type. The adult-onset variety is characterized by slowly progressing dementia, spasticity, and a protracted course. Most are labeled as schizophrenia or multiple sclerosis, unless other family members are known to be affected. Occasional cases present with neuropathy. The sulfatide lipidoses are uniformly fatal and there is no specific therapy.

Diagnosis is usually established by the determination of leukocyte or fibroblast arylsulfatase A levels. This test is not fully reliable but is ulitized for heterozygote detection. Prenatal diagnosis of sulfatide lipidosis is now possible, allowing selective termination of pregnancy. However, there is an overlap between the enzyme levels for homozygotes and heterozygotes.[1]

The most striking pathologic change is widespread degeneration of white matter of the central nervous system, accompanied by the accumulation of masses of sulfatide (metachromatic-staining) material in macrophages and in certain groups of neurons.[2] Deposits of metachromatic material are also present in Schwann cells, renal epithelium, gall bladder, pancreas, and anterior pituitary. Ultrastructurally, the sulfatide deposits display a characteristic lamellated pattern.[3]

Pathology and Pathogenesis of Neuropathy

Segmental demyelination with little alteration in axons is characteristic of this neuropathy. Metachromatic granular inclusions in the perinuclear region of Schwann cells of myelinated and unmyelinated nerve fibers is pathognomonic.[4] This material is composed of sulfatide, and on ultrastructural examination displays a lamellated pattern identical to the CNS inclusions. It is likely that these inclusions indicate abnormal storage within Schwann cells and do not merely represent myelin breakdown products.[5]

The pathogenesis of this demyelinative neuropathy presumably is related to the generalized disorder of lipid metabolism. Myelin breakdown probably results from a metabolic disturbance that affects the ability of the Schwann cell to maintain its myelin segment. The mechanism underlying myelin loss is unclear, as is its relationship to sulfatide storage. The degree of demyelination correlates poorly with the amount of inclusion material present.[5]

Clinical Features of Neuropathy

Diffuse limb weakness, hypotonia, and diminished tendon reflexes are early findings in the infantile and juvenile conditions. Muscle cramps and extremity pain are occasional complaints in the initial stages. Signs of peripheral neuropathy are always present from the outset in these forms, and occasionally dominate the early clinical profile. As CNS dysfunction progressively develops, a curious mixture of hypertonicity, ataxia, and areflexia appears. In the adult form signs and symptoms of neuropathy are usually few, and often are obscured by severe dementia and spasticity.[4,5]

The CSF protein is usually elevated to 100 to 200 mg per dl. Motor nerve conduction velocity is frequently profoundly slowed, characteristic of a demyelinating neuropathy. Nerve biopsy is almost always diagnostic for sulfatide lipidosis, and prior to the development of serum enzyme assays, sural nerve biopsy was considered one of the most reliable tests.

GALACTOSYLCERAMIDE LIPIDOSIS (GLOBOID CELL LEUKODYSTROPHY, KRABBE'S DISEASE)

Biochemical Abnormality

The enzyme galactosylceramide β-galactosidase is deficient in all cases, leading to the accumulation of galactocerebroside in CNS and PNS. This diagnosis can now be established by enzymatic assay in affected individuals, fetuses, and heterozygous carriers.[6]

General Features

This is an autosomal recessive condition and occurs equally in both sexes. Onset is usually in the first year of life, rarely juvenile. Typically, the affected child, apparently normal during the first months of life, becomes irritable, hypersensitive to sounds, and may have a seizure. Within a few months motor and mental deterioration becomes apparent and hypertonicity appears. Eventually the child becomes blind, mute, and quadriplegic. The duration of the illness is usually two years and most clinical phenomena reflect CNS involvement. Visceral enlargement or skin changes are not part of this illness. The sole indications of peripheral nerve dysfunction are hyporeflexia and abnormal nerve conduction.[7]

The most striking pathologic change is widespread degeneration of CNS white matter, accompanied by profuse clusters of characteristic cells (globoid cells) with abundant cytoplasm and one or more nuclei. Globoid cells are macrophages, contain galactocerebroside, and occur throughout CNS white matter. Ultrastructurally, they are characterized by abnormal, intracellular tubular profiles that have a crystalloid appearance in cross-section. Injection of galactocerebroside into a rat's brain produces typical globoid cells with identical ultrastructural features.[6]

The PNS is affected in nearly every case.[5,8] Segmental demyelination may be prominent, presumably related to a primary metabolic disorder in Schwann cells. Globoid cells do not occur in the PNS, but similar ultrastructural inclusions are present in Schwann cells and in perivascular histiocytes.[5] Usually there is a mild or moderate degree of nerve fiber loss, and nonspecific axonal changes occasionally occur.[9]

LIPOPROTEIN DEFICIENCIES

Two hereditary lipoprotein-deficiency states are associated with nervous system dysfunction. One is deficiency of beta-lipoprotein, with principal involvement of the CNS together with moderate PNS dysfunction; the other is deficiency of high-density lipoprotein (HDL), prominently featured by peripheral neuropathy.

ABETALIPOPROTEINEMIA (BASSEN-KORNZWEIG DISEASE)

Biochemical Abnormality

The specific metabolic deficit in abetalipoproteinemia is unknown. Reduced synthesis of very low-density lipoprotein, low-density lipoprotein and chylomicrons are all characteristic of this disorder. Consequently, triglycerides accumulate in intestinal mucosa, fat-soluble vitamins (A and E) are not absorbed, and plasma cholesterol levels are reduced.[10]

Pathology and Pathogenesis

Although it has been suggested that peripheral neuropathy of distal axonopathy type is a feature of this disorder, this has not been adequately documented morphologically. Autopsy and nerve biopsy studies have revealed segmental demyelination and predominant large fiber axonal loss.[11-14] Electrophysiologic studies do not support the notion of primary demyelination. One postmortem study depicts diffuse fiber loss in gracile and cuneate tracts and in the ascending spinocerebellar systems.[11] These changes are compatible with primary neuronal dysfunction in these systems (neuronopathy). Unfortunately, the dorsal root ganglia and Clarke's column neurons were not adequately described.

The pathogenesis of the nervous system dysfunction is unknown. Two hypotheses are current.[10] One is that malabsorption of fat-soluble vitamins at an early age results in this widespread disorder. The other holds that absent low-density lipoprotein impairs cholesterol synthesis and affects the content of sterols in membranes of many cell types, leading to early dysfunction and eventual disappearance of these cells.

Clinical Features

This is an autosomal recessive disorder that occurs equally in males and females. Onset is in infancy and the clinical picture is dominated by intestinal malabsorption. Growth retardation is soon apparent, accompanied by clumsiness and limb ataxia. Subsequently, tremor and dysarthria indicate cerebellar system abnormality, while hyporeflexia and diffuse proprioceptive dysfunction imply large-fiber sensory malfunction.[11,12] The clinical profile is thus similar in some aspects to that of Friedreich's ataxia.[13] Stocking-glove sensorimotor loss, distal muscle atrophy, and occasional spasticity may occur. Motor conduction velocity is moderately reduced and sensory action potentials are reduced or absent. Retinitis pigmentosa appears in adolescence, accompanied by night blindness and diminished visual acuity. Myocardial fibrosis associated with congestive heart failure, ventricular enlargement, and arrhythmias has been described.[14] Individuals may live until middle age, but are usually incapacited by neurologic involvement. Clinical laboratory evaluation is usually diagnostic and is featured by low plasma cholesterol, absent chylomicrons, abnormal levels of low-density lipoprotein, and bizzare erythrocytes with spiny processes (acanthocytes).[10] Recent reports have implicated vitamin E deficiency secondary to intestinal malabsorption in the causation of the retinal and neurologic changes, indicating that dietary fat restriction and high doses of vitamins A and E may prevent or arrest these complications.[15]

HIGH-DENSITY LIPOPROTEIN DEFICIENCY (TANGIER DISEASE)

Biochemical Abnormality

The nature of the fundamental biochemical defect is unknown; presumably there is either decreased synthesis or increased catabolism of high-density lipoprotein (HDL).[10] The cardinal biochemical features of Tangier disease are the virtual absence of serum HDL, a low serum cholesterol, and massive deposition of cholesterol esters within tissues. The latter accounts for some of the most striking clinical signs in this illness. The biochemical disturbance underlying cholesterol ester deposition remains obscure, but may relate to instability of chylomicrons leading to the uptake of their contents by reticuloendothelial cells throughout the body.

General Features

HDL deficiency is autosomal recessive and occurs equally in both sexes. There is a considerable spectrum both in degree and variety of clinical phenomena in this condition. Some experience only mild enlargement of the tonsils throughout life, while others become incapacitated with neuropathy, have severe hepatosplenomegaly, and corneal opacities. In general, it is not a life-threatening condition. Tonsilar enlargement is dramatic and the condition may be first suspected on discovering large, yellow multilobular glands on oropharyngeal examination. Evidence of PNS dysfunction is present in most cases, and peripheral neuropathy may be the initial manifestation of the condition (vide infra). Splenomegaly secondary to cholesterol-ester deposits occurs in two thirds of the cases and may produce anemia and thrombocytopenia. Lymph nodes, cornea, and rectal mucosa are also frequently distorted by cholesterol ester deposition.[10]

Pathology and Pathogenesis

The CNS is normal.[16] PNS changes are reported from several nerve biopsies and one postmortem study.[16-22] Diminished numbers of small myelinated and unmyelinated fibers occur in both radial and sural nerves, without evidence of segmental demyelination or active axonal degeneration. A variable number of small lipid droplets are present in Schwann cells. The postmortem study demonstrates abnormal foamy histiocytes in the distal segments of cutaneous nerves, but does not document such changes in large nerve trunks.[16] In sum, the morphologic studies of the PNS in HDL deficiency provide little insight into the pathogenesis of this condition. Both clinical and pathologic data are consistent with a primary degeneration of motor and sensory axons. The lipid droplets within Schwann cells are probably derived from nerve-fiber breakdown, but the reason for the failure of these cells to dispose of the lipid, as occurs during Wallerian degeneration for example, is unknown. Presumably, it is related in some way to the HDL deficiency.[23]

Clinical Features

A curious variety of symptoms and signs has been reported in cases of HDL deficiency. Some resemble a multiple mononeuropathy[18] and others a progressive loss of small myelinated and unmyelinated fibers.[22]

The multiple mononeuropathy may affect cranial or limb nerves, be permanent or transient, occur several times in the same individual, and occasionally give rise to changes so subtle as to escape detection by the patient.[24] Nerve biopsies or detailed electrophysiologic studies are not available in these cases.

The other pattern, suggestive of small myelinated and unmyelinated fiber loss, has been carefully documented in three individuals. The initial clinical profile may superficially resemble syringomyelia, with severe impairment of pain and temperature sense over the face and the proximal portions of the limbs, and wasting of the small hand muscles.[22] Gradually, over 10 or more years, disability progresses, other muscles become weak, and the tendon reflexes diminish. Nerve biopsies from such cases reveal predominant loss of small myelinated and nonmyelinated fibers, corresponding to the pattern of sensory loss.

PHYTANIC ACID STORAGE DISEASE (REFSUM'S DISEASE)

Biochemical Abnormality

The biochemical abnormality is defective oxidative catabolism of phytanic acid derived from ingested phytol. The initial alpha oxidation of phytanic acid to yield alpha-hydroxyphytanic acid does not occur, and it has been proposed that a deficiency of phytanic acid alphahydroxylase underlies this disorder. Biochemical investigations now permit heterozygote identification, and suggest treatment by a diet low in phytol.[25]

General Features

This is an extremely rare autosomal recessive condition, clearly related to inability to degrade ingested phytanic acid. The diet of affected individuals is not unusual, nor is absorption of phytanic acid. Dairy products, fish oils, and ruminant fats appear to be the major sources of dietary phytanic acid. Serum levels of phytanic acid are elevated in every case, with excessive storage throughout the body. Dietary restriction of phytol can reduce plasma levels of phytanic acid to normal, and may improve neurologic signs and symptoms. Attempts to produce the disease in experimental animals by feeding large amounts of phytanic acid have not been successful, and it remains to be established just how tissue accumulation of phytanic acid relates to clinical manifestations.[26]

The illness is usually first manifest before age 20. Cardinal clinical features are atypical retinitis pigmentosa, peripheral neuropathy, and ataxia.[27] Most individuals initially experience failing night vision, followed by gradual deterioration of visual function, and eventually near-blindness. Pigmentary degeneration of the retina is of the "salt and pepper" variety. Cataracts appear in one third of cases, further compromising visual function. Evidence of PNS dysfunction is present at some time in most cases (*vide infra*). Anosmia, deafness, and disordered cardiac function are common; cardiomyopathy is the most frequent cause of death.[28] Dry, scaly skin or diffuse ichthyosis is especially frequent in children.

Few postmortem studies are available, none has ultilized modern histopathologic techniques and, in general, the findings do not satisfactorily account for the clinical phenomena.[29] Liver and kidneys contain increased lipid, and myocardial fibrosis is common. The medulla oblongata displays degeneration and atrophy of the inferior olive, the olivocerebellar fibers, and medial leminiscus. In the spinal cord, axonal reaction of anterior horn cells and degeneration of the gracile fasciculi occur.[29]

Pathology and Pathogenesis of Neuropathy

The salient gross morphologic feature of this condition is enlargement of peripheral nerves and proximal nerve trunks, related to the predominance of hypertrophic changes in these areas.[29] Microscopically, fibers are reduced in number, and surviving myelinated axons are often surrounded by concentric layers of Schwann cell processes. Such 'onion bulbs' may completely enclose demyelinated axons. Segmental demyelination and remyelination are evident in teased fibers. Nonspecific crystalline inclusions are present in some Schwann cells and may originate within mitochondria.[30]

In sum, the few pathologic descriptions of the PNS in phytanic acid storage disease provide little insight into either the basic pathologic process or its pathogenesis. Onion-bulb formation is a nonspecific process associated with chronic myelinopathy or axonopathy.[31] Changes in the gracile fasciculi suggest the presence of a distal axonopathy (see Chapter 2), but further postmortem studies are needed to verify this notion.

Clinical Features of Peripheral Neuropathy

Initial manifestations of peripheral neuropathy are symmetrical distal weakness and reflex loss in the lower limbs.[27] This is accompanied by diminished position and vibration sense, and paresthesias. Atrophy of the lower leg and intrinsic foot muscles is common, and pes cavus may occur. Generally, weakness and sensory loss appear in the hands as well. With time, all tendon reflexes are lost, all sensory modalities become impaired, and proximal weakness develops. This is accompanied by electrophysiologic evidence of denervation in affected muscles and profoundly slowed nerve conduction. The cerebrospinal fluid is acellular and the protein concentration markedly elevated. Initially, most experience a gradual progression of neurologic deficit.[28] In over half there is dramatic, unexplained remission of signs. Eventually, exacerbations occur which, in turn, may be followed by partial remissions. Most individuals are disabled and eventuate with moderate to severe peripheral nervous system dysfunction, in combination with ataxia, impaired vision, and poor hearing.[28]

ALPHA-GALACTOSIDASE A DEFICIENCY (FABRY'S DISEASE, ANGIOKERATOMA CORPORIS DIFFUSUM)

Biochemical Abnormality

Defective activity of the lysosomal enzyme alpha-galactosidase characterizes this disorder, resulting in progressive deposition of neutral glycosphingolipids in most visceral tissues and fluids.[32] Globotriosylceramide is the predominant lipid stored in this condition. Elucidation of the specific enzymatic defect has permitted accurate diagnosis of affected individuals, asymptomatic carriers of unborn fetuses, and allowed trials of enzyme replacement therapy.[33,34]

General Features

This disorder is inherited in an X-linked recessive fashion, and usually first appears in childhood or adolescence. The course is steadily progressive and the mean age at death is 41 years. In general, there is an excellent correlation between the clinical manifestations and progressive deposition of glycosphingolipids.[33] In addition to signs of neurologic dysfunction, dermatologic, ocular, cardiovascular, and renal disease, are prominent.[34]

The characteristic skin lesion is a cluster of punctate, red angiectasis usually located between the umbilicus and the knees. Corneal opacities and tortuous conjunctival and retinal vessels are common.[33] Cardiovascular and renal failure account for most of the deaths in Fabry's disease. Renal failure is an especially disabling feature: many individuals become uremic, require hemodialysis, and transplantation is occasionally necessary.[34]

In hemizygous males, failure of each organ system can be directly linked with deposition of lipid within the malfunctioning tissue: angiokeratomas reflect lipid storage in vessel walls resulting in aneurysm formation; ocular findings are secondary to lipid infiltrates in the cornea and conjunctival vessels; cardiac failure results from deposits within the myocardium and valves; and glomerular and distal tubular epithelial lipid infiltration produce renal failure. Lipid deposits in endothelial cells may occlude the lumen of arterioles in any tissue, including the CNS, thereby producing a variety of signs. This phenomenon probably accounts for the dissimilarity among cases in the same sibship. Heterozygous females may show less obtrusive manifestations, most frequently corneal opacification.[33]

Treatment of Fabry's disease has centered around relief of pain and management of renal failure. Circulating enzyme replacement is currently being attempted in affected individuals, and preliminary results are encouraging.[35,36] Hopefully, a method of delivering exogeneous alpha-galactosidase A to affected target organs can be devised.

Pathology and Pathogenesis

This condition most probably represents a sensory and autonomic neuronopathy. The primary morphologic event is lipid storage in neurons, presumably reflecting local metabolic disorder. This process results in cell loss and disappearance of their processes. Study of postmortem and nerve biopsy material reveals selective loss of small neurons in lumbar dorsal root ganglia, and lipid incusions in others.[37] Correlating with the neuronal changes are moderate fiber loss in the gracile fasciculi of the spinal cord, and selective loss of small myelinated fibers and unmyelinated fibers in peripheral nerves. Segmental demyelination and distal axonal degeneration are not prominent features.[38] Abnormal lipid inclusions are described in perineurial cells and vascular endothelial cells, but not in Schwann cells. There are no studies of the peripheral autonomic ganglia, but lipid-distended neurons are present both in the intermediolateral columns of the thoracic spinal cord and in Onuf's (parasympathetic) nucleus in the sacral cord.[39]

Neuronal changes, apparently asymptomatic, are present in scattered loci in the CNS, including the substantia nigra, amygdala, hypothalamus, and nucleus ambiguus.

Clinical Features of Neuropathy

Pain is probably the single most debilitating symptom of Fabry's disease. Two types of pain occur: episodic bouts and constant acral discomfort. The episodic bouts ("Fabry crises") consist of periods of excruciating burning pain over hands and feet, often spreading to other areas. Crises may occur spontaneously, are sometimes triggered by fatigue, temperature change and exercise, increase in frequency with age and may be severe enough to cause the afflicted individual to contemplate suicide.[33] Most patients also experience constant, low-level burning discomfort in the hands and feet between crises. Curiously, there are usually no objective signs of sensory impairment, reflex loss, or weakness in this condition. Motor and sensory conduction velocities are normal, as are sensory amplitudes.[32]

Episodic diarrhea, nausea, vomiting, abdominal pain, and diminished sweating in the legs are generally attributed to involvement of autonomic ganglia.[40]

REFERENCES

1. DULANEY, JT AND MOSER, HW: *Sulfatide lipidosis: metachromatic leukodystrophy.* In STANBURY, JB, WYNGAARDEN, JB AND FREDRICKSON, DS (EDS): The Metabolic Basis of Inherited Disease, ed 4, McGraw-Hill, New York, 1978, p 770.

2. TERRY, RD, SUZUKI, K AND WEISS, M: *Biopsy study in 3 cases of metachromatic leukodystrophy.* J Neuropathol Exp Neurol 25:141, 1966.

3. SUZUKI, K, SUZUKI, K AND CHEN, G: *Metachromatic leukodystrophy: isolation and chemical analysis of metachromatic granules.* Science 151:1231, 1966.

4. WEBSTER, H DEF: *Schwann cell alterations in metachromatic leukodystrophy. Preliminary phase and electron microscopic observations.* J Neuropathol Exp Neurol 21:534, 1962.

5. BISCHOFF, A: *Neuropathy in leukodystrophies.* In DYCK, PJ, THOMAS, PK AND LAMBERT, EH (EDS): *Peripheral Neuropathies,* Vol II, WB Saunders, Philadelphia, 1975, p 891.

6. SUZUKI, K AND SUZUKI, Y: *Galactosylceramide lipidosis: globoid cell leukodystrophy.* In STANBURY, JB, WYNGAARDEN, JB AND FREDRICKSON, DS (EDS): The Metabolic Basis of Inherited Disease, ed 4, McGraw-Hill, New York, 1978, p 747.

7. HOGAN, GR, GUTMANN, L AND CHOU, SM: *The peripheral neuropathy of Krabbe's (globoid) leukodystrophy.* Neurology (Minneap) 19:1094, 1969.

8. DUNN, HG, ET AL: *The neuropathy of Krabbe's infantile cerebral sclerosis (globoid cell leukodystrophy).* Brain 92:329, 1969.

9. SUZUKI, K AND GROVER, WD: *Krabbe's leukodystrophy (globoid cell leukodystrophy): An ultrastructural study.* Arch Neurol 22:385, 1970.

10. HERBERT, PN, GOTTO, AM AND FREDRICKSON, DS: *Familial lipoprotein defiency.* In STANBURY, JB, WYNGAARDEN, JB AND FREDRICKSON, DS (EDS): The Metabolic Basis of Inherited Disease, ed 4, McGraw-Hill, New York, 1978, p 544.

11. SOBREVILLA, LA, GOODMAN, ML AND KANE, CA: *Demyelinating central nervous system disease, macular atrophy and acanthocytosis (Bassen-Kornzweig syndrome).* Am J Med 37:821, 1964.

12. YUILL, GM, SCHOLZ, C AND LASCELLES, RG: *Abetalipoproteinemia: A case report with pathological studies.* Postgrad Med J 52:713, 1976.

13. MILLER, R., ET AL: *The neurology of abetalipoproteinemia.* Neurology (Minneap.) 30:1286, 1980.

14. DISCHE, MR AND PORRO, RS: *The cardiac lesions in Bassen-Kornzweig syndrome.* Am J Med 49:568, 1970.

15. AZIZI, E, ET AL: *Abetalipoproteinemia treated with parenteral and oral vitamins A and E, and with medium chain triglycerides.* Acta Pediatr Scand 67:797, 1978.

16. BALE, PM ET AL: *Pathology of Tangier disease.* J Clin Pathol 24:609, 1971.

17. ENGEL, WK, ET AL: *Neuropathy in Tangier disease: alpha lipoprotein deficiency manifesting as familial recurrent neuropathy and intestinal lipid storage.* Arch Neurol 17:1, 1967.

18. KOCEN, RS, ET AL: *Familial alpha-lipoprotein deficiency (Tangier disease) with neurologic abnormalities.* Lancet 1:1341, 1967.

19. KOCEN, RS, ET AL: *Nerve biopsy findings in two cases of Tangier disease.* Acta Neuropathol 26:317, 1973.

20. HAAS, LF, AUSTAD, WI AND BERGIN, JD: *Tangier disease.* Brain 97:351, 1974.

21. FERRANS, VJ AND FREDRICKSON, DS: *The pathology of Tangier disease. A light and electron microscopic study.* Am J Pathol 78:101, 1975.

22. DYCK, PJ, ET AL: *Adult-onset of Tangier disease: I. Morphometric and pathologic studies suggesting delayed degradation of neurtral lipids after fiber degeneration.* J Neuropathol Exp Neurol 37:119, 1978.

23. YAO, JK, ET AL: *Biochemical studies in a patient with a Tangier syndrome.* J Neuropathol Exp Neurol 37:138, 1978.

24. SPIESS, H, LUDIN, HP AND KUMMER, H: *Polyneuropathie bie familiare Analphalipoproteinamie (Tangier disease).* Nervenarzt 40:191, 1969.

METABOLIC
NEUROPATHY:
HEREDITARY
DISORDERS
OF LIPID
METABOLISM

25. STEINBERG, D: *Phytanic acid storage disease: Refsum's syndrome.* In STANBURY, JB, WYNGAARDEN, JB AND FREDRICKSON, DS (EDS): The Metabolic Basis of Inherited Disease, ed 4, McGraw-Hill, New York, 1978, p. 688.

26. STOKKE, O: *Alpha oxidation of fatty acids in various mammals, and a phytanic acid feeding experiment in an animal with low alpha oxidation capacity.* Scand J Clin Lab Invest 20:305, 1967.

27. REFSUM, S: *Heredopathia atactica polyneuritiformis: A familial syndrome not hitherto described. A contribution to the clinical study of the hereditary diseases of the nervous system.* Acta Psychiatr Scand Suppl 38:1, 1964.

28. REFSUM, S: *Heredopathia atactica polyneuritiformis.* In VINKEN, PJ AND BRUYN, GE (EDS): Handbook of Clinical Neurology, *Vol 21,* North Holland Publishing, New York, 1975, p 181.

29. CAMMERMEYER, J: *Pathology of Refsum's disease.* In VINKEN, PJ AND BRUYN, GW (EDS): Handbook of Clinical Neurology, *Vol 21,* North Holland Publishing, New York, 1975, p 234.

30. FARDEAU, M AND ENGEL, WK: *Ultrastructural study of a peripheral nerve biopsy in Refsum's disease.* J Neuropathol Exp Neurol 28:278, 1969.

31. ASBURY, AK AND JOHNSON, PC: Pathology of Peripheral Nerve. WB Saunders, Philadelphia, 1978, p 136.

32. BRADY, RO, ET AL: *Enzymatic defect in Fabry's disease: ceramidetrihexosidase deficiency.* N Eng J Med 276:1163, 1967.

33. DESNICK, RJ, KLIONSKY, B AND SWEELEY, CC: *Fabry's disease (x-galactosidase A deficiency).* In STANBURY, JB, WYNGAARDEN, JB AND FREDRICKSON, DS (EDS): The Metabolic Basis of Inherited Disease, ed 4, McGraw-Hill, New York, 1978, p 810.

34. BRADY, RO AND KING, FM: *Fabry's disease.* In DYCK, PJ, THOMAS, PK AND LAMBERT, EH (EDS): Peripheral Neuropathy, *Vol 11,* WB Saunders, Philadelphia, 1975, p 914.

35. BRADY, RO, ET AL: *Replacement therapy for inherited enzyme deficiency. Use of purified ceramidetrihexosidase in Fabry's disease.* N Eng J Med 289:9, 1973.

36. DESNICK, RJ, THORPE, SR AND FIDDLER, MB: *Towards enzyme therapy for lysosomal storage disease.* Physiol Rev 56:57, 1976.

37. OHNISHI, A AND DYCK, PJ: *Loss of small peripheral sensory neurons in Fabry disease.* Arch Neurol 31:120, 1974.

38. KOCEN, RS AND THOMAS, PK: *Peripheral nerve involvement in Fabry's disease.* Arch Neurol 22:81, 1970.

39. SUNG, JH: *Autonomic neurons affected by lipid storage in the spinal cord in Fabry's disease: distribution of autonomic neurons in the sacral cord.* J Neuropathol Exp Neurol 38:87, 1979.

40. BANNISTER, R AND OPPENHEIMER, DR: *Degenerative diseases of the nervous system associated with autonomic failure.* Brain 95:457, 1972.

Chapter 10

HEREDITARY MOTOR
AND SENSORY NEUROPATHIES

Studies in recent years have indicated that cases diagnosed clinically as peroneal muscular atrophy, Charcot-Marie-Tooth disease and Déjerine-Sottas disease are genetically heterogeneous. Some of these have been shown to consist of a distal spinal muscular atrophy (spinal form of Charcot-Marie-Tooth disease); the remainder display both motor and sensory involvement. Since no specific biochemical changes have been identified, the latter have been given the general title of hereditary motor and sensory neuropathies (HMSN), with a numerical subdivision into types I, II, and III to replace the previous confusing eponyms.[1-3] Tables 4 and 5 outline the principal conditions, include the old and new nomenclatures, summarize the clinical and pathologic features, and highlight the current theories of pathogenesis. Although this classification is generally accepted,[4-7] it is still subject to modification[8-10] and controversy continues over proposed intermediate forms.[10-13] Their pathogenesis is uncertain.[14-20]

HMSN TYPE I

Definition

This is a slowly progressive, relatively benign, motor and sensory polyneuropathy. Most cases display autosomal dominant inheritance, but kinships with probable autosomal recessive inheritance are reported.[10] HMSN type I includes the majority of individuals previously labeled as either having peroneal muscular atrophy, Charcot-Marie-Tooth disease, or Roussy-Levy syndrome.[10,21]

Pathology and Pathogenesis

PATHOLOGY. Abnormalities are confined to the spinal cord and peripheral nerves. The most prominent spinal cord alteration is loss of myelinated

TABLE 4. The Principal Hereditary Motor and Sensory Neuropathies (HMSN)

MAYO NOMENCLATURE	ALTERNATIVE NAMES	INHERITANCE	CLINICAL AND ELECTROPHYSIOLOGIC FEATURES	PATHOLOGY	PATHOGENETIC HYPOTHESIS	COMMENTS
HMSN Type I	Hypertrophic form of peroneal muscular atrophy (PMA). Hypertrophic form of Charcot-Marie-Tooth (CMT) disease. Roussy-Levy syndrome (some cases).	Usually autosomal dominant (linked to Duffy locus on chromosome 1), rarely autosomal recessive. Recessive cases are more severely affected. Marriage of two affected individuals has produced children resembling recessively inherited HMSN Type I.	Not an uncommon condition. Many mild, asymptomatic cases. Onset in childhood, adolescence or later. Slowly progressive distal atrophy and weakness. Little sensory loss. Nerves often enlarged. Pes cavus common, scoliosis unusual. Essential tremor in some individuals. Sensory and motor conduction diffusely affected, motor may be extremely slow. Abnormal visual and auditory evoked potentials indicate optic and acoustic nerve involvement in some cases. Normal active life span common.	Distal segmental demyelination, remyelination and onion bulbs. Fewer myelinated axons of large diameter in distal nerves. CNS normal except for dorsal columns.	Pathology and morphometry suggest primary axonal disorder (distal axonopathy). Xenograft studies and abnormal axonal transport of dopamine beta-hydroxylase support this hypothesis.	The "classic" form of CMT disease or PMA. Mild cases widely misdiagnosed as orthopedic foot disorders. Rare variants associated with optic atrophy, deafness, or spastic paraplegia.

HMSN Type II	Neuronal form of PMA. Neuronal form of CMT disease.	Usually autosomal dominant, rarely autosomal recessive; recessive cases more severely affected.	Less common than HMSN type I. Onset most often in 2nd decade. Progressive distal weakness and atrophy similar to HMSN Type I. Sensory and motor nerve conduction only mildly abnormal.	Nerves not enlarged. Fewer myelinated axons of large diameter in distal nerves. Rare demyelination, few onion bulbs. No reliable autopsy report.	Generally held to represent disease of motor and sensory neurons. Not a variant of spinal muscular atrophy (SMA), although a distal form of SMA with features resembling other types of CMT disease but without sensory involvement exists.	Often clinically indistinguishable from HMSN Type I. Nerve conduction study usually essential for differential diagnosis. Intermediate forms between types I and II proposed but not established.
HMSN Type III	Déjerine-Sottas disease. Hypertrophic neuropathy of infancy. Congenital hypomyelination neuropathy.	Autosomal recessive. Probably genetically heterogeneous.	Rare. Onset in infancy, or from birth. Slowly progressive motor and sensory loss, and ataxia. Scoliosis and pes cavus frequent. Enlarged nerves. Patients often severely disabled in adult life. Occasional pupillary abnormality. Motor nerve conduction velocity severely reduced, sensory action potentials unrecordable.	Enlarged nerves. Hypomyelination. Long demyelinated axon segments and many onion bulbs.	One case with decreased nerve cerebroside and increased liver ceramide monohexoside sulfate. Primary Schwann-cell disorder possible.	Need for confirmation of disordered lipid metabolism.

TABLE 5. The Principal Hereditary Sensory Neuropathies (HSN)

MAYO NOMENCLATURE	ALTERNATIVE NAMES	INHERITANCE	CLINICAL AND ELECTROPHYSIOLOGIC FEATURES	PATHOLOGY	PATHOGENETIC HYPOTHESIS	COMMENTS
HSN Type I	Dominantly inherited sensory neuropathy. Hereditary sensory neuropathy of Denny-Brown.	Autosomal dominant.	Rare. Onset in second decade. Progressive distal extremity sensory loss. Mutilation of feet. Pain and temperature sense more affected than touch-pressure. Occasional lancinating pain. Sweating impaired in distal extremities. Motor nerve conduction normal. Preserved sensory action potentials (A-alpha component) in earlier stages with abnormal A-delta and C-fiber potentials. Proximal tendon reflexes and autonomic function spared (except sweating). Life expectancy normal with good foot care.	Proximal-to-distal gradient of fiber loss. Unmyelinated and small myelinated fibers more depleted than myelinated large fibers.	Pathology and clinical data support hypothesis of slowly progressive sensory distal axonopathy.	Firm correlation of sensory deficit with fiber-type loss on morphologic and electrophysiologic studies. Sparing of proximal autonomic function helpful in differentiating from amyloid neuropathy. Increased synthesis of immunoglobulin A in one kinship.
HSN Type II	Congenital sensory neuropathy. Recessive hereditary sensory neuropathy. Morvan's disease.	Autosomal recessive	Rare. Onset in early childhood or at birth. Progression poorly documented. Hands and feet mutilated, pathologic fracture common. Distal touch-pressure may be affected earlier; eventually all modalities involved. Sensory loss not confined to extremities. All tendon reflexes lost. Distal sensory conduction profoundly affected. Motor nerve conduction near normal. Prognosis not known.	Mild proximal to distal gradient of fiber loss. Myelinated fibers severely depleted, unmyelinated fibers less so. Occasional degenerating fiber present on biopsy. Some distal segmental demyelination and remyelination.	Morphologic evidence somewhat supports hypothesis similar to HSN 1. Xenograft studies indicate no disorder of Schwann cells.	Morphology supports notion of a progressive, degenerative condition; clinical state often seems static.

HSN Type III	Riley-Day syndrome. Familial dysautonomia.	Autosomal recessive. Predominantly in Jewish families.	Rare. Onset in infancy. Autonomic dysfunction prominent: absent lachrymation, labile sweating, blood pressure, and temperature. Loss of taste. Generalized diminution of pain-temperature sensation. Preserved touch sensation. Short stature. Hyporeflexia. Decreased amplitude of sensory action potentials, mild slowing of motor conduction. Mutilation unusual. Decreased life expectancy.	Sural nerve has near-total absence of unmyelinated axons and reduced numbers of myelinated axons. Slow progression with age. Reduced number of neurons in sympathetic, dorsal root, gasserian, and spheno-palatine ganglia. Ciliary ganglia normal. No CNS change aside from progressive dorsal column degeneration, and depletion of preganglionic sympathetic neurons.	Congenital absence of autonomic and sensory ganglia and peripheral processes indicates disorder of embryogenesis, with mild progressive degenerative disease of neurons. Role for diminished Nerve Growth Factor in embryo and postnatal period has been postulated. Relationship of abnormal levels of catecholamine metabolites and low serum dopamine β-hydroxylase to the labile autonomic clinical phenomena unclear. Diagnosis usually established shortly after birth; may be initially misdiagnosed as HSN Type IV.
HSN Type IV	Congenital insensitivity to pain. Congenital sensory neuropathy with anhidrosis.	Autosomal recessive	Very rare. Onset in infancy. Widespread absence of pain-temperature sensation. Strength normal. Episodic fever. Absent sweating. Mental retardation. Mutilation usual. Short stature.	PNS incompletely studied. Reduced number of smaller neurons in dorsal root ganglia.	Pathogenesis may resemble that of HSN Type III, but insufficient data to support this notion firmly. Mental retardation and lack of sweating help distinguish from HSN III. More clinical, pathologic and basic studies needed.

axons in the gracile fasciculi at upper cervical levels. Shrunken anterior horn cells in the lumbar cord are occasionally present. PNS changes are prominent in this condition and usually include (1) enlargement of nerves, "hypertrophic neuropathy" (2) abundant segmental demyelination, remyelination, and onion-bulb formation in distal nerves, and (3) reduced numbers of axons in distal nerves. It has been suggested that many of the surviving distal axons are atrophic. Ultrastructural examination of advanced cases reveals "onion bulbs" frequently devoid of axons, and occasionally vacuolated endoneurial fibroblasts and an abundant fibrillar material in the endoneurial spaces.[18,21]

PATHOGENESIS The pathogenesis is unknown. Xenograft studies of HMSN type I have indicated no evidence of an inherent Schwann cell abnormality.[15] Slowed axonal transport of dopamine beta hydroxylase has been demonstrated.[22] Taken in conjunction with the pathologic findings, these studies suggest that a distal axonal change is the primary event, and that segmental demyelination and remyelination are secondary. It is possible that this disorder results from an inherited abnormality of neuronal or axonal metabolism, but no study of human or an appropriate experimental animal has indicated the nature or existence of a metabolic disorder.

Clinical Features

INCIDENCE AND HEREDITY. HMSN type I remains undiagnosed in many instances, and therefore most studies of prevalence are inaccurate. It appears to be a fairly common disorder with a world-wide occurrence.[21] The inheritance pattern is usually autosomal dominant, and this has been linked to the Duffy locus on chromosome 1;[41] families with a probable recessive inheritance also have been identified.[10] Variable expression of this genetic disorder probably accounts for the presence of individuals with slightly deformed feet as the sole manifestation of disease in kinships with advanced cases.[9] Slightly affected individuals often first become aware of their disease when it appears, in a more serious form, in their children.

SYMPTOMS AND SIGNS. HMSN type I may be most simply described as a chronic polyneuropathy featured by weakness and wasting of distal limb muscles and foot deformity.

Common initial complaints are weakness of the distal lower extremities beginning in the first or second decade. The disorder may be present from birth. Subsequently, a gait disorder is noted, usually a nonspecific "unsteady ankle" sensation while walking; eventually foot-drop and a steppage gait may occur. Weakness and wasting of the hands usually begin some years after the lower extremities are involved. Mild paresthesias of the feet are occasionally present. Frequently, the only complaint is progressive deformity of the feet accompanied by atrophy of the legs. Such individuals may seek orthopedic consultation early in the illness. Kyphoscoliosis occurs in some cases, particularly severer cases with an early onset. In some families, distal sensory loss may be prominent and may lead to persistent foot ulceration.

The progression of neurologic signs in a fully developed case is stereotyped.[10,21] Individuals display initial weakness in the extensor hallucis and digitorum longus and the anterior tibial and peroneal muscles, before the calf muscles are affected. Fasciculations may occur in weakened muscles. Foot-drop and contracture of the calf muscles may result from the unopposed flexor action of the posterior compartment muscles; eventually they too undergo atrophy, sometimes resulting in a stork-legged or "inverted champagne bottle" appearance of the lower limbs. This pattern of weakness is occasionally accompanied by progressive pes cavus and clawed toes. The typical pes cavus deformity is a foreshortened, high-arched foot attributable to weakness of the intrinsic foot muscles and the unequal action of long toe flexors and extensors (Figure 16). Atrophy seldom extends above the midthigh, and weakness only very rarely involves the girdle muscles. Absence of the Achilles tendon reflex is an early sign, and generalized tendon areflexia is usual in established cases. Sensory involvement, although present in all individuals, is generally not a prominent feature of this condition, and may be difficult to elicit on routine clinical examination. In advanced cases, careful analysis of pin, touch, and thermal sense will usually demonstrate some disorder, but in mild cases may only be detectable from sensory nerve conduction studies. Discolored skin, edema, and cold extremities probably result from inactivity, diminished blood flow, and muscle loss, rather than autonomic dysfunction, which is not a feature of HMSN I.

The hands usually do not become weak until years after the condition has become advanced in the lower extremities.[21] Occasionally, the intrinsic hand muscles may atrophy to an extreme degree, resulting in a "claw hand" deformity, analogous to pes cavus. Weakness of forearm muscles occurs in the more severe cases. Mild involvement of upper arm or shoulder girdle muscles is detectable in severe cases. Mild sensory loss may accompany the hand weakness.

Firm, thickened nerves can be palpated in about 50 percent of the cases.

There is considerable variation in atrophy, weakness, and distal skeletal deformity. Individuals may frequently be profoundly weak with only slight atrophy and minimal pes cavus. Contrary to popular belief, the majority of cases do *not* display the triad of pes cavus, "champagne bottle" legs and claw hands, but rather manifest a mild degree of weakness, atrophy, or foot deformity. In children, slowed nerve conduction may be the sole manifestation of disease. Such cases are usually only detected in genetic screening of relatives of severe cases.[21]

Essential tremor accompanies the neuropathy in members of some kinships. Since the features of the illness in these instances are otherwise

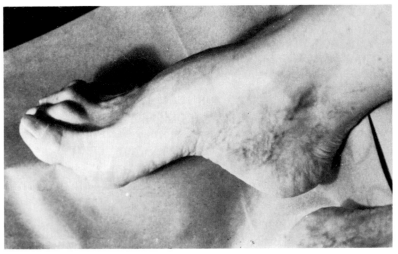

FIGURE 16. Pes cavus deformity in a middle-aged female with chronic peripheral neuropathy. The foot appears foreshortened with a high arch and bowed instep.

identical to HMSN type I, there seems little justification for not including them under this classification.[10] Previously, such cases were designated as the Roussy-Levy syndrome.

Pupillary abnormalities,[23] optic atrophy,[24] and deafness[25] are rare associations. In the absence of optic atrophy, optic nerve involvement may be demonstrable from visual-evoked-potential studies.

Laboratory Studies

ROUTINE LABORATORY AND CEREBROSPINAL FLUID. Usually normal, although the CSF protein may be mildly elevated.

ELECTRODIAGNOSIS. Profoundly slow motor nerve conduction is a hallmark of this condition; velocities as low as 10 to 20 m per sec are common. Sensory nerve conduction in digital and sural nerves is also slowed, and the potential amplitude decreased. Frequently, sensory action potentials are not detectable by routine recording techniques.

Slowed motor nerve conduction may be abnormal in cases with few neurologic findings; for this reason, electrodiagnosis has been a useful tool in genetic counseling.[21]

BLOOD-GROUP STATUS. HLA linkage of hereditary neuropathy has recently been suggested;[26] if confirmed, this may also prove to be helpful in genetic counseling.

NERVE BIOPSY. Nerve biopsy in most cases reveals fiber loss, segmental demyelination, and sometimes "onion-bulb" formation. These findings are characteristic but not pathognomic of HSMN type I, since they may occur in other chronic neuropathies characterized by repeated episodes of segmental demyelination and remyelination.

Course, Prognosis and Treatment

Progression is gradual and individuals may appear to plateau for many years before worsening again. HMSN type I is frequently a benign condition, and need not seriously handicap affected individuals. Even in severe cases there is no evidence that it shortens life expectancy, and most working individuals remain employed until retirement age. Preservation of proximal strength often enables even seriously involved cases to remain ambulatory if aided by braces, special shoes, and surgery to correct deformity, and occasionally by tibialis posterior tenodesis to reduce foot-drop.

There is no specific treatment. Genetic counseling is usually mandatory, especially in small communities where, unknowingly, mildly affected individuals have intermarried and produced severely affected homozygous offspring.[27]

Differential Diagnosis

The differential diagnosis of a fully developed case is usually simple. The principal conditions misdiagnosed as HMSN I are:

Friedreich's Ataxia: Excluded by severely reduced nerve conduction in HMSN type I.

HMSN type II: Excluded by severely abnormal nerve conduction tests and usually earlier onset in HMSN type I (although motor conduction velocities may overlap between the two forms).

Hereditary distal spinal muscular atrophy: Excluded by abnormal motor and sensory nerve conduction studies and presence of sensory loss in HMSN type I.

Refsum's disease: Excluded by absence of pigmentary retinal degeneration and elevated serum phytanic acid levels in HMSN type I.

Chronic inflammatory idiopathic polyneuropathy: A markedly fluctuating course, absence of family history and foot deformity, and a substantially elevated CSF protein level will suggest this condition. Differential diagnosis in chronic progressive cases may be difficult. The presence of inflammatory infiltrates in nerve biopsies from some cases of chronic inflammatory idiopathic polyneuropathy may be helpful.

Case History and Comment

CASE HISTORY. A fifty-year-old accountant was admitted to hospital because of urinary frequency and hesitancy. He underwent surgery for prostatic hyperplasia and made an uneventful recovery. During his hospitalization he slipped on a wet floor and sustained a mild concussion. The neurologist was called and noted, in addition to a postconcussive state, mild pes cavus, moderate atrophy on the calf and anterior compartment muscles, 4/5 (MRC scale) strength, and fasciculations in the extensors and flexors of toes and feet, 4/5 strength of the intrinsic hand muscles, tendon areflexia and slightly diminished pinprick and position sense in toes and fingers. Walking barefoot was difficult because of ankle instability. Walking while wearing high-topped shoes was normal. The remainder of the examination was unremarkable. There was no palpable nerve enlargement. Motor nerve conduction velocity in the peroneal nerves was 10 to 15 m per sec, and in the ulnar, 20 to 25 m per sec. Median nerve sensory conduction was 30 to 40 m per sec.

The patient had been unaware of his neurologic illness, and attributed the weakness of his extremities, first noted at age 40, to advancing age. He had worn special shoes "because of club feet" since childhood, and had never been a swift runner; however, he was a member of his high school swimming team.

Both parents died in middle age in an accident. One of his three older brothers had used short-leg braces since age 30. Examination of the patients' two male adolescent children revealed that the 18-year-old had absent Achilles reflexes and peroneal motor conduction velocities of 30 m per sec.

COMMENT. This man had a mild hereditary polyneuropathy of early onset with deformed feet and marked slowing of nerve conduction. The diagnosis of HMSN type I was apparent to the neurologist, but had been overlooked by other physicians. The patient was either unaware of his illness or wished to deny it, and was distressed that his 18-year-old son also was affected. This case emphasizes the insidious course of the condition and the need for genetic counseling.

HMSN TYPE II

Definition

This is less common than HMSN type I and displays similar clinical features. Inheritance is usually autosomal dominant. Factors that separate this disorder from type I are normal or only moderately reduced nerve conduction velocity, later onset, and absent or minimal hypertrophic changes on nerve biopsy.[2,3,5]

Pathology and Pathogenesis

PATHOLOGY. There has been no postmortem report on this disorder; all pathologic material is from nerve biopsies. The most striking finding is a decreased number of myelinated fibers in distal nerves. In contrast to type I, there is little segmental demyelination or "onion-bulb" formation.[21]

PATHOGENESIS. The pathogenesis of this disorder is unknown. Xenograph studies indicate no primary abnormality of Schwann cells.[16] It is generally held that this condition represents a primary disorder of neuron or axon, and it is commonly referred to as the "neuronal form" of peroneal muscular atrophy.[10,21]

Clinical Features

The onset of symptoms of this disorder is most often in the second decade, but many cases begin in the first decade and the onset may be delayed until middle or even late life. Clinical features, including signs, symptoms, course, and prognosis are similar to those of HMSN type I, except that upper extremities are less severely affected, sensory loss and tremor are less prominent,[10] widespread tendon areflexia is less common, foot deformity tends to be less severe, and nerve thickening does not occur.

Motor and sensory nerve conduction velocities are within normal limits or only moderately reduced, in contrast to the usually profoundly slowed conduction of type I. Indeed, clinical electrophysiology and nerve biopsy are the cardinal means of distinguishing between these disorders (see Table 4). There is some overlap for motor conduction velocity between the two forms, but not for sensory conduction.

HMSN TYPE III

Definition

The status of this condition is confused. It is a rare, probably genetically heterogeneous, slowly progressive, debilitating peripheral neuropathy, beginning in infancy or present from birth. It includes examples of progressive childhood onset hypertrophic neuropathy of autosomal recessive inheritance that have been categorized as Déjerine-Sottas disease,[21] and others, also probably of autosomal inheritance with hypotonic weakness present from birth.[28] Both are characterized by severe hypomyelination and demyelination in peripheral nerves and by severely reduced nerve conduction velocity.[10]

Pathology and Pathogenesis

PATHOLOGY. Changes are confined to the peripheral nervous system and the dorsal columns of the spinal cord. Salient features are gross enlargement of distal peripheral nerves, loss of myelinated axons, segmental demyelination and remyelination, and "onion-bulb" formation. Myelin sheaths of normal thickness are not present (hypomyelination) and many fibers lack myelin sheaths (amyelination). Particularly in the congenital cases, the onion bulbs may be composed mainly of concentric layers of basal lamina with few Schwann cell processes.[28]

PATHOGENESIS. The pathogenesis is unknown. One patient has demonstrated a decrease in peripheral nerve cerebrosides and an increase in liver ceramide monohexoside sulfate.[18] The relationship of this biochemical abnormality to the peripheral neuropathy is unknown.

Clinical Features

INCIDENCE AND HEREDITY. This is a rare condition with a worldwide incidence. Most cases are isolated, or if multiple, confined to a single sibship, suggesting autosomal recessive inheritance.

SIGNS AND SYMPTOMS. Cases identifiable as Déjerine-Sottas disease begin in infancy. Early motor landmarks, such as walking, are often delayed. Initially, weakness appears in the distal lower extremities. Soon afterwards, the upper extremities become involved. Proximal extremity muscles are eventually affected in most cases, resulting in severe disability. Areflexia is the rule and, in almost all cases, enlarged peripheral nerves can be easily palpated. Sensory loss may be severe, usually affecting touch, position, and vibration sense more than pain. Pseudoathetosis and sensory ataxia may occur. Autonomic function is spared. Hearing loss is common and occasional patients are nearly deaf. Abnormal pupillary responses to light occasionally occur.

Other cases (congenital hypomyelination neuropathy) present with hypotonic weakness from birth and display the features described above in more severe degree.[28,42]

A distinguishing feature of HMSN type III is the frequency of skeletal abnormality. Many affected individuals are of short stature, kyphoscoliotic, and have severe deformities of hands and feet.

Laboratory Data

CEREBROSPINAL FLUID. The CSF protein content is often elevated, presumably because lumbar roots are involved.

ELECTROPHYSIOLOGY. Motor conduction velocity is extremely slow, often less than 10 m per sec. Sensory nerve action potentials are unrecordable by standard techniques.

NERVE BIOPSY. The nerve biopsy findings are characteristic and have been detailed above.

Course and Prognosis

This illness progresses more rapidly and is generally more disabling than HMSN type I; many are confined to a wheelchair by the time of adulthood. There is no study of longevity in this illness.

Differential diagnosis

Diagnosis of this disorder is rarely difficult. The congenital or infantile onset, recessive inheritance, and skeletal deformities, distinguish it from most cases of HMSN types I and II, the usual absence of CNS signs and the severely reduced nerve conduction velocity from Friedreich's ataxia, and normal serum phytanic acid levels from Refsum's disease. The rare recessively inherited instances of HMSN type I are distinguishable on nerve biopsy, where some of the myelinated fibers possess myelin sheaths of normal thickness.

HSN TYPE I
(DOMINANTLY INHERITED SENSORY NEUROPATHY)

Definition

This is a rare, dominantly-inherited, sensory neuropathy primarily affecting the distal lower extremities. The onset is in the second decade and progression is slow. Loss of unmyelinated fibers and mutilated feet usually occur. This disorder was previously labelled *hereditary sensory radicular neuropathy of Denny-Brown,* and was one cause of *lumbosacral syringomyelia* and *Morvan's disease.*[29,30]

Pathology and Pathogenesis

PATHOLOGY. There is a marked loss of unmyelinated axons in distal nerves and a moderate loss of small myelinated fibers. Histometric studies of sensory nerves have demonstrated a progressive depletion of small myelinated fibers at distal levels. Large myelinated axons are usually spared, and vacuolated fibroblasts are prominent in the endoneurium.[31] Postmortem examination has revealed reduced numbers of lumbar dorsal root ganglion neurons. Nerves are not enlarged, segmental demyelination and remyelination are not present, and onion-bulb formation is not a feature of this illness.[29] There are no CNS changes other than loss of axons in the gracile fasciculi.

PATHOGENESIS. The pathogenesis is unknown. It is generally held that this disorder results from slowly progressive distal axonal atrophy and degeneration, and that dorsal root ganglion cells degenerate after years of centripetal spread of axonal disease. The histopathology is suggestive of a distal axonopathy.

Clinical Features

INCIDENCE. This is an uncommon condition and occurs throughout the world. Its inheritance is autosomal dominant.[32]

SYMPTOMS AND SIGNS. The onset is usually in the second decade or later. Individuals initially notice painless injuries to the sole of the foot. Calluses often form on the base of the toes, become discolored and then ulcerate. Frequently, the ulcers become infected and cellulitis develops or purulent drainage occurs. Repeated trauma to the anesthetic feet may result in joint destruction, pathologic fractures, and grossly deformed feet. Mild denervation of distal muscles may be present and pes cavus may occur in rare cases. It is always accompanied by severe sensory loss in the feet. Episodes of lancinating pain of the feet or arms are an intermittent phenomenon in about one half of the cases. Occasional kinships with features similar to those of HSN type I have shown hearing loss,[30] and others, spastic paraparesis.[33]

Neurologic examination in the early stages of disease usually reveals a striking dissociated pattern of sensory change, featured by a profound loss of pain and temperature sense with only slight loss of touch, pressure, and position sense. Such cases display a diminished Achilles reflex and intact strength. This pattern of sensory loss correlates with histometric and physiologic studies that have demonstrated a loss of myelinated fibers and greatly diminished C and A-delta action potentials. With time, the entire foot and lower leg become anesthetic and ankle deformities develop. The Achilles reflex disappears and the quadriceps reflex is depressed. Atrophy of the small muscles of the feet is common, and mild weakness for toe extension and for dorsiflexion and eversion at the ankles may occur. It is frequently difficult to evaluate the motor findings because of severe limitation of movement at toe and ankle joints. In any event, the sensory loss always dominates the clinical profile.[29,34]

Upper-extremity sensory loss is usually mild and, when present, confined to the fingers. Infection of the fingers or mutilation of the hand is rare in this disorder. Many individuals are unaware of sensory changes in the hands, and strength and tendon reflexes are usually preserved in the upper limbs.

Autonomic dysfunction is not a feature of this illness. HSN-type-I patients retain bladder and sexual function, and do not experience postural hypotension.[29]

Laboratory Data

ROUTINE. The cerebrospinal fluid is usually normal. Increased serum levels of immunoglobulin A may occur.

ELECTROPHYSIOLOGY. Sensory nerve conduction studies of the sural nerve show diminished amplitude but near-normal velocites in early cases. Peroneal and tibial motor nerve conduction velocities are normal. Advanced cases may display slightly prolonged motor and sensory latencies in the lower extremities. Sensory and motor conduction studies in the upper extremities are usually normal.

NERVE BIOPSY. Sural nerve biopsy in early cases reveals a grossly normal specimen which, on light microscope examination, has a normal complement of large-diameter myelinated fibers and moderate reduction of small myelinated fibers. Electron microscope examination will usually display a striking depletion in the number of unmyelinated fibers.[31]

Course, Prognosis and Treatment

The course is a gradual, proximal progression of the sensory loss in the feet, usually to a level below the knee. The proximal lower extremities are not affected and the hands are usually spared, or sustain only a minor sensory loss. Life expectancy is normal in this condition with proper treatment, and many patients remain gainfully employed.

There are two concerns for the physician. One is genetic counseling on the probability and nature of the illness. Treatment revolves around proper foot care. The chief disability in this illness stems from bone and joint deformity and repeated infected ulcerations of the feet. Occasionally, amputation is necessary. These complications are probably largely preventible by scrupulous maintainence of foot hygiene and skilled podiatric management.

Differential Diagnosis

Conditions that are occasionally misdiagnosed as HSN type I include:

HEREDITARY AMYLOIDOSIS. In contrast to HSN type I, this condition is usually featured by prominent autonomic dysfunction.

SYRINGOMYELIA. In contrast to HSN type I, this condition usually begins in the cervical segments, is not hereditary and involvement of the lower extremities is extremely rare.

DIABETIC POLYNEUROPATHY. In contrast to HSN type I, diabetes mellitus is not dominantly inherited, the onset is usually later in life, the upper extremities are commonly involved, and abnormalities of carbohydrate metabolism are present.

HSN TYPE II. In contrast to HSN type I, this condition has an early onset, is recessively inherited, and the upper extremities are usually involved. The differential diagnosis between HSN types I and II may be impossible, on occasion, since the clinical features appear to overlap in some kinships.

Case History and Comment

CASE HISTORY. A thirty-five-year-old clerk was admitted to hospital with septicemia from an infection of the left foot. Ten years earlier, she first noticed painless bruises of the metatarsal pads and recurrent calluses of the dorsum of the great toe. A podiatrist informed her that she had hammer toes and peripheral neuropathy. She declined to see a neurologist and continued to work as a filing clerk. In the ensuing ten years, repeated infections of the soles of both feet occurred and a nonhealing ulcer developed on the 1st metatarsal pad on the left. Her gait had become uneven and bony deformities gradually developed in both feet.

The sepsis responded to a three-week course of antibiotics. Neurologic consultation revealed bilateral hammer-toe deformities and grossly deformed feet with limitation of motion at the ankles. There was a partially healed ulcer at the base of the left metatarsal. The toes of both feet were shortened, with only remnants of toenails. Sensory examination revealed anesthesia to pin and markedly diminished thermal sensation over the plantar surfaces bilaterally. There was no weakness of dorsiflexion or plantar flexion of the ankle. The intrinsic muscles of the feet and long toe flexors and extensors could not be tested because of limitation of movement. The Achilles reflex was very poor while other reflexes were brisk. There were no abnormalities of mental status and the cranial nerves were intact. Urinary bladder function was normal and there was no orthostatic hypotension.

Routine laboratory evaluation, including serum globulins and a glucose tolerance test, were normal. X-rays of the feet showed healed bilateral osteomyelitis of the tarsal and metatarsal bones, with fusion of the tarsal bones. Electromyography of the muscles of upper and lower extremities was normal. Sensory conduction in the sural and median nerves was normal. Nerve biopsy was declined.

The patient's mother had developed recurrent foot ulcers in the 6th decade and wore orthopedic shoes until her death from a myocardial infarct at age 60. The patient is married and has two adolescent daughters who are neurologically normal.

COMMENT. This case demonstrates many of the salient features of HSN type I: probable dominant inheritance, late onset, dissociated sensory loss confined to the feet, and recurrent pedal infections with bony deformity; of the only serious alternate diagnoses, diabetes mellitus was ruled out by tests of carbohydrate metabolism; amyloid neuropathy was unlikely as tests of autonomic function were normal.

HSN II
(RECESSIVELY INHERITED SENSORY NEUROPATHY)

Definition

This is a rare, recessively-inherited disorder, characterized by a sensory neuropathy present at birth or with an onset in infancy. Absence of myelinated sensory fibers is correlated with anesthesia and mutilation of the extremities. This disorder was previously labelled *Morvan's disease, infantile syringomyelia*, or *congenital sensory neuropathy*. The clinical criteria for HSN type II are based on detailed studies of relatively few patients.[29,34]

Pathology and Pathogenesis

PATHOLOGY. There are no autopsy reports of this condition. The following features are prominent in nerve biopsies: a striking decrease in myelinated axons of all diameters, more pronounced at distal levels; a moderate decrease in the number of unmyelinated fibers; some evidence of segmental demyelination and remyelination; occasional degenerative change in myelinated axons; and vacuolated endoneurial fibroblasts.[29]

PATHOGENESIS. The pathogenesis is unknown. It is generally held that this disorder, like HSN type I, is associated with distal axonal changes. Xenograft studies have suggested that the Schwann cell does not have a primary role.[35] The evidence that this disorder is degenerative stems solely from observation of scattered fiber breakdown in nerve biopsies; the clinical illness appears static, and it has been suggested that HSN II represents a failure in differentiation of primary sensory neurons or their prenatal degeneration. A recent study of an experimental animal model of sensory neuropathy suggests that there is progressive axonal loss with aging.[35]

Clinical Features

INCIDENCE AND HEREDITY. HSN type II is a very rare condition and has a worldwide distribution. It is inherited in an autosomal recessive manner.

SYMPTOMS AND SIGNS. Almost all cases are recognized in infancy and, in some, the disorder appears to have been present at birth. Ulcerating wounds develop on the fingers and feet at an early age, and painless fractures of the fingers may occur in falls. At an age when a reliable sensory examination can be performed, there is usually a total absence of position, touch, and pressure sensation over the hands and feet, moderate-to-severe loss of pain and thermal sense in these areas, absence of all tendon reflexes, and normal muscle strength. Commonly, there are similar sensory abnormalities over the proximal extremities, trunk, and forehead. Mental status, cranial nerves, and autonomic function are usually preserved.

Laboratory Tests

Routine laboratory tests are usually unremarkable.

ELECTROPHYSIOLOGY. Electromyography is usually normal, although occasionally, fibrillation potentials are present in the intrinsic foot muscles. Motor nerve conduction velocities are generally normal or in the low-normal range. Unobtainable sensory action potentials from either digital or sural nerves are characteristic of this condition.

NERVE BIOPSY. See *Pathology,* above.

Course Prognosis and Treatment

Unequivocal evidence of progression is lacking in most cases. Children grow into adolescence and accomodate to severe sensory loss of the extremities. Most have deformed, shortened, ulcerated fingers and toes. The problems and therapies for foot care are identical to those outlined for HSN type I, compounded by severe limitation imposed by deformed and deafferented hands. Unless exceptional parental care is afforded these children at a young age, and self-care instruction given during adolescence, they may become severely handicapped. There are no data on longevity in this condition.

Differential Diagnosis

Conditions occasionally misdiagnosed as HSN type II include:

HSN TYPE I. This condition is dominantly inherited, usually confined to the lower extremities, and has a later onset than HSN type II.

HSN TYPE III. This condition is also present in infancy, but its prominent autonomic phenomena readily distinguish it from HSN type II.

HSN TYPE IV. This condition is characterized by high fevers and mental retardation, but initially may be confused with HSN type II since both are present in infancy and featured by mutilation of the extremities.

HSN TYPE III (FAMILIAL DYSAUTONOMIA; RILEY-DAY SYNDROME)

Definition

This rare, autosomally recessive condition is probably a disorder of embryogenesis. Congenital absence of autonomic and sensory ganglion cell results in a characteristic clinical syndrome.

Pathology and Pathogenesis

PATHOLOGY. There are diminished numbers of sympathetic ganglion cells throughout, with a corresponding decrease in peripheral sympathetic terminals. Degenerative changes have not been described, but older individuals have fewer neurons.[36] The preganglionic sympathetic neurons in the intermediolateral columns of the thoracic spinal cord are reduced in number. Parasympathetic neurons are strikingly depleted in some ganglia (sphenopalatine), but normal in others (ciliary).[37]

Sensory neurons in dorsal root ganglia are fewer than normal in young individuals, and depletion continues with aging. There is a corresponding progressive loss of axons in the dorsal columns and sensory nerves.[38]

PATHOGENESIS. The pathogenesis is unknown. Since the neuronal deficits are present at birth and degeneration slowly continues, an antenatal deficit of some trophic mechanism has been proposed.[38] Presumably this trophic mechanism is inadequate during life to sustain the remaining neurons; thus, degeneration continues. A congenital abnormality of nerve growth factor (NGF) is currently being investigated.[39]

Clinical Features

INCIDENCE AND HEREDITY. This is a rare disorder. It is inherited in an autosomal recessive fasion and the majority of cases have been Jewish.

SIGNS AND SYMPTOMS. Many of the clinical manifestations of HSN type III correlate well with the congenital absence of autonomic and sensory neurons.

In infancy, poor sucking, crying without tears (alachrima), vomiting crises, blotchy skin, and unexplained fluctuating body temperatures are diagnostic hallmarks. Sweating is usually normal. Older children are noted to have postural hypotension and absence of taste. Sensory dysfunction is prominent, featured by absent corneal reflexes, diminished sensation of pain and temperature, and areflexia. Touch-pressure sensation is relatively spared and strength is often normal. Mutilation of the extremities is rare. Seizures may occur. Intelligence is usually normal. Short stature and scoliosis are common; the tongue is smooth and fungiform papillae are lacking.[38]

Laboratory Studies

ROUTINE LABORATORY STUDIES. Usually normal.

SPECIAL BIOCHEMICAL STUDIES. Norepinephrine and epinephrine catabolite excretion is diminished; dopamine products are excreted in normal amounts. A block in epinephrine synthesis has not been demonstrated.

ELECTROPHYSIOLOGY. Electromyography is usually normal. Motor nerve conduction may be slightly slowed. Sensory nerve action potentials are strikingly diminished in amplitude.

NERVE BIOPSY. Sural nerve biopsies in young patients have demonstrated a marked decreased number of unmyelinated fibers and lesser depletion of myelinated fibers. Segmental demyelination and onion-bulb formation are not features of this condition.

Course Prognosis and Treatment

This is a serious illness associated with a diminished life expectancy. Many die in infancy or childhood from multiple causes related to autonomic dysfunction: aspiration during incoordinated sucking, severe postural hypotension, abnormal responses to hypoxia, or dehydration following vomiting. Occasional individuals survive to middle age, but have limited activity because of autonomic lability and sensory dysfunction. There is no treatment aside from symptomatic care during crises. Pharmacologic manipulation of autonomic dysfunction is not indicated because of the unpredictable response of denervated receptors.[38]

Differential Diagnosis

The correct diagnosis is usually rapidly established in infancy. Few syndromes in pediatric neurology are as dramatic and precise as HSN type III. On occasion, a diagnosis of HSN type IV may be entertained; however, mental retardation and absence of sweating (prominent in type IV) are not features of HSN type III.

HSN TYPE IV (CONGENITAL SENSORY NEUROPATHY WITH ANHIDROSIS)

Definition

This extremely rare, autosomal recessive disorder is manifested in infancy by bouts of high fever. Older children display absence of pain sensation, absent sweating, and mental retardation. This disorder was previously labelled *congenital insensitivity to pain*.[29,34,40] The salient features of this condition are presented in Table 5.

REFERENCES

1. DYCK, PJ: *Definition and basis of classification of hereditary neuropathy with neuronal atrophy and degeneration.* In DYCK, PJ, THOMAS, PK AND LAMBERT, EH (EDS): Peripheral Neuropathy, Vol II, WB Saunders, Philadelphia, 1975, p 755.
2. DYCK, PJ AND LAMBERT, EH: *Lower motor and primary sensory neuron disease with peroneal muscular atrophy. I. Neurobiologic, genetic and electrophysiological findings in hereditary polyneuropathy.* Arch Neurol 18:603, 1968.
3. DYCK, PJ AND LAMBERT, EH: *Lower motor and primary sensory neuron disease with peroneal muscular atrophy. II. Neurobiologic, genetic and electrophysiological findings in hereditary polyneuropathy.* Arch Neurol 18:619.
4. THOMAS, PK AND CALNE, DB: *Motor nerve conduction velocity in peroneal muscular atrophy: evidence for genetic heterogeneity.* J Neurol Neurosurg. Psychiatry 37:68, 1974.
5. THOMAS, PK, CALNE, DB AND STEWART, G: *Hereditary motor and sensory polyneuropathy (peroneal muscular atrophy).* Ann Human Genet 38:111, 1974.
6. BUCHTHAL, F AND BEHSE, F: *Peroneal muscular atrophy and related disorders. I. Clinical manifestations as related to biopsy findings, nerve conduction and electromyography.* Brain 100:41, 1977.
7. BEHSE, F AND BUCHTHAL, F: *Peroneal muscle atrophy and related disorders. 2. Histological findings in sural nerves.* Brain 100:67, 1977.
8. HARDING, AE AND THOMAS, PK: *Autosomal recessive forms of hereditary motor and sensory neuropathy.* J Neurol Neurosurg Psychiatry 43:669, 1980.

9. HARDING, AE AND THOMAS, PK: *Genetic aspects of hereditary motor and sensory neuropathy (Types I and II)*. J Med Genet 17:329, 1980.

10. HARDING, AE AND THOMAS, PK: *Clinical features of hereditary motor and sensory neuropathy Types I and II*. Brain 103:259, 1980.

11. HUMBERSTONE, PM: *Nerve conduction studies in Charcot-Marie-Tooth disease*. Acta Neurol Scand 48:176, 1972.

12. SALISACHS, P: *Wide spectrum of motor conduction velocity in Charcot-Marie-Tooth disease. An anatomico-physiological interpretation*. J Neurol Sci 23:25, 1974.

13. BRADLEY, WG, MADRID, R AND DAVIS, CJF: *The peroneal muscular atrophy syndrome. III. Clinical, electrophysiological and pathological correlations*. J Neurol Sci 32:123, 1977.

14. AGUAYO, AJ, BRAY, GM AND PERKINS, CS: *Axon-Schwann cell relationships in neuropathies of mutant mice*. Ann NY Acad Sci 317:512, 1978.

15. DYCK, PJ, LAIS, AC AND LOW, PA: *Nerve xenographs to assess cellular expression of the abnormality of myelination in inherited neuropathy and Friedreich's ataxia*. Neurology 28:261, 1978.

16. DYCK, PJ, ET AL: *Nerve xenographs to apportion the role of axon and Schwann cell in myelinated fiber absence in hereditary sensory neuropathy, type II*. Neurology 29:1215, 1979.

17. WAXMAN, SG AND OUELLETE, EM: *Ultrastructural and cytochemical observations in a case of dominantly inherited hypertropic (Charcot-Marie-Tooth neuropathy.)* J Neuropathol Exp Neurol 38:586, 1979.

18. DYCK, PJ, ET AL: *Histologic and lipid studies of sural nerves in inherited hypertrophic neuropathy: preliminary reports of a lipid abnormality in nerve and liver in Dejerine-Sottas disease*. Mayo Clin Proc 45:286, 1970.

19. YAO, JK AND DYCK, PJ: *Lipid abnormalities in hereditary neuropathy. 2. Serum phospholipid*. J Neurol Sci 36:234, 1978.

20. WILLIAMS, LL: *Pyruvate oxidation in Charcot-Marie-Tooth disease*. Neurology 29:1492, 1979.

21. DYCK, PJ: *Inherited neuronal degeneration and atrophy affecting peripheral motor, sensory and autonomic neurons*. In DYCK, PJ, THOMAS, PK AND LAMBERT, EH (EDS): Peripheral Neuropathy, *Vol. II*, WB Saunders, Philadelphia, 1975, p 825.

22. BRIMIJOIN, S, CAPEK, P AND DYCK, PJ: *Axonal transport of dopamine-B-hydroxylase by human sural nerves in vitro*. Science 180:1295, 1973.

23. SALISACHS, P AND LAPRESLE, J: *Argyll-Robertson-like pupils in the neural type of Charcot-Marie-Tooth disease*. Eur Neurol 16:172, 1977.

24. ROSENBERG, RN AND CHUTORIAN, A: *Familial opticoacoustic nerve degeneration and polyneuropathy*. Neurology 17:827, 1967.

25. SATYA-MURTI, S, CACACE, AT AND HANSON, PA: *Abnormal auditory evoked potentials in hereditary motor-sensory neuropathy*. Ann Neurol 5:445, 1979.

26. WILLIAMS, LL: *HLA in Charcot-Marie-Tooth Disease*. Ann Neurol 8:452, 1980.

27. KILLIAN, JM AND KLOEPFER, WH: *Homozyzous expression of a dominant gene for Charcot-Marie-Tooth neuropathy*. Ann Neurol 5:515, 1979.

28. KENNEDY, WR, SUNG, JH AND BERRY, JF: *A case of cogenital hypomyelination neuropathy. Clinical, morphological and chemical studies*. Arch Neurol 34:337, 1977.

29. DYCK, PJ AND OHTA, M: *Neuronal atrophy and degeneration predominantly affecting peripheral sensory neurons*. In DYCK, PJ, THOMAS, PK AND LAMBERT, EH (EDS): Peripheral Neuropathies, *Vol II*, WB Saunders, Philadelphia, 1975, p 791.

30. DENNY-BROWN, D: *Hereditary sensory radicular neuropathy*. J Neurol Neurosurg Psychiatry 14:237, 1951.

31. SCHOENE, WC, ET AL: *Hereditary sensory neuropathy, a clinical and ultrastructural study*. J Neurol Sci 11:463, 1970.

32. DYCK, PJ, ET AL: *A Virginia kinship with hereditary sensory neuropathy: peroneal muscular atrophy and pes cavus*. Mayo Clin Proc 40:685, 1965.

33. CAVANAGH, NPC, ET AL: *Hereditary sensory neuropathy with spastic paraplegia*. Brain 102:79, 1979.

34. THOMAS, PK: *Peripheral Neuropathy*. In MATTHEWS, WB (ED): Recent Advances in Clinical Neurology, No 1, Churchill Livingston, Edinburgh, 1975, pp 253.

35. JACOBS, JM ET AL: *A new neurological rat mutant 'mutilated foot.'* J Anat 132:525, 1981.

36. PEARSON, J, AXLEROD, F AND DANEIS, J: *Current concepts of dysautonomia: neuropathologic defects*. Ann NY Acad Sci 228:288, 1974.

37. PEARSON, J AND PYTEL, B: *Quantitative studies of ciliary and sphenopalatine ganglia in familial dysautonomia*. J Neurol Sci 39:123, 1978.

38. PEARSON, J: *Familial dysautonomia (a review).* J Auton Nerv Syst 1:119, 1979.
39. BREAKFIELD, X: *Altered nerve growth factor in familial dysautonomia: discovering the molecular basis of an inherited neurologic disease.* Neurosci Newsletter 12:28, 1981.
40. THRUSH, DC: *Congenital insensitivity to pain—a clinical, genetic and neurophysiological study of four children from the same family.* Brain 96:369, 1973.
41. GUILOFF, RJ, ET AL: *Linkage of autosomal dominant type 1 hereditary motor and sensory neuropathy to the Duffy locus on chromosome 1.* J Neurol Neurosurg Psychiatry 45:669, 1982.
42. GUZZETTA, F, FERRIERE, G, AND LYON, G: *Congenital hypomyelination polyneuropathy.* Brain 105:395, 1982.

Chapter 11

TOXIC NEUROPATHY: PHARMACEUTICAL AGENTS

New pharmaceutical agents are constantly being identified or implicated as causes of human peripheral neuropathy; most such drugs appear to produce distal axonopathy, usually after prolonged use. Except for isoniazid and vincristine, there are few careful experimental studies of the neurotoxicity of these substances. Clinical reports are often the sole basis for many of the alleged drug-induced peripheral neuropathies. Some instances doubtless reflect PNS dysfunction secondary to other, coincident conditions. This chapter discusses pharmaceutic agents that consistently appear associated with neuropathy.

CHLORAMPHENICOL

This antibiotic produces a distal symmetrical neuropathy, usually accompanied by optic neuropathy.[1] Most instances occur in children and young adults receiving prolonged, high-level therapy, and it is generally held that the incidence of neuropathy parallels both dose and duration. Chloramphenicol is now given in short courses to avoid other, more serious hematologic complications, and peripheral neuropathy is extremely rare.

The neuropathy is heralded by numbness of the feet, followed by moderate calf pain and tenderness.[2] Objective signs are few, save for diminution of pain and touch sensation, and loss of Achilles and patellar reflexes. The upper extremities are usually spared. Complete recovery of peripheral neuropathy and optic neuritis occurs if chloramphenicol therapy is stopped soon after initial sensory symptoms appear. Treatment with high doses of B vitamins is advocated, although its rationale is questionable.[3]

There is no animal model of this neuropathy and few morphologic studies of the human PNS disease. An instance of fiber loss in the gracile fasciculi is recorded in an individual without evidence of neuropathy.[4]

CLIOQUINOL

Clioquinol, iodochlorohydroxyquin, is an oral intestinal amebicide. Formerly, it was widely used as therapy or prophylaxis for diarrhea, and its abuse produced an outbreak of a subacute myelo-optic neuropathy (SMON) syndrome in Japan between 1956 and 1972.[5] Human postmortem studies and experimental animal investigations clearly document optic nerve and spinal cord degeneration (central distal axonopathy) following prolonged high-level exposure to clioquinol.[6,7] However, experimental animal studies in several species have repeatedly failed to document degeneration in the PNS.[7] The notion that clioquinol therapy produces neuropathy stems from clinical observations of numbness and sensory loss in the feet and absent Achilles reflexes.[8] Japanese reports claim occasional slowing of motor and sensory nerve conduction velocities, and further allege that both axonal degeneration and segmental demyelination are present in some sural nerve biopsies.[9] Most cases of human clioquinol neurotoxicity occurring outside of Japan have been dominated by signs of myelopathy or optic neuropathy, and only slight slowing of nerve conduction is evident on careful electrophysiologic testing.[10] At this time, existence of clinically significant peripheral neuropathy as part of the clioquinol neurotoxicity syndrome is *sub judice*.[8]

DAPSONE

Dapsone, Avlosulfon, is a sulfone derivative used in treating leprosy and dermatologic conditions. Nine instances of reversible neuropathy have been reported, most occurring after prolonged use.[11,12] Weakness is the predominant feature in all cases, and it is widely held that dapsone may produce a predominantly motor neuropathy. Weakness is symmetrical and usually begins in distal extremities. Eventually, atrophy occurs. Electrophysiologic studies consistently reveal slowed motor conduction velocity and denervation of distal muscles, with no abnormalities of sensory conduction.[12]

It is suggested that dapsone primarily affects the axons of motor neurons, and its sporadic occurrence reflects variable acetylation, as with isoniazid *(vide infra)*.[13] There is no morphologic study of human dapsone neuropathy, and despite two attempts, no experimental animal model.[14]

DIPHENYLHYDANTOIN

Diphenylhydantoin (phenytoin, Dilantin), a drug widely used in the treatment of epilepsy and pain, is stated to cause peripheral neuropathy and cerebellar degeneration. Acute administration of phenytoin to experimental animals causes decreased nerve action potential amplitude and decreased nerve conduction velocity.[15] The evidence for human peripheral neuropathy stems primarily from one report describing absent lower limb reflexes, mild sensory loss, slightly slowed motor and sensory conduction in distal limb nerves, and electromyographic evidence of denervation in the muscles of the hands and feet.[16] Abnormalities occurred most often in individuals taking diphenylhydantoin for many years. It is generally considered that while prolonged diphenylhydantoin therapy may result in diminished reflexes and minor electrophysiologic abnormalities, clinically significant peripheral neuropathy does not occur or is extremely rare.[17,73]

DISULFIRAM

Disulfiram (Antabuse) is used as an adjunct in treatment of motivated, chronic alcoholic patients. The principal neurotoxic syndrome associated with disulfiram is peripheral neuropathy of the distal axonopathy type.[18] Most cases occur at standard therapeutic doses (250 to 500 mg daily) and commence within several months of starting treatment. Tingling paresthesias in the feet, followed shortly by unsteady gait, are initial complaints. Signs of diminished pain, temperature, and position sense in the feet, absent reflexes and weakness of foot dorsiflexion are present in most cases. Eventually, distal upper extremities are involved. Cranial nerve palsies are not a feature of disulfiram neuropathy. Optic neuritis may occur independently of peripheral neuropathy. Drug withdrawal is followed by remission of signs within months in most cases.[18-20]

Mild slowing of motor nerve conduction, diminished amplitude of sensory action potentials, and electromyographic evidence of denervation in distal muscles are characteristic of disulfiram neuropathy. Sural nerve histologic changes include loss of myelinated fibers and nonspecific axonal degeneration.[20] The few experimental animal studies are compatible with distal axonopathy,[21] and one report describes local axonal degeneration related to local injection of the drug.[22]

ETHIONAMIDE

Ethionamide is used in the treatment of tuberculosis. Its role is limited because of serious gastrointestinal, dermatologic, and CNS side effects. Several clinical reports describe progressive, moderate distal symmetrical sensory polyneuropathy; paresthesias of the feet, loss of Achilles reflex and gradual recovery suggest that this is a distal axonopathy.[23-25] Neither electrophysiologic nor nerve biopsy studies are available, and there is no experimental animal model of ethionamide neuropathy.

GOLD

Organic gold compounds are employed in the treatment of rheumatoid arthritis, but potentially severe toxic reactions limit their use. Cutaneous and renal side effects are common; peripheral neuropathy is rare. None of the toxic side effects appears to be dose related.

Peripheral neuropathy is often heralded by intermittent numbness in the legs, followed within months by progressive distal weakness, diminished pain and temperature sense, and areflexia in the distal extremities.[26-28] Onset is usually subacute and may be accompanied by diffuse myokymia and muscle pain. Following drug withdrawal, gradual recovery occurs, the degree of residual dysfunction usually being proportionate to the maximum disability. Motor and sensory nerve conduction velocities are moderately slowed, and cerebrospinal fluid protein elevated. Nerve biopsies reveal a mixture of axonal degeneration and segmental demyelination.[27,28] Neither vasculitis nor endoneurial inflammatory cells are histologic features of this illness. Lymphocyte transformation studies are negative.

The nature and pathogenesis of this neuropathy are unclear. Neither the morphologic studies of nerve biopsies, nor an experimental animal study clearly indicate whether the primary change is axonal or demyelinative.[28] It is also undecided if the PNS dysfunction results from a direct toxic effect of gold or has an allergic basis. Review of the experimental data and clinical phenomena does not strongly support either position, and the nature of gold neuropathy remains elusive.

GLUTETHIMIDE

Glutethimide (Doriden) is a sedative-hypnotic drug that shares many of the pharmacologic properties of thalidomide, a structurally similar compound. Glutethimide neuropathy is rare, and usually follows long-term, high-dose therapy. The clinical pattern suggests a distal axonopathy: slowly progressive distal sensory impairment, bilateral symmetrical leg and foot paresthesias, and cramping and tenderness of the calf muscles.[29] All sensory modalities are diminished in the feet, Achilles reflexes are lost and mild ataxia occurs. Signs gradually remit within six months of drug withdrawal. There are no detailed clinical descriptions of the neuropathy or reports of nerve biopsies, and no experimental animal model.

HYDRALAZINE

Hydralazine (Apresoline) is widely used in the treatment of hypertension. It rarely produces peripheral neuropathy, presumably of the distal axonopathy type. Manifestations of neuropathy appear after widely varying intervals of treatment. In the few case reports, symptoms of distal-extremity numbness and paresthesias predominate; leg weakness is mild and less frequent.[30,31] Following withdrawal of the drug, neurologic dysfunction gradually subsides and recovery is usually complete. There exist neither morphologic studies of human nerve nor an animal model of hydralazine neuropathy.

It is likely that hydralazine-induced PNS dysfunction is related to pyridoxine deficiency. Two factors strongly support this notion. One is the similarity both in chemical structure and in clinical manifestations, the other is that both cause increased excretion of xanthurenic acid (*vide infra*) following a tryptophan load in humans.[31]

ISONIAZID

General

Isoniazid (INH) is one of the cheapest and most effective antituberculous drugs. Peripheral neuropathy of the distal axonopathy type is the most common toxic side effect. The primary route of INH metabolism is by acetylation. Individuals unable to acetylate normally (slow acetylators) maintain prolonged high blood levels of INH, and are more susceptible to neuropathy than are rapid acetylators. The basis for slow acetylation is genetic, inherited as an autosomal recessive trait.[32,33]

INH exerts most of its toxic actions by interference in several ways with compounds of the vitamin B_6 group (pyridoxine, pyridoxal and pyridoxamine). Most important for the pathogenesis of neuropathy is probably its inhibition of pyridoxal phosphokinase, the enzyme which phosphorylates pyridoxal to yield a coenzyme essential for several metabolic reactions.[33]

Pathology and Pathogenesis

Studies of human postmortem material, nerve biopsies, and experimental animal models, strongly support the view that INH neuropathy is a distal axonopathy. Degeneration of myelinated and unmyelinated axons has been carefully documented in sural nerve biopsies;[34] while distal PNS axonal degeneration, denervation muscle atrophy, and fiber loss in dorsal columns are present at autopsy.[33] Peripheral neuropathy is readily produced in rats and its pattern closely mimics that seen in man.[35,36] Both sensory and motor nerves undergo dose-dependent, distal axonal degeneration, and fiber loss is also present in the rostral gracile fasciculi.[35] INH intoxication in other species (dog, chicken) produces widespread vacuolation of white matter, presumably reflecting a primary effect on the oligodendrocyte.[33]

The pathogenesis of peripheral neuropathy is clearly related to the overall interference with B_6 metabolism, and axonal degeneration can be prevented by the administration of vitamin B_6. The primary event which leads to axonal degeneration is uncertain, since the role of pyridoxal phosphate-dependent enzymes in axonal integrity is not known.[33] The overall pattern of axonal change in INH distal axonopathy is widely held to be similar to that of other metabolic axonopathies (see Chapter 2).

Clinical Features

Peripheral neuropathy is a dose-related effect, allegedly more likely to occur in malnourished individuals,[37] and slow acetylators.[33] Common doses (3 to 5 mg per kg daily) are associated with a 2 percent incidence of neuropathy, 6 mg per kg daily with 17 percent incidence and, with higher doses, the incidence increases still more. Symptoms of neuropathy may appear within three weeks in the latter group, conventional doses cause neuropathy after six months. Initial symptoms are tingling paresthesias in the feet, usually followed by complaints of weakness or unsteady gait. Rarely, paresthesias commence in the fingers. Loss of vibration, pain, and temperature sense is usually greater than position and deep pain. Aching cutaneous pain in the calf muscles is an especially common complaint, and often accompanies distal leg weakness and reflex loss. The neuropathy evolves gradually with continued INH administration; such cases eventually develop distal muscle atrophy, ataxia and profound sensory loss.[38]

Recovery usually commences within weeks of drug withdrawal and is gradual, taking months in mild cases and years with advanced involvement. Pyridoxine administration does not affect the rate of recovery.[33]

Peripheral neuropathy can be prevented in most instances by daily administration of 100 mg of pyridoxine. Fortunately, pyridoxine does not affect the antituberculous action of INH.

METRONIDAZOLE AND MISONIDAZOLE

Metronidazole (Flagyl), used in the treatment of anaerobic bacterial and protozoan infections, and the related compound misonidazole, used as a cell sensitizer for cancer radiotherapy, are reported to cause peripheral neuropathy of the distal axonopathy type.[39,40,41] Nerve biopsy in a case of metronidazole neuropathy has revealed axonal degeneration.[40] Misonidazole, a radio-sensitizing agent, produces a distal symmetrical, predominantly sensory polyneuropathy, often associated with painful paresthesias.[41] Experimental animal studies of misonidazole intoxication reveal distal axonal degeneration in intramuscular hind-foot nerves, accompanied by widespread necrotic changes in the CNS, somewhat resembling experimental thiamine deficiency.[42]

NITROFURANTOIN

Nitrofurantoin (Furadantin) is a synthetic antimicrobial agent used to treat urinary tract infections. Peripheral neuropathy of the distal axonal type is among the most serious toxic effects of nitrofurantoin.[43,44] It is suggested that two factors predispose individuals with renal failure to nitrofurantoin neuropathy. One is the excessive tissue concentrations of nitrofurantoin, normally excreted by the kidney,[43] that occur with renal failure; the other is the presence of subclinical neuropathy in uremia (see Chapter 6). Although neither suggestion is experimentally proven, it is considered prudent to avoid using this drug in uremic patients. Nitrofurantoin neuropathy also occurs in individuals without pre-existing renal failure. Normal adults, treated with nitrofurantoin for two weeks, may develop asymptomatic neuropathy with slowed nerve conduction.[45] Experimental animal studies have also demonstrated that intoxication can produce axonal degeneration in normal animals.[46,47]

Peripheral neuropathy usually commences within months, sometimes weeks, of beginning therapy.[43,44] Numbness distally in the legs is usually the initial symptom, followed by subacute onset of severe distal weakness in the limbs and profound sensory loss. All reports stress the rapidity of development of this neuropathy, almost unique among the distal axonopathies. Occasionally, a predominantly motor syndrome appears[48] and, in view of the subacute onset, it may superficially resemble the Guillain-Barré syndrome. Electrophysiologic studies usually display mild slowing of motor nerve conduction, suggesting an axonopathy. The course is variable: If the drug is withdrawn immediately following initial symptoms, only mild impairment occurs and recovery is complete. Should severe changes occur before therapy is stopped, recovery is slow and incomplete.

Experimental animal studies[46,47] and a human postmortem report[49] describe distal axonal degeneration. Postmortem changes in an especially advanced case include dorsal root degeneration and chromatolysis in dorsal root ganglion and anterior horn neurons.[49] Spinal tract degeneration has not been convincingly demonstrated. The observations of axonal degeneration as far proximal as spinal roots and neuronal chromatolysis may correlate with poor recovery in advanced cases. The biochemical lesion underlying this unusual distal axonopathy is unknown, although it is suggested that nitrofurans may disrupt metabolism by competitive inhibition of pyruvate oxidation.[50]

NITROUS OXIDE

Nitrous oxide, widely used as a dental anesthetic and a food propellant, was until recently held to be an inert, harmless substance. It is now recognized to cause a toxic myeloneuropathy. Its abuse as a euphoriant occurs among young people and dentists in North America. Moderate abuse may result in signs of mild, distal, symmetrical sensory polyneuropathy.[51,52] Prolonged, high-level abuse also produces signs of myelopathy.[53] The most common initial symptom is numbness in the distal arms and legs, often combined with poor finger dexterity, leg weakness, and gait imbalance. Signs of PNS dysfunction at this early stage include depressed tendon reflexes, and slight impairment of vibration and pain sensation in the hands and legs. Lhermitte's sign also occurs. Mild slowing of motor and sensory nerve conduction may accompany this early clinical stage. More severe cases develop lower extremity spasticity, severe loss of vibration, position and pain sense in all extremities, hyperreflexia, and Babinski responses.[53] Sural nerve histology and cerebrospinal fluid are normal.

The overall pattern and evolution of the early stage of the clinical profile suggest a toxic, predominantly central distal axonopathy; and the fully developed syndrome somewhat mimics clioquinol myeloneuropathy (vide supra) and combined system disease (see Chapter 5). The well known megaloblastic effect of this substance[54] somewhat reinforces the latter view, as does the demonstration of spongy degeneration in the dorsal and lateral columns in monkeys exposed to nitrous oxide.[55] Animal experiments indicate that nitrous oxide may give rise to this myelopathy by an interference with vitamin B_{12} metabolism (see Chapter 5).

PERHEXILINE MALEATE

Perhexiline maleate (Pexid) is a drug used in the treatment of angina pectoris. Peripheral neuropathy is its principal toxic effect.

Initial complaints occur after treatment for months or years, and are not clearly dose-related. Numbness appears in the distal extremities, rapidly followed by diminution of all sensory modalities. Weakness affects proximal and distal muscles, the latter more severely. Facial diplegia and perioral numbness occasionally occur and dysphagia can be an early feature.[56] Autonomic neuropathy, including postural hypotension, may coexist and may be the presenting symptom. Reflexes are absent or diminished throughout. Recovery occurs slowly after discontinuing therapy. Motor and sensory nerve conduction velocities are markedly slowed, and cerebrospinal fluid protein values moderately elevated. Considerable weight loss may occur, and as the erythrocyte sedimentation rate is sometimes elevated, confusion with a paraneoplastic neuropathy can arise.

Muscle biopsy reveals denervation atrophy. Nerve biopsies demonstrate extensive segmental demyelination, remyelination and axonal degeneration. Osmiophilic inclusions are abundant in Schwann cells, fibroblasts and endothelial cells.[57] Pathologic changes are accompanied by locally increased ganglioside levels of uncertain significance.[58] In sum, the clinical profile, electrophysiologic studies, and nerve biopsy findings indicate a combination of segmental demyelination and axonal degeneration. The nature of the primary event is unclear. Elucidation of the pathogenesis of perhexiline maleate neuropathy awaits development of an appropriate experimental animal model; attempts so far have proved unsuccessful, apart from producing the lamellated cellular inclusions.[57]

PLATINUM (CIS PLATINUM)

Cis-diamine-dichlorplatinum 11 (cis-platinum) is a new, widely used antineoplastic agent. Several preliminary reports describe progressive distal symmetrical sensory neuropathy associated with its use.[59,60] Weakness is mild, if present at all. Sensory nerve conduction velocity is not markedly altered and motor conduction is near normal. Axonal loss is described in a sural nerve biopsy, and experimental animal studies reveal axonal changes at multiple sites in the PNS and CNS. The overall pattern and pathogenesis of cis-platinum axonal degeneration is uncertain.

PYRIDOXINE

Pyridoxine is an essential, water-soluble vitamin (B_6) and a coenzyme for many decarboxylation and transamination reactions. The recommended human daily requirement of pyridoxine is 2.5 mg per day. A recent report describes persistent distal symmetrical sensory loss in the limbs of two individuals who consumed large quantities (over 2 grams daily) of pyridoxine.[74] This is accompanied by severe slowing of distal sensory nerve conduction and normal motor conduction and electromyograms. Neither patient is weak. It is suggested that the human sensory neuropathy (neuronopathy?) may reflect pyridoxine-induced dysfunction in sensory neurons, analogous to the degeneration in dorsal root ganglion cells of dogs maintained at megavitamin levels.[75]

SODIUM CYANATE

Sodium cyanate was formerly used to treat sickle-cell anemia. Peripheral neuropathy is a serious toxic effect and commonly occurs following prolonged, conventional levels of therapy. A study of 27 randomly chosen patients receiving sodium cyanate described nerve conduction abnormalities in 16, sensory symptoms in 5 and signs consistent with PNS dysfunction in 10. All improved following drug withdrawal.[61] Severe neuropathy also may occur and is characterized by gradual development of distal lower extremity sensory loss and foot-drop. Morphologic studies of human sural nerve biopsies[62] and experimentally intoxicated primates and rodents are consistent with distal axonopathy, although proximal demyelination has been a prominent feature late in the experimental disease.[63]

THALIDOMIDE

Thalidomide, formerly used as a sedative-hypnotic, is featured by serious side effects of peripheral neuropathy and embryopathy. Its current pharmaceutic use is confined to the treatment of erythema nodosum leprosum. Thalidomide neuropathy is characterized by unusual clinical features that may reflect widespread nervous system degeneration.[64-66]

Initial symptoms are always sensory, usually consisting of numbness and tingling in the feet, then in the hands. Sensory loss to pain and touch is more profound than to vibration or for joint position, and usually progresses proximally to yield a sizable stocking-glove pattern. Weakness develops subsequently, and may be proximal or distal. Tendon reflexes may be depressed or increased, and Babinski responses are occasionally present. Characteristic somatic findings of brittle nails and palmar erythema appear together with the neuropathy. Electrophysiologic studies reveal absent or reduced amplitude of sensory potentials and normal motor conduction. Recovery of sensory function may not commence for years following drug withdrawal, is generally poor, may take years, and some patients have residual dysesthesias. Motor recovery is usually satisfactory.[66]

The human and experimental animal material is limited and does not satisfactorily account for the clinical features. Widespread loss of fibers in peripheral nerves and dorsal columns of the spinal cord, and diminished number of dorsal root ganglion cells are described.[67] These changes possibly reflect, in part, primary degeneration of ganglion cells (sensory neuronopathy).[68] This would correlate with poor recovery of sensation in some cases. Unexplained clinical features include proximal weakness, hyperreflexia, and sparing of vibration and position sense.

VINCRISTINE

General

Vincristine (Oncovin), an alkaloid derived from the periwinkle plant *Vinca rosea*, is widely employed in the treatment of leukemia, lymphoma, and some solid tumors. Peripheral neuropathy and gastrointestinal dysfunction constitute the principal toxic effects and may limit its use[69,70]

Gastrointestinal dysfunction, constipation and adynamic ileus, and bladder atony, occasionally occur. All are widely held to result from dysfunction of the autonomic nervous system;[69] however, there is neither morphologic nor electrophysiologic support for this notion.

Pathology

Human nerve biopsies consistently display axonal degeneration as the prominent feature; segmental demyelination is rare.[69] Regenerating axons are present in recovering cases. Biopsies of distal muscles reveal denervation changes; proximal muscles contain mild, primarily myopathic, alterations. There is no satisfactory postmortem study of the human nervous system. Reports of animal studies contain descriptions of changes in widely varied areas of both the CNS and the neuromuscular system, and correlate poorly with the clinical findings. Species variation and differing experimental protocols may account for some of these discrepancies. Proximal axonal swelling, neuronal neurofilamentous proliferation, and primary diffuse myopathy are all described.[66,71]

PATHOGENESIS. Vinca alkaloids function as mitotic spindle inhibitors by binding to tubulin, the microtubule subunit protein. It is proposed that tubulin binding impairs axonal transport and results in nerve-fiber breakdown. Experimental animal studies that demonstrate abnormalities in fast axoplasmic transport afford some support for this view.[71]

Clinical Features

Vincristine neuropathy occurs in a stereotyped manner, is manifest to some extent in most treated patients, and has clinical features that suggest an unusual distribution and evolution of axonopathy.[69,70]

Paresthesias, often starting in fingers before feet, are the most common initial symptom, and antecede sensory signs by several weeks. Sensory loss is usually mild and remains confined to the most distal parts of the extremities. Weakness, clumsiness, and muscle cramps subsequently appear, may evolve rapidly to severe motor impairment, and are occasionally most pronounced in distal, upper-limb muscles.[70] Eventually, distal leg weakness occurs. Motor signs dominate vincristine polyneuropathy and may seriously disable affected individuals. Tendon reflexes are absent or diminished in most cases; loss of Achilles reflexes may precede the first sensory symptoms, probably reflecting involvement of afferent fibers from muscle spindles.[72] Numbness and sensory loss in the trigeminal distribution may occur, and jaw pain of obscure etiology is present in 5 to 10 percent of cases.

Electromyographic findings reflect denervation in distal muscles, and sensory nerve conduction studies demonstrate reduced action potential amplitudes.[70]

The prognosis of vincristine neuropathy varies. Withdrawal from therapy at the early stage leads to rapid disappearance of sensory symptoms. Weakness also wanes, but more slowly. Mild residual weakness, impairment of superficial sensation, and absent Achilles reflexes persist in severe cases. Neuropathy may also improve if the dose is reduced, enabling some patients to continue therapy without this disabling side effect.[70]

REFERENCES

1. WALLENSTEIN, L AND SNYDER, J: *Neurotoxic reaction to Chloromycetin.* Ann Int Med 36:1526, 1952.

2. JOY, RJT, SCALETTAR, R AND SODEE, DB: *Optic and peripheral neuritis. Probable effect of prolonged chloramphenicol therapy.* JAMA 173:1731, 1960.

3. WILSON, W: *Toxic amblyopia due to chloramphenicol.* Scot Med J 7:90, 1962.

4. COGAN, G, TRUMAN, JT AND SMITH, TR: *Optic neuropathy, chloramphenicol and infantile agranulocytosis.* Invest Ophth 12:534, 1973.

5. TSUBAKI, T, HONMA, Y AND HOSHI, J: *Neurobiological syndrome associated with clioquinol.* Lancet 1:696, 1971.

6. SOBUE, I, ET AL: *Myeloneuropathy with abdominal disorders in Japan. Neuropathologic findings in seven autopsied cases.* Neurology (Minneap) 22:1034, 1972.

7. KRINKE, G, ET AL: *Clioquinol and 2,5-hexanedione induce different types of distal axonopathy in the dog.* Acta Neuropathol 47:213, 1979.

8. SCHAUMBURG, HH AND SPENCER, PS: *Clioquinol.* In SPENCER, PS AND SCHAUMBURG, HH (EDS): Experimental and Clinical Neurotoxicology, Williams & Wilkins, Baltimore, 1980, p 395.

9. TSUKAGOSHI, H, TOHGI, H AND TOYOKURA, Y: *The peripheral nerve in cases of SMON. II. Clinico-pathological study of sural nerve.* Clin Neurol 11:400, 1971 (JAP).

10. BAUMGARTNER, G, ET AL: *Neurotoxicity of halogenated hydroxyquinolines: clinical analysis of cases reported outside Japan.* J Neurol Neurosurg Psychiatry 42:1073, 1979.

11. RAPOPORT, AM AND GUSS, SB: *Dapsone-induced peripheral neuropathy.* Arch Neurol 27:184, 1972.

12. GUTMANN, L, MARTIN, JD AND WALTON, W: *Dapsone motor neuropathy—an axonal disease.* Neurology (Minneap) 26:514, 1976.

13. GELBER, R, ET AL: *The polymorphic acetylation of dapsone in man.* Clin Pharmacol Ther 12:225, 1971.

14. WILLIAMS, MH AND BRADLEY, WG: *An assessment of dapsone toxicity in the guinea pig.* Br J Dermatol 86:650, 1972.

15. MARCUS, D, SWIFT, T AND MCDONALD, T: *Acute effects of phenytoin on peripheral nerve function in the rat.* Muscle and Nerve 4:48, 1981.

16. LOVELACE, RE AND HORWITZ, SJ: *Peripheral neuropathy in long term diphenylhydantoin therapy.* Arch Neurol 18:69, 1968.

17. SWIFT, TR, ET AL: *Peripheral neuropathy in epileptic patients.* Neurology (Minneap) 31:826, 1981.

18. BRADLEY, WG AND HEWER, RL: *Peripheral neuropathy due to disulfiram.* Br Med J 2:449, 1966.

19. MODDEL, G, ET AL: *Disulfiram neuropathy.* Arch Neurol 35:658, 1978.

20. MORKI, B, OHNISHI, A AND DYCK, PJ: *Disulfiram neuropathy.* Neurology (Minneap) 31:730, 1981.

21. ANZIL, AP AND DUZIC, S: *Disulfiram neuropathy: an experimental study in the rat.* J Neuropathol Exp Neurol 37:585, 1978.

22. ZUCCARELLO, M AND ANZIL, AP: *Localized model of experimental neuropathy by topical application of disulfiram.* Exp Neurol 64:699, 1979.

23. POOLE, GW AND SCHNEEWEISS, J: *Peripheral neuropathy due to ethioniamide.* Annual Review of Respiratory Diseases 84:890, 1961.

24. LEGGAT, PO: *Ethionamide Neuropathy.* Tubercule 43:95, 1962.

25. TALA, E AND TEVOLA, K: *Side effects and toxicity of ethionamide and prothionamide.* Ann Clin Res 1:32, 1969.

26. DOYLE, JB AND CANNON, EF: *Severe polyneuritis following gold therapy for rheumatoid arthritis.* Ann Intern Med 33:1468, 1950.

27. WALSH, JC: *Gold neuropathy.* Neurology (Minneap) 20:455, 1970.

28. KATVAK, SM, ET AL: *Clinical and morphological features of gold neuropathy.* Brain 103:671, 1980.

29. STERMAN, AB AND SCHAUMBURG, HH: *Neurotoxicity of selected drugs.* In SPENCER, PS AND SCHAUMBURG, HH (EDS): Experimental and Clinical Neurotoxicology, Williams & Wilkins, Baltimore, 1980, p 593.

30. KIRKENDALL, WM AND PAGE, EB: *Polyneuritis occurring during hydralazine therapy.* JAMA 167:427, 1962.

31. RASKIN, NH AND FISHMAN, RA: *Pyridoxine-deficiency neuropathy due to hydralazine.* N Eng J Med 273:1182, 1965.

32. EVANS, DAP: *Pharmacogenetics.* Am J Med 34:639, 1963.

33. BLAKEMORE, WF: *Isoniazid.* In SPENCER, PS AND SCHAUMBURG, HH (EDS): Experimental and Clinical Neurotoxicology, Williams & Wilkins, Baltimore, 1980, p 476.

34. OCHOA, J: *Isoniazid neuropathy in man: quantitative electron microscope study.* Brain 93:831, 1970.

35. KLINGHARDT, GW: *Arzneimittelschadigungen des peripheren Nervensystems unter besonderer Berucksichtigung der Polyneuropathie durch Isonicotinsaurehydrazid (experimentelle und human pathologische Untersuchungen).* Proc Vth Int Congr Neuropath Exerpta Medica Found Int Cong Series No 100, 1966, p 292.

36. CAVANAGH, JB: *On the pattern of change in peripheral nerves produced by isoniazid intoxication in rats.* J Neurol Neurosurg Psychiatry 30:219, 1964.

37. MONEY, GL: *Isoniazid neuropathies in malnourished tuberculous patients.* J Trop Med 62:198, 1959.

38. GAMMON, GD, BURGE, FW AND KING, G: *Neural toxicity in tuberculous patients treated with isoniazid (isonicotinic acid hydrazide)* Arch Neurol Psychiatry 70:64, 1953.

39. COXON, A AND PALLIS, CA: *Metronidazole neuropathy.* J Neurol Neurosurg Psychiatry 39:403, 1977.

40. BRADLEY, WG, KARLSSON, IJ AND RASSO, ICG: *Metronidazole neuropathy.* Br Med J 2:610, 1977.

41. MELGAARD, B, ET AL: *Misonidazol neuropathy, a clinical electrophysiological and histological study.* Ann Neurol (in press).

42. GRIFFIN, JW, ET AL: *Neurotoxicity of misonidazol in rats. I. Neuropathology.* Neurotoxicology 1:299, 1979.

43. LOUGHRIDGE, LW: *Peripheral neuropathy due to nitrofurantoin.* Lancet 2:1133, 1962.

44. ELLIS, FG: *Acute polyneuritis after nitrofurantoin therapy.* Lancet 2:1136, 1962.

45. TOOLE, JF, ET AL: *Neural effects of nitrofurantoin.* Arch Neurol 18:860, 1968.

46. KLINGHARDT, GW: *Schadigungen des Nervensystems durch Nitrofurane bei der Ratte.* Acta Neuropathol (Berl) 9:18, 1967.

47. BEHAR, A., ET AL: *Experimental nitrofurantoin polyneuropathy in rats.* Arch Neurol 13:160, 1965.

48. MORRIS, JS: *Nitrofurantoin and peripheral neuropathy with megaloblastic anemia.* J Neurol Neurosurg Psychiatry 29:22, 1966.

49. LHERMITTE, R, ET AL: *Polynevrites au cours de traitements par la nitrofurantoine.* Presse Medicale 71:767, 1963.

50. PAUL MF, ET AL: *Inhibition by furacin of citrate formation in testis preparations.* J Biol Chem 206:491, 1954.

51. LAYZER, RB, FISHMAN, RA AND SCHAFER, JA: *Neuropathy following abuse of nitrous oxide.* Neurology (Minneap) 28:504, 1978.

52. SAHENK, Z, MENDELL, JR, COURI, D AND NACHTMAN, J: *Polyneuropathy from inhalation of nitrous oxide cartridges through a whipped cream dispenser.* Neurology (Minneap) 28:485, 1978.

53. LAYZER, RB: *Myeloneuropathy after prolonged exposure to nitrous oxide.* Lancet 11:1227, 1978.

54. AMESS, JAL, ET AL: *Megaloblastic haemopoiesis in patients receiving nitrous oxide.* Lancet 1:339, 1978.

55. DINN, JJ, ET AL: *Animal model for subacute combined degeneration.* Lancet 11:1154, 1978.

56. SAID, G: *Perhexiline neuropathy: a clinicopathological study.* Ann Neurol 3:259, 1978.

57. FARDEAU, M, TOME, FMS AND SIMON, P: *Muscle and nerve changes induced by perhexiline maleate in man and mice.* Muscle Nerve 2:24, 1979.

58. POLLET, S, ET AL: *Analysis of the major lipid classes in human peripheral nerve biopsies.* J Neurol Sci 41:199, 1979.

59. CLARK, A, ET AL: *Neurotoxicity of cis-platinum: pathology of the central and peripheral nervous systems.* Neurology (Minneap) 30:429, 1980.

60. HEMPHILL, M, ET AL: *Sensory neuropathy in cis-platinum chemotherapy.* Neurology (Minneap) 30:429, 1980.

61. PETERSEN, CM, ET AL: *Sodium cyanate induced polyneuropathy in patients with sickle-cell disease.* Ann Intern Med 81:152, 1974.

62. OHNISHI, A, PETERSEN, CM AND DYCK, PJ: *Axonal degeneration in sodium cyanate-induced neuropathy.* Arch Neurol 32:530, 1975.

63. TELLEZ-NAGEL, I, ET AL: *An ultrastructural study of chronic sodium cyanate-induced neuropathy.* J Neuropathol Exp Neurol 36:351, 1977.

64. FULLERTON, PM AND KREMER, M: *Neuropathy after intake of thalidomide (Distaval).* Br Med J 2:855, 1961.

65. FULLERTON, PM AND O'SULLIVAN, DJ: *Thalidomide neuropathy: a clinical, electrophysiological and histological follow-up study.* J Neurol Neurosurg Psychiatry 31:543, 1968.

66. LEQUESNE, PM: *Neuropathy due to drugs.* In DYCK, PJ, THOMAS, PK AND LAMBERT, EH (EDS): Peripheral Neuropathy, Vol II, WB Saunders, Philadelphia, 1975, p 1263.

67. KLINGHARDT, GW: *Ein Beitrag der experimentellen Neuropathologie zür Toxizitatsprufung neuer Chemotherapeutica.* Mitt Max-Planck-Ges 3:142, 1965.

68. STERMAN, AB AND SCHAUMBURG, HH: *Neurotoxicity of Selected Drugs.* In SPENCER, PS AND SCHAUMBURG, HH (EDS): Experimental and Clinical Neurotoxicology, Williams & Wilkins, Baltimore, 1980, p 593.

69. BRADLEY, WG, ET AL: *The neuromyopathy of vincristine in man: clinical, electrophysiological and pathological studies.* J Neurol Sci 10:107, 1970.

70. CASEY, EB, ET AL: *Vincristine neuropathy: clinical and electrophysiological observations.* Brain 96:69, 1973.

71. GREEN, LS, ET AL: *Axonal transport disturbances in vincristine induced peripheral neuropathy.* Ann Neurol 1:255, 1977.

72. MCLEOD, JG AND PENNY, R: *Vincristine neuropathy: an electrophysiological and histological study.* J Neurol Neurosurg Psychiatry 32:297, 1969.

73. SHORVON, SD AND REYNOLDS, EH: *Anticonvulsant peripheral neuropathy: a clinical and electrophysiological study of patients on single drug treatment with phenytoin, carbamazepine or barbiturates.* J Neurol Neurosurg Psychiatry 45:620, 1981.

74. SCHAUMBURG, HH, ET AL: *Pyridoxine megavitaminosis produces sensory neuropathy (neuronopathy?) in humans.* Ann Neurol 12:107, 1982.

75. KRINKE, G, ET AL: *Pyridoxine megavitaminosis produces degeneration of peripheral sensory neurons (sensory neuronopathy) in the dog.* Neurotoxicology 2:13, 1980.

Chapter 12

TOXIC NEUROPATHY: OCCUPATIONAL, BIOLOGICAL AND ENVIRONMENTAL AGENTS

An enormous number of potentially toxic chemicals is deployed in the workplace and general environment. Many have been identified or implicated as causes of peripheral neuropathy, usually of the distal axonopathy type. Except for acrylamide, thallium, the hexacarbons and organophosphates, there are few careful experimental studies of these substances. Clinical reports, often isolated, are the sole basis for some of the alleged, chemically-induced peripheral neuropathies. Agents consistently associated with neuropathy are included in this chapter. Specifically excluded are chemicals such as the polyhalogenated biphenyls, inorganic mercury, carbon monoxide, DDT, and carbon tetrachloride, whose link with neuropathy seems tenuous. Diphtheritic neuropathy is included in this chapter as the sole example of a biologic toxin consistently associated with neuropathy.

ACRYLAMIDE

General

Acrylamide monomer is important in several industries. Polymerization of the monomer produces substances that are useful flocculators and grouting agents. Acrylamide monomer is neurotoxic, while the polymer is not. The monomer is a white powder, soluble in water, and can be absorbed readily by inhalation, ingestion, or through the skin. Most instances of neuropathy have occurred via dermal contact in industrial or occupational settings.[1] Episodic contact dermatitis of the hands usually antedates neuropathy, indicating that significant exposure has occurred. The population at large probably has little risk of neurotoxic exposure, except for rare instances when the monomer has contaminated well water.

Pathology and Pathogenesis

PATHOLOGY. Acrylamide monomer clearly produces distal axonopathy in experimental animals,[2] and sural nerve biopsies from two humans recovering from acrylamide neuropathy revealed axonal degeneration predominantly affecting large fibers.[3] Detailed morphologic and electrophysiologic studies have been performed in various experimental species intoxicated with acrylamide, and it is widely held that acrylamide-induced changes are a valid model for the pattern of distal axonopathy induced by many neurotoxic agents.[4] The fundamental axonal change is accumulation of 10 nm neurofilaments. These accumulations initially appear in the distal regions of large-diameter myelinated axons of the PNS and CNS in the pattern outlined in Chapter 2. In cats, the earliest morphologic changes have been detected in Pacinian corpuscles of the hind and forefeet, primary annulospiral endings of muscle spindles, and in preterminal axons of the gracile nucleus.[2] With continued intoxication, proximal segments of peripheral nerves undergo change and widespread tract-oriented degeneration occurs in the corticospinal, spinocerebellar, and optic tracts. Electrophysiologic studies of experimental animals confirm the pattern of PNS vulnerability.[5]

PATHOGENESIS. The metabolism of acrylamide is poorly understood; it is rapidly distributed throughout the body and some may persist in nervous tissue for 14 days. Small changes in the acrylamide molecule result in loss of neurotoxicity, and many analogues appear innocuous.[6] The primary mechanism of neurotoxic damage is unknown, despite considerable experimental study. Presumably the pathogenesis of this toxic distal axonopathy is associated with a disorder of axonal or neuronal metabolism.

Clinical Features

SYMPTOMS, SIGNS AND COURSE. Numbness and excessive sweating of feet and fingers and an unsteady gait are usual initial complaints.[7] Difficulty in walking is frequently disproportionate to the mild initial weakness. This characteristic of acrylamide neurotoxicity may reflect either muscle-spindle or cerebellar dysfunction. Excessive sweating is sometimes accompanied by skin peeling in the hands and other signs of exfoliative dermatitis.

Objective signs are present in all symptomatic individuals and reflect the distal PNS motor, sensory and, possibly, CNS cerebellar dysfunction.[4] Early on, weakness of the hands and feet is usually combined with an unusually diffuse loss of tendon reflexes, unlike most toxic neuropathies which are featured by early selective loss of the Achilles' reflex. Sensory change inevitably includes depression of vibration sense. Other modalities are variously affected. Clumsiness and occasional intention tremor may be present in the upper extremities, and broad-based swaying gait is a common early finding.[7,8] Cranial-nerve palsy and autonomic dysfunction (aside from increased sweating) are not features of this condition.

Removal from exposure in the early stages results in gradual, complete functional recovery from both PNS and CNS involvement. Careful examination may reveal persistent depression of vibration sense as the sole abnormality.[4] In more severely affected individuals, improvement usually continues for many months, but frequently there is residual distal weakness, gait ataxia, and vibration-sense loss. There is no specific treatment for acrylamide neurotoxicity.

Laboratory Investigation

ROUTINE CLINICAL TESTS. Routine laboratory tests are unremarkable.

CEREBROSPINAL FLUID. The CSF is acellular and the protein content either normal or slightly elevated.

CLINICAL ELECTROPHYSIOLOGY. Electromyography of distal limb muscles usually reveals ample evidence of denervation.[8] Motor nerve conduction velocities characteristically are normal or only slightly reduced. Sensory nerve action potentials are almost always abnormal, and are suggested as a sensitive electrophysiologic screening test for early or subclinical neuropathy. Reduction in amplitude is the most common abnormality, and is present early even in distal portions of upper-extremity nerves.[9]

Differential Diagnosis

The diagnosis is not difficult in an individual with proven industrial or occupational exposure. The presence of gait, ataxia, moist, peeling hands, and peripheral neuropathy in such individuals leaves little room for doubt.[8] A detailed occupational history is probably the most important diagnostic procedure, since acrylamide neurotoxicity almost never stems from unrecognized environmental sources.

ARSENIC (INORGANIC)

General

Human neurotoxicity from arsenic is now usually associated with ingestion of arsenic trioxide. Arsenic compounds are not mined as such, but occur principally as by-products of smelting of copper and lead ores. Workers in smelting industries are at risk for chronic arsenic intoxication, as are miners and individuals whose wells are adjacent to mines containing arsenic-rich ores.[10] Arsenic trioxide remains a popular vehicle for homicide and suicide, and survivors may develop a subacute neuropathy.[11]

Pathology and Pathogenesis

PATHOLOGY. Axonal degeneration is the predominant change in nerve biopsies from patients with arsenic neuropathy,[11] and it is probable that inorganic arsenic intoxication produces distal axonopathy. One autopsy report of a severe case of arsenic neuropathy, utilizing limited histologic techniques, describes changes in peripheral nerves and the dorsal columns of the spinal cord.[12] Unfortunately, there is no reasonable experimental animal model of inorganic arsenic neurotoxicity, and the nature and distribution of axonal changes remain to be elucidated.

PATHOGENESIS. The pathogenesis of arsenical distal axonopathy is unknown. It is suggested that the interaction of arsenic with the thiol group of lipoic acid is a link between arsenic neuropathy and the clinically similar axonopathy of thiamine deficiency.[13] It is assumed that arsenic acts on the lipoic acid component of the pyruvate dehydrogenase complex, inhibiting the conversion of pyruvate to acetyl CoA. The affinity of arsenic trioxide for keratin of hair and nail is attributed to similar thiol binding.

Clinical Features

Peripheral neuropathy is the predominant neurologic complication of exposure to inorganic arsenic.[10,11,14,15,16] Two varieties exist: a subacute type that appears within weeks of a massive overdose (unsuccessful suicide, homicide),[11] and an insidiously developing type following prolonged low-level exposure in industry.[10] Many reports of arsenic neuropathy do not differentiate between the two types of exposure, and this distinction is not widely appreciated.

CHRONIC EXPOSURE TYPE. Chronic low-level exposure to organic arsenic produces a consistent chronologic triad of conditions.[13] The initial phase is characterized by weakness, malaise, anorexia, and vomiting. The second stage is featured by mucous membrane irritation, hyperkeratosis, darkened skin, white striae of the nails (Mees' lines), and pitting edema. It is likely that many individuals in this stage have subclinical neuropathy. The third stage is overt peripheral neuropathy whose onset is heralded by numbness and burning sensations of the hands and feet. Diminished vibration and position sensation in the lower extremities is usually present and may result in a tabetic syndrome. Other modalities are less consistently affected. Weakness is usually mild and confined to extensors of the feet and intrinsic hand muscles. Continued exposure may result in severe distal, stocking-glove, sensorimotor neuropathy. Recovery is usually excellent in mildly affected individuals, and less satisfactory in the more rare cases with severe involvement.[13]

SINGLE EXPOSURE TYPE. A single large dose of arsenic produces vomiting within minutes or hours. This may be followed by tachycardia, diarrhea, hypotension, vasomotor collapse, and death within a day. Survivors may develop neuropathy within ten days to three weeks. Sensory symptoms appear first: usually these consist of numbness and intense paresthesias distally in the limbs. Weakness in the distal lower extremities soon follows and may involve the upper extremities as well. The illness has a subacute progression, usually evolves within two to five weeks and the degree of impairment varies considerably. Some experience only mild, predominantly sensory neuropathy, others (probably the majority) develop severe distal sensorimotor polyneuropathy.[11] Impairment of position and vibration sense may be especially profound. Systemic signs of arsenic intoxication (skin, nails) are often not pronounced in this variety. Recovery is gradual and, in the mild cases, usually complete. Individuals with pronounced atrophy and severe sensory loss recover to some degree over a two-year period, but these often stabilize in a permanently disabled state.

Treatment of both varieties involves chelation therapy with either British Anti Lewisite or penicillamine. There is little evidence that treatment of fully-developed neuropathy affects its course. It is suggested that chelation therapy be continued for months following exposure.[11]

Laboratory Studies

CLINICAL LABORATORY. Routine laboratory studies are usually unremarkable. Analysis of hair, fingernail clippings, and urine for arsenic reveal markedly elevated levels in chronic cases. Tissue arsenic levels are not consistently elevated in the subacute neuropathy following a single dose.

CEREBROSPINAL FLUID. The CSF is acellular and the protein level normal.

CLINICAL ELECTROPHYSIOLOGY. Electromyography usually reveals evidence of denervation in distal lower-limb muscles. Motor nerve conduction is only mildly or moderately slowed, while the amplitude of sensory action potentials is profoundly depressed.[11]

Differential Diagnosis

Cases that follow massive single exposure are usually obvious. Arsenical neuropathy following chronic low-level exposure may pose a formidable diagnostic problem. The neurologic syndrome is similar to those of uremia, nutritional disorders, or other nonspecific sensorimotor neuropathies. Furthermore, the systemic manifestations of arsenic intoxication are often mild and readily overlooked. Hair, urine, and fingernail arsenic levels are justified in evaluating polyneuropathies of obscure etiology.

CARBON DISULFIDE

Carbon disulfide (CS_2) is used in the production of viscose rayon fibers and cellophane films. CS_2 neurotoxicity is inevitably a result of airborne industrial exposure, and has been a persistent problem in Scandanavia, Japan, and Southern Europe. Subacute exposure of humans to high concentrations produces profound psychologic disturbance, while chronic low-level intoxication produces peripheral neuropathy of the distal axonopathy type in man and experimental animals.[17]

Chronic exposure to low airborne levels (10 to 40 ppm) is reported to result in prolonged motor nerve conduction in the lower limbs, presumably evidence of subclinical neuropathy.[18] Exposure to levels of 170 ppm for four to six months produces symptoms of numbness and weakness distally in the lower extremities. Weakness, loss of Achilles and patellar reflexes, and diminished sensation to pin, touch, and vibration sense accompany these symptoms.[19] Upper-limb involvement follows continued exposure. Moderate slowing of motor and sensory nerve conduction and evidence of denervation of distal muscles are features of this neuropathy.[20] Recovery is slow and, in severe cases, frequently incomplete. There are no detailed clinical studies of individuals who remain impaired after prolonged recovery, and it is possible that residual spinal cord damage may account for some of this disability. This notion is supported by experimental animal studies which demonstrate tract-oriented distal axonal degeneration in the spinal cord as well as changes in distal fibers of the PNS. There are no reliable reports of the morphologic changes in human CS_2 distal axonopathy. Experimental animal studies describe axonal swellings with accumulations of 10 nm neurofilaments, similar to the changes in acrylamide and hexacarbon neuropathies.[17]

CYANIDE

General

Acute cyanide intoxication is usually lethal, due to the rapid reaction of cyanide ion with trivalent iron of cytochrome oxidase. Chronic cyanide intoxication is not fatal, and may result in widespread CNS and PNS degeneration. Chronic cyanide poisoning from occupational sources is rare;

however, environmental exposure may result from consumption of the seeds of certain stone fruits (apricot, peach, wild cherry). This condition is extremely rare in Europe and North America; however, ingestion of large quantities of the cassava plant has been linked with a debilitating neurologic condition in Nigeria (Nigerian neuropathy), and cyanogenic plants are also implicated in other tropical neurologic disorders.[21] Affected Nigerians have significantly elevated plasma thiocyanate levels, are riboflavin-deficient and generally in poor health.[22]

Clinical Features

Initial symptoms of Nigerian neuropathy are painful paresthesias of the feet, followed by numbness of the hands. Subsequently, weakness develops in the distal lower limbs, along with a broad-based ataxic gait. Loss of sensation and weakness frequently display a stocking-glove distribution, with an especially severe impairment of proprioception in the legs. Severe atrophy of the lower legs, similar to HSMN type I, occasionally is present. Tendon reflexes are usually exaggerated and hypertonicity may occur. Lower extremity ataxia is attributed to sensory impairment rather than cerebellar involvement. Motor nerve conduction may be moderately slowed in the lower extremities.

Signs of CNS dysfunction are present in most cases. Optic atrophy and visual impairment are prominent features of this illness, and sensorineural hearing loss may occur. Many of the sensory symptoms are attributed to dorsal column dysfunction, and hyperreflexia and hypertonicity probably reflect corticospinal involvement.[21]

The condition is slowly progressive and rarely fatal. There are no reports describing the effect of change of diet, nerve biopsies, postmortem examination, or a suitable animal model of this condition.

DIMETHYLAMINOPROPIONITRILE (DMAPN)

General

DMAPN, an effective catalyst in polymerization reactions, was introduced into the manufacture of polyurethane foams in 1967. A toxic distal axonopathy syndrome with atypical features occurred in many workers following its deployment.[23,24] DMAPN was soon recognized as the cause, withdrawn from use, and no new cases developed. Striking and unusual features accompanying DMAPN axonopathy are urinary hesitancy and sexual dysfunction. These antedate the usual symptoms of polyneuropathy, and affected individuals have been erroneously diagnosed as having prostatic hypertrophy.[25]

Pathology and Pathogenesis

Results of human nerve biopsy and experimental animal studies indicate that DMAPN produces distal axonal degeneration. Axonal swellings filled with neurofilaments and nonspecific organelles are described. Although the clinical profile suggests selective involvement of small nerve fibers, morphologic data do not strongly support this notion.[23] There are no reports describing DMAPN-induced changes in the autonomic nervous system of man or animals. Reversible changes in autonomic function occur after short periods of exposure to DMAPN, suggesting that urinary and sexual dysfunction may, in part, be pharmacologic. The pathophysiology of distal axonal degeneration is unknown. Presumably, it shares features with other metabolic and toxic axonopathies (see Chapter 2).

Clinical Features

SYMPTOMS, SIGNS AND PROGNOSIS. The latency between first exposure to DMAPN and appearance of symptoms varies with the concentrations or amounts used. Initial symptoms are usually urinary hesitancy and abdominal discomfort, followed by decreased stream, reduced frequency of urination, and occasional incontinence. Partial or complete impotence develops subsequent to the urinary dysfunction, and is often accompanied by numbness of the feet. Subsequently, proximal numbness and paresthesias develop in the legs and hands, accompanied by weakness in the legs. A distinctive feature of DMAPN neurotoxicity is diminished pain, temperature and touch sensation in the lower sacral dermatomes.[25] Vibration sense is diminished in the feet. Weakness occurs in the distal extremities, and is most severe in the toe and foot extensors. Atrophy is unusual. The tendon reflexes are usually preserved, an atypical feature for a distal axonopathy. Cranial nerve and autonomic functions, other than urinary and sexual, are spared. It is suggested that the unusual constellation of autonomic and sensory symptoms, together with relative sparing of tendon reflexes, indicate that DMAPN axonopathy selectively affects small nerve fibers.[25]

The prognosis is good for young individuals with mild or moderate involvement. Some older individuals have experienced persistent sexual and urinary dysfunction.

Laboratory Studies

CLINICAL LABORATORY. Values of most routine laboratory tests are normal.

CEREBROSPINAL FLUID. The CSF is usually normal.

ELECTRODIAGNOSTIC STUDIES. Motor nerve conduction is usually normal; occasionally slight slowing is present in severely affected patients. Sensory nerve action potentials have diminished amplitudes. Sacral nerve latencies in three reported patients were prolonged.[25]

URODYNAMIC STUDIES. Cystometrograms may demonstrate a flaccid urinary bladder with increased residual volume, and intravenous pyelography usually reveals significant postvoiding residual.

Differential Diagnosis

The fully developed syndrome of DMAPN intoxication resembles no other neurotoxic condition. This constellation of findings, combined with epidemic occurrence in an industrial setting, readily establishes its presence. Isolated cases in the early stages, when urinary symptoms predominate, are difficult urologic diagnoses. Isolated cases in later stages may suggest diabetic autonomic and sensory neuropathy, amyloid neuropathy, or a lesion of the cauda equina.

DICHLOROPHENOXYACETIC ACID (2,4-D)

2,4-D was introduced as a herbicide in the early 1950s. Instances of distal symmetrical polyneuropathy are described in workers with extensive dermal contact.[26,27] One week following exposure, pain and numbness appear in the distal legs. Subsequently mild distal weakness and sensory impairment is detectable. The Achilles reflexes are lost. Electromyography reveals partial denervation in weakened muscles, and motor nerve conduction velocity is normal. Complete recovery occurs within a few months. There are no reports of nerve biopsies and no experimental animal models of 2,4-D polyneuropathy.

DIPHTHERITIC NEUROPATHY (POLYRADICULOPATHY)

Definition and Etiology

Diphtheria is an acute infectious disease produced by *Corynebacterium diphtheriae,* and is usually a local inflammatory infection confined to the upper respiratory tract or sometimes the skin. The organism produces a protein exotoxin responsible for the cardiomyopathy and polyradiculopathy occurring in approximately 20 percent of cases. Diphtheritic neuropathy is now rare in North America and Europe, but remains a significant problem in countries without compulsory vaccination.

Pathology and Pathogenesis

PATHOLOGY. Meticulous human postmortem and abundant experimental animal studies indicate that diphtheritic neuropathy results from widespread, noninflammatory demyelination of nerve roots and adjacent portions of somatic nerves.[28] The distribution of demyelinative lesions in individuals who die during an acute neuritic illness is consistently in the dorsal root ganglia and adjacent ventral and dorsal roots. Among cranial nerves, only the nodose ganglion of the vagus is consistently affected. Peripheral portions of spinal nerves appear to be largely spared in the acute illness. The distribution of lesions corresponds to zones of high permeability of the blood-nerve barrier. Dorsal root ganglia are vulnerable in several neurotoxic conditions (Adriamycin, methyl mercury), presumably because their capillaries are fenestrated. Experimental studies with isotope-labeled diphtheria toxin strongly support this localization, and may explain why the central nervous system and much of the PNS is spared.[29] Both human and experimental pathologic studies suggest that the demyelinative lesion is a direct effect of toxin on myelin or Schwann cell, and is not immunologically mediated.[30,33] Local injection of diphtheria toxin produces focal demyelination in many fibers, following a latent period, without accumulation of lymphocytes or plasma cells. Demyelination begins in the paranodal zones.[31] Once focal demyelination is complete, remyelination promptly begins. Axonal change is usually slight unless large doses of toxin are administered.

PATHOGENESIS. An *in vitro* biochemical study suggests that diphtheria toxin does not directly degrade myelin, but inhibits myelin protein synthesis by the Schwann cell.[32] Since diphtheritic lesions undergo prompt remyelination, some Schwann cells remain viable. Once the toxin gains access to myelinated fibers, it is rapidly bound and its effect is not neutralized by antitoxin.

The close relationship of the loci of lesions to areas of permeable intraneural blood vessels has provided a key to understanding the pathogenesis of the diffuse polyneuropathy that appears five to eight weeks following the initial throat infection with *C. diphtheriae*. However, several of the most striking features of the clinical illness remain unexplained.[33] One is the prolonged latency following the initial faucial inflammation; exotoxin is released at this time but does not produce diffuse polyneuropathy. Another is the local pharyngeal and accomodation paralysis that appears early after faucial diphtheria. It seems likely that this reflects a local effect of exotoxin on peripheral nerve, but the mechanism is obscure and there are no adequate pathologic studies. Local paralysis may occur with cutaneous diphtherial infection.

Clinical Features

There are two distinct PNS syndromes associated with faucial diphtheria, a local pharyngeal-palatal neuropathy occurring soon after throat infection, and a diffuse sensorimotor neuropathy that develops after five to eight weeks. Presumably both conditions are caused by the exotoxin, one resulting from a local reaction on peripheral nerve, the other a blood-borne diffuse effect on somatic and autonomic ganglia and spinal roots. The overall incidence of local neuropathy is approximately 15 percent, generalized neuropathy about 10 percent. Individuals with local pharyngeal neuropathy are allegedly at greater risk of subsequently developing the generalized condition, and the frequency is proportionate to the intensity of the faucial infection. Prompt administration of antitoxin in faucial diphtheria sharply reduces the incidence of neuropathy.

LOCAL NEUROPATHY. Palatal paralysis, with nasal speech accompanied by impaired pharyngeal and laryngeal sensation, develops between 20 and 30 days of onset of the throat infection. Poor pharyngeal sensation and a weak cough may further compromise the respiratory status of individuals with inflammatory upper-respiratory lesions. Within another week, paralysis of ocular accommodation often appears, resulting in blurred vision. Pupillary reflexes to light are spared. Rarely, diaphragmatic, laryngeal, pharyngeal, facial, and oculomotor muscles then become weak; death from failure of respiration has occurred at this stage. Focal neuropathy in the limbs may appear with cutaneous diphtheria. A consistent feature of the early local neuropathy is the prevalence of weakness over sensory signs; this is predominantly a cranial motor neuropathy. Usually the condition gradually worsens for two or three weeks then rapidly improves. The prognosis for complete recovery is excellent.[33]

GENERALIZED NEUROPATHY. The generalized neuropathy develops within 8 to 12 weeks following the onset of the infective illness, although it may occur as early as three weeks. It is a mixed sensorimotor neuropathy of rapid onset with a predominantly distal distribution of weakness, paresthesias, and sensory loss. Tendon reflexes are depressed or lost. Occasionally, position sense is markedly impaired with relative preservation of muscle strength, giving rise to a sensory ataxia ('diphtheritic pseudotabes'). Recovery is usually complete, and begins within days or weeks of the onset of paralysis.[33]

Myocardial involvement may occur, resulting in cardiac failure or dysrhythmias, and may be fatal. It usually develops at about the third week of illness.

Laboratory Investigations

BACTERIOLOGIC. Culture of *C. diphtheriae* from the fauces or from a cutaneous ulcer will establish the diagnosis.

CEREBROSPINAL FLUID. The protein content is often moderately elevated and a lymphocyte pleocytosis may be present.

CLINICAL ELECTROPHYSIOLOGY. There are no reports of clinical electrophysiology of human diphtheria using contemporary techniques. Diphtheria toxin is widely used as an experimental model of PNS demyelination, and there is considerable knowledge about its electrophysiologic effects in experimental animals.[33]

ETHYLENE OXIDE

Ethylene oxide is a gas widely used in industry, especially in sterilizing heat-sensitive biomedical materials. A recent report describes distal symmetrical polyneuropathy in two individuals exposed to ethylene oxide from a leaking sterilizer.[34] Symptoms of distal-extremity numbness and weakness are accompanied by evidence of diminished sensation in the feet and hands. Tendon reflexes are diminished throughout and ankle jerks are absent. Motor nerve conduction velocity is mildly diminished. Encephalopathic symptoms may accompany the peripheral neuropathy. There are no reports of nerve biopsies or postmortem findings in humans with ethylene oxide intoxication. Experimental animals develop hindlimb weakness and atrophy after prolonged exposure, but nervous system tissue from these animals has not been examined.[35] In sum, it appears likely that ethylene oxide can produce nervous system disease of the distal axonopathy type.

HEXACARBONS (*n*-HEXANE, METHYL *n*-BUTYL KETONE)

General

n-Hexane and methyl *n*-butyl ketone are considered together in this section because each is metabolized to 2,5-hexanedione (2,5-HD),[36] the agent responsible for most, if not all, of the neurologic effects that accompany repetitive exposure to these compounds.[37,38]

 n-Hexane is widely used as an inexpensive solvent and is a component of lacquers, glues, and glue thinners. Worldwide human neurologic disease has been associated both with occupational exposures[39] and following deliberate inhalation of vapors containing *n*-hexane (glue sniffers).[40,41] Methyl *n*-butyl ketone (MnBK) has a greater neurotoxic potential than *n*-hexane, and was enjoying increasing use as solvent until implicated in the 1973 outbreak of peripheral neuropathy in Ohio.[42] Methyl ethyl ketone (MEK) is also present in some neurotoxic solvent mixtures and thinners containing either *n*-hexane or MnBK. Although some reports of human neuropathy have identified MEK as the causative agent, this solvent does not cause neuropathy in animals. However, MEK is able to potentiate hexacarbon neuropathy in animals, and may have accelerated development of neurotoxicity in individuals exposed to *n*-hexane and MnBK.[37]

Pathology and Pathogenesis

PATHOLOGY. The neurotoxic hexacarbons produce distal axonopathy in man and experimental animals. Human nerve biopsies and postmortem nervous system tissue display massively swollen axons filled with 10 nm neurofilaments both in distal nerve fibers and in the rostral gracile fasciculi.[4] A distal axonopathy-type distribution of giant axonal swellings is apparent in experimental animals exposed to these compounds, and in cord-ganglion-muscle combination tissue cultures exposed to 2,5-HD.[38] Axonal swellings in the PNS appear to develop on the proximal side of nodes of Ranvier in distal, nonterminal regions of affected fibers. Organelles accumulate in these regions and may contribute to the breakdown of nerve fibers distal to the swollen region.[43] Axonal swellings develop more proximally with time.[4,38,44] They are associated with myelin retraction and focal demyelination to a degree that is unusual in an axonopathy. This demyelination may correlate with the marked distal slowing of nerve conduction characteristic of human hexacarbon neuropathy.[40]

PATHOGENESIS. There is strong evidence to suggest that the neurotoxic property of *n*-hexane and M*n*BK is largely attributable to the common gamma-diketone metabolite 2,5-HD. Other gamma-diketones such as 2,5-heptanedione and 3,6 octanedione cause neuropathy, whereas related compounds (2,4-hexanedione, 2,3-hexanedione and 2,6-heptanedione) which lack the 1,4 spacing of the carbonyl groups, fail to produce experimental neuropathy.[36] Presumably, circulating 2,5-HD disrupts neuronal axonal function and results in focal, massive accumulations of neurofilaments in distal regions of certain axons (see Chapter 2). Recent experimental animal studies suggest that 2,5-HD can directly affect axonal metabolism.[45] The mechanism of toxic action is not known.

Clinical Features

GENERAL. Sensory and motor dysfunction usually develops insidiously with occupational exposure.[4,39] Individuals sometimes consult an orthopedist on the erroneous assumption that instability of the knees reflects a joint disorder. Individuals deliberately inhaling high concentrations of solvent vapors containing *n*-hexane and MEK have experienced a subacute onset of motor neuropathy.[41] Weight loss, malaise and abdominal pain frequently accompany the development of hexacarbon neuropathy.

SIGNS AND SYMPTOMS. The most common initial complaint, both in industrial cases and among glue sniffers, is numbness of the toes and fingers. This type of distal sensory neuropathy may be the only clinical illness in the least severe industrial cases.[39] The pattern of sensory abnormality is characteristically symmetrical and involves only the hands and feet, rarely extending as high as the knee. A moderate loss of touch, pin, vibration, and thermal sensation is usually prominent and may be accompanied by loss of the Achilles reflex. In mild cases, other tendon reflexes are spared and there is preservation of position sense and no sensory ataxia, cranial nerve abnormalities, autonomic dysfunction, or periosteal pain.[39] In the more severely involved industrial cases, weakness and weight loss occur, occasionally accompanied by anorexia, abdominal pain, and cramps in the lower extremities. Reflex loss is usually less than that observed in other polyneuropathies, and even in the moderate-to-severe cases, may be confined to the Achilles reflex and finger-jerks.[38] Weakness most commonly involves intrinsic muscles of the hands and long extensors or flexors of the digits. A common complaint in these individuals is difficulty with pinching movements, grasping objects, and stepping over curbs.[42] Pure motor neuropathy is unusual in industrial cases. Vibration and position sense are only mildly impaired and sensory loss for pinprick and touch is usually confined to the hands and feet. As the neuropathy becomes more severe, weakness and atrophy dominate the clinical picture and extend to involve proximal extremity muscles. Some glue-sniffing cases display a subacute, distal-to-proximal progression of weakness early in the course of the disease. Glue sniffers with prolonged high exposure may display signs of "bulbar" or phrenic-nerve paralysis.[41] Blurred vision is an occasional complaint, but objective evidence of visual loss has not been documented. No predisposing conditions have been proven to exist for hexacarbon neurotoxicity. Slowed motor nerve conduction is described in "normal" workers in a factory with documented cases of solvent neuropathy.[42] This strengthens the notion that subclinical and readily reversible nerve damage may be an unrecognized industrial problem.

Autonomic disturbances have been reported among the glue sniffers, but not in the industrial cases. Prominent among these disturbances is hyperhidrosis of the hands and feet, occasionally followed by anhidrosis.[41] Blue discoloration of the hands and feet, reduced extremity temperature, and Mees' lines are sometimes present in these patients. Impotence has occasionally occurred among glue sniffers with a moderate or severe neuropathy, but its relationship to nervous system dysfunction has not been established.

Laboratory Studies

CLINICAL LABORATORY. Routine clinical laboratory tests are normal.

CEREBROSPINAL FLUID. In the majority of cases of hexacarbon neuropathy, the cerebrospinal fluid contains a normal amount of protein, and cells are absent. The rare case with elevated cerebrospinal fluid protein may reflect nerve fiber degeneration which has ascended to the spinal roots.

ELECTRODIAGNOSTIC STUDIES. The electromyographic abnormalities are usually symmetrical and greater in distal than in proximal muscles. In patients with minimal involvement, sparse fibrillation and abnormal motor unit potentials are often the only findings. Nerve conduction times and clinical examination are usually normal at this stage.[42]

More severe cases generally display more frequent fibrillation potentials and positive sharp waves, and a reduced motor unit recruitment pattern on volition. With recovery or stabilization of the condition, the electromyographic changes disappear.

In cases with minimal involvement, motor and sensory nerve conduction is usually normal or at the low-normal range of velocity. As the clinical illness intensifies, a progressive slowing of conduction occurs,[40] and in the most extreme cases, distal peroneal nerve conduction cannot be elicited. Severe slowing of distal motor nerve conduction frequently appears disproportionate to the moderate weakness. Such profound slowing is characteristic of demyelinating neuropathies (see Chapter 2), and may reflect paranodal demyelination associated with the giant axonal swellings.[40] A recent visual evoked potential study describes abnormal amplitude and latency, interpreted as consistent with axonal degeneration in the CNS visual pathways.[46] This finding may correlate with distal axonal degeneration observed in the optic tracts of animals experimentally intoxicated with 2,5-HD.[47,48]

NERVE BIOPSY. Nerve biopsies from mild cases may be normal, even when examined by electron microscopy. Occasionally, muscle biopsy from such cases may reveal abnormalities of neuromuscular junctions or of intramuscular nerve twigs.[39] The most informative nerve biopsy results are usually obtained from moderately or severely involved individuals; in these cases, teased myelinated nerve fiber preparations have clearly illustrated paranodal giant axonal swellings accompanied by myelin retraction.[40]

Course and Prognosis

Insidious onset and slow progression are the hallmarks of the industrial cases. In most instances, this is a reflection of low-level, intermittent exposure.[39,42] In some of the glue sniffers, especially those with excessive abuse, a subacute course develops, leading in the severe cases to quadriplegia within two months of the first symptom. The Guillain-Barré syndrome has been a serious diagnostic contender in these patients.[41]

A universal feature of hexacarbon neurotoxicity is the continuous progression of disability after removal from toxic exposure. Progression ("coasting") usually lasts for one to four months and often occurs in the hospital. The degree of recovery in most cases correlates directly with the intensity of the neurologic deficit. Individuals with a mild or moderate sensorimotor neuropathy usually recover completely within 10 months of cessation of exposure.[4] Severely affected industrial cases also improve, but sometimes retain mild-to-moderate residual neuropathy on follow-up examination as long as three years after exposure. Such individuals have, on occasion, developed hyperactive knee jerks and lower-extremity spasticity.[4,40,41] This reflex change probably reflects degeneration in the corticospinal tracts that accompanied the peripheral neuropathy.

Glue sniffers who sustain an extreme degree of distal atrophy may never recover full strength, and persistent hyperpathia and autonomic dysfunction are described.

Differential Diagnosis

The clinical features of hexacarbon neuropathy do not help to distinguish this condition from many other toxic or metabolic distal axonopathies. Profound slowing of motor nerve conduction disproportinate to moderate weakness, and nerve biopsy demonstration of paranodal giant axonal swellings strongly suggest hexacarbon neuropathy. The most useful diagnostic test is a detailed occupational and social history, specifically inquiring about solvent exposure and inhalant abuse.

Case History and Comment

A 22-year-old female worked long hours in a small, poorly ventilated factory. She handled rags saturated with a solution containing *n*-hexane and inhaled large amounts of *n*-hexane vapor for two years before developing anorexia, weight loss, and a cramping sensation in the hands. Two weeks later, she noticed cramping in the calves and an unsteady gait that was improved by the use of high-heeled boots. Two months later, her legs felt much weaker and she noted numbness of the toes. These symptoms steadily increased in intensity over the next two months until she was unable to walk to work. She was admitted to hospital. Neurologic examination revealed no abnormalities of cranial nerves or mental status. There was diffuse, symmetrical, distal, flaccid weakness of all extremities. The intrinsic muscles of the hands and dorsiflexors of the feet were 2/5 MRC scale. Proximal limb muscles were 3/5 MRC scale, and abdominal muscles were also severely weak. The vital capacity was normal. No tendon reflexes could be elicited. There was a moderate-to-severe loss of pin sensation in a stocking-glove distribution, with only a slight diminution in position and vibration sense. After four months in this state she gradually began to improve, was discharged from the hospital, and steadily regained strength over the next 18 months. Since that time, she noticed no further improvement of strength but began to walk again, although in an abnormal fashion. Neurologic examination two years after discharge from the hospital revealed a slow, stiff-legged, waddling gait. She could stand on a narrow base and Romberg's sign was not present. Rapid alternating movements of the upper extremities were performed well, as were finger-to-nose movements. Distal and proximal upper-extremity muscles were 4/5 MRC scale; distal lower-extremity muscles were 4/5 MRC scale. Many large, proximal lower limb muscle groups (hamstrings, glutei, quadriceps) were 4/5 MRC scale. She was unable to rise from a chair without using her hands for support, and unable to sit up from a supine position without rolling to one side and using her arms for assistance. There was a moderate diminition of pinprick and touch sensation below the ankle and wrist, but position and vibration sensation were normal. The tendon reflexes were brisk in the arms and very brisk in the legs, with bilateral Babinski signs present. There was increased resistance to rapid passive movements of the lower limbs, and she displayed a spastic catch.

Comment

This patient demonstrates two cardinal features associated with occupational axonal neuropathies: poor working conditions and gradual onset of symptoms. She developed a neuropathy of unusual severity with quadriparesis and near-total paralysis of the distal extremities because of the prolonged, high-level exposure to the hexacarbon toxicant. Motor impairment was far more severe than the sensory deficit, perhaps reflecting high levels of ambient *n*-hexane in the final months of exposure. Signs of corticospinal tract degeneration did not appear until the peripheral nerves regenerated.

LEAD

General

Symptomatic lead polyneuropathy is now rare in North America and Europe. There is disagreement as to whether subclinical nerve damage, defined by abnormal nerve conduction in asymptomatic individuals, occurs in lead-exposed workers.[49,50] Occupational exposure especially occurs in smelting industries, battery manufacture, demolition work, and in automobile radiator repair. Common environmental sources are paint ingestion and consumption of moonshine whiskey.[51] Lead is unusual among human neurotoxins as its neuropathy so far resists the classification outlined in

Chapter 2. Lead clearly can produce a demyelinating neuropathy in experimental animals, yet the pathologic changes of the human neuropathy are poorly characterized. Furthermore, neither the experimental nor the available human neuropathologic material explain some of the bizarre clinical features of lead neuropathy.

Pathology and Pathogenesis

Wallerian-type axonal degeneration is the only well-described pathologic alteration in reports of *human* nerves from individuals with lead neuropathy.[51] Postmortem reports of cases in the older literature include descriptions of spinal-root degeneration, chromatolysis of anterior horn cells, and fiber-tract degeneration in the spinal cord. Inadequate descriptions and contradictory findings in these early reports, combined with the absence of contemporary postmortem data, have added to the confusion surrounding the neuropathology of lead neuropathy. Clinical features of some cases suggest primary dysfunction of anterior horn cells,[52] but neither human nor experimental animal studies firmly support this notion. There exists one contemporary report of a sural nerve biopsy from an individual with lead neuropathy, describing loss of large myelinated fibers.[50] The morphologic changes in the early stages of human neuropathy have not been reported; most descriptions apparently represent advanced stages of this condition.[51] Segmental demyelination is not a prominent feature in any reported case, but its existence has not been ruled out by these limited studies. In contrast, segmental demyelination is clearly the predominant change in most models of *experimental* chronic lead neuropathy.[53] Several events occur prior to demyelination: there is an early rapid accumulation of lead in nerve, the blood-nerve barrier is abnormally permeable,[55] endoneurial pressure is increased,[54] nerves become grossly swollen, and intranuclear inclusions appear within Schwann cells. The role of these events in the pathogenesis of segmental demyelination is unclear. There are two leading hypotheses. One is that lead has an early direct toxic effect on Schwann cells[56] and accumulation of fluid has no primary role in demyelination; the second states that primary injury to the blood-nerve barrier leads to an accumulation of lead-containing edema fluid and elevated endoneurial pressure, producing an abnormal, lead-rich endoneurial environment, eventuating in Schwann cell injury.

The cellular distribution of lead in the PNS is not known. In certain other organs it is selectively accumulated in nuclei and mitochondria; and lead-containing intranuclear inclusion bodies appear, similar to the inclusions recently described in Schwann cells. This lends support to the hypothesis that lead directly affects Schwann cells.[56]

Clinical Features

GENERAL. Symptomatic lead neuropathy usually develops after prolonged exposure and is usually preceded by weight loss, anorexia, fatigue, constipation, and episodic abdominal pains.

SYMPTOMATIC NEUROPATHY. Lead intoxication results in predominantly motor neuropathy of unusual variability. Sensory complaints and findings are minimal. Five distinct patterns of weakness are described in the older literature. In order of frequency they are:

(1) extensors of the fingers and wrists ("wrist-drop type")
(2) proximal shoulder girdle muscles
(3) intrinsic hand muscles
(4) peroneal muscles
(5) paralysis of the larynx.

Cases displaying such focal patterns of weakness are now rare.[52] The few recent studies of probable adult lead neuropathy describe progressive generalized weakness, mild distal atrophy, reflex loss, and occasional fasciculations.[49] Lower-limb weakness is prominent in childhood cases. Electromyography of weakened muscles usually reveals abundant fibrillation potentials.[52] Motor nerve conduction is normal. Sensory amplitudes in weakened extremities may be strikingly reduced. One contemporary report of sural nerve biopsy describes loss of myelinated fibers.[49]

ASYMPTOMATIC NEUROPATHY. Electrophysiologic studies of neurologically normal, asymptomatic individuals with chronic occupational exposure to lead claim significant slowing of nerve conduction. Abnormal electromyographic findings, indicative of denervation, are also described. The degree of electrophysiologic abnormality sometimes correlates with elevated blood lead levels.[50] The interpretation of these studies has been seriously challenged in a recent careful study of Danish lead workers,[49] and the prevalence of subclinical lead neuropathy remains controversial.

Laboratory Studies

CLINICAL LABORATORY. Mild anemia, basophilic stippling of erythrocytes, and elevated urine coproporphyrin are characteristic of plumbism. Determination of urine lead is helpful, and levels in excess of 0.2 mg per liter are usually regarded as significant.

Diagnosis can be confirmed after promoting lead excretion by dosing with a chelating agent and measuring the subsequent rise in urine lead levels. Excretion of over 500 μg in 24 hours indicates excessive lead stores in soft tissue. Blood levels are less helpful and, when low, may be misleading, because lead is rapidly cleared from the circulation. Elevated blood levels per se do not indicate intoxication, and controversy surrounds the "safe" level allowed in individuals with occupational exposure.[50] Mean blood levels in North American children are reportedly 15 μg/dl-28 μg/dl.[51]

CEREBROSPINAL FLUID. The CSF is acellular and the protein level normal.

ELECTRODIAGNOSTIC STUDIES. Described in Clinical Features, *vide supra*.

Treatment and Prognosis

The most important single feature of treatment is eliminating further exposure to lead. Once abnormal intake of lead is ended, much of the lead in soft tissue is gradually shifted into bone. As long as significant quantities of lead remain in bone, any illness associated with demineralization may mobilize it. This lead again circulates, becomes stored in soft tissues, and may exacerbate plumbism. The aim of chelation therapy is to bind the lead in soft tissue so that it can then be excreted. Either penicillamine (favored in mild cases) or calcium-disodium EDTA may be used as chelating agents.

Chelating agents are administered in short courses, each associated with a rise in urine lead levels. Recovery may begin within two weeks following the initiation of therapy.[52] Strength gradually improves over a prolonged period, frequently over a year. Complete recovery is usual except in extremely advanced cases.

Differential Diagnosis

Symptomatic lead neuropathy usually is readily identified in exposed workers or consumers of moonshine whiskey who become diffusely weak or develop wrist-drop.

Clinical distinction of lead neuropathy from motor neuron disease is sometimes difficult, and may require urine lead levels with a chelation challenge. In general, lead intoxication should be suspected both in individuals with a generalized predominantly motor neuropathy, and in idiopathic plexus or isolated nerve lesions (especially the radial and peroneal).

METHYL BROMIDE

Methyl bromide has found use as a fumigant, fire extinguisher, refrigerant, and insectide. Chronic exposure to high levels of methyl bromide may result in a syndrome characterized by signs of pyramidal tract, cerebellar, and peripheral nerve dysfunction. One report describes distal symmetrical polyneuropathy in eight individuals following chronic low-level exposure.[57] The overall pattern of the clinical illness strongly suggests that methyl bromide polyneuropathy represents a distal axonopathy. This notion is unproven, as there are neither morphologic reports of human PNS tissue nor an adequate experimental animal study.

Symptoms of numbness and weakness distally in the legs appear after several months exposure. These symptoms gradually increase and are then accompanied by an unsteady gait and clumsy hands. Signs include variable flaccid weakness of lower-leg muscles, and moderately diminished sensation to pin and touch in a stocking-glove distribution. Tenderness of the calf muscles is usually prominent and may erroneously suggest the diagnosis of myositis. The Achilles reflex is usually diminished or absent. The CSF is normal. Electrophysiologic studies reveal denervation in distal muscles and delayed sensory conduction. Gradual improvement and complete recovery occurs within a year following withdrawal from exposure.[57]

ORGANOPHOSPHORUS ESTERS

General

Organophosphorus (OP) esters have three major industrial applications: insecticides, petroleum additives, and modifiers of plastics. Most OP esters inhibit acetylcholinesterase, a property exploited in their use as pecticides, helminthicides, and war gases.[58]

Some OP esters, additionally, can produce distal axonopathy characterized by widespread CNS and PNS degeneration. This effect does *not* involve inhibition of acetylcholinesterase, often has a curiously delayed onset following single exposure, and has been responsible for devastating epidemics of neurotoxic injury.[59] The most infamous is triorthocresyl phosphate (TOCP). Other organophosphates known to be responsible for human distal axonopathy are leptophos, mipafox, and trichlorphon, while diisopropyl phosphorofluridate haloxon, butafox, and haloxon produce similar changes in experimental animals. Distal axonopathy has been generally held to be a relatively uncommon neurotoxic result of exposure to organophosphorus compounds, which number more than 50,000, especially when compared with the well known anticholinesterase effects. Recent experimental studies indicate that distal axonopathy may be fairly pervasive among the organophosphate esters,[60] and many compounds previously regarded as innocuous may be capable of producing axonopathy after prolonged exposure under suitable conditions. The biochemistry and pharmacology of the OP esters is complex, beyond the scope of this volume, and recently reviewed elsewhere.[58] Of all the organophosphorus compounds, TOCP has produced the most instances of neuropathy in man, is extensively studied in animals, and will be discussed in this section as a paradigm for the other compounds of this class.

TOCP

TOCP is an oily substance, lipid soluble, readily absorbed through skin and mucous membranes, and usually produces only mild cholinergic symptoms in humans. It is valued as a softener in the plastics industry and as a high-temperature lubricant. Many instances of neuropathy have resulted from the adulteration or misuse of TOCP in food, drink or cooking oil. Prominent outbreaks occurred in the United States from drinking adulterated Jamaica ginger extract (Jake Leg Paralysis),[61] and in Morroco due to cooking with contaminated cooking oil.[62]

Pathology and Pathogenesis

PATHOLOGY. TOCP is conclusively demonstrated to produce a distal axonopathy in man and experimental animals. There are no contemporary morphologic studies of the human illness. Postmortem studies from the 1930 Jake Leg Paralysis revealed Wallerian degeneration in the PNS. CNS alteration in these cases included changes in the cervical levels of the gracile fasciculi and the lumbar levels of the corticospinal tracts, indicative of distal axonopathy.[61] Experimental animal studies in a variety of species have repeatedly confirmed this distribution of CNS findings, and clearly demonstrate a pattern of distal axonal degeneration in the PNS. Large diameter, heavily myelinated nerve fibers appear most vulnerable, and lower extremity nerves are most affected.[63,64] Ultrastructural studies of the axonal alterations demonstrate proliferation of smooth endoplasmic reticulum, but provide little insight into the pathogenesis of this condition.[64]

PATHOGENESIS. The biochemical mechanism underlying the most common form of OP neurotoxicity—inhibition of acetylcholinesterase—involves phosphorylation of the esterase. Since OP compounds are good phosphorylating agents, it is proposed that phosphorylation of additional nervous system esterases (other than acetylcholine esterase) may account for the delayed distal axonopathy produced by TOCP.[65] There are many esterases in the nervous system, and the physiologic function of most is unknown. Considerable biochemical evidence indicates that there is a specific nervous system esterase affected by TOCP. This esterase, "neurotoxic esterase" (an unfortunate name since the esterase is the target of the neurotoxin and is not itself neurotoxic as the name implies), is found throughout the PNS and CNS, and is irreversibly inhibited by TOCP and the OP compounds that produce distal axonopathy.[66] Furthermore, it is suggested that its selective inhibition might provide an *in vitro* assay for screening the more than 50,000 OP compounds for their ability to produce distal axonopathy. This would be a tremendous advantage over current laborious and inaccurate bioassay techniques. The role of "neurotoxic esterase" in TOCP distal axonopathy remains clouded, since its metabolic function is unknown.[58]

There is no valid hypothesis to explain the one-to-three week interval between a single intoxication with TOCP and onset of symptoms and signs of neuropathy.

Clinical Features

GENERAL. The considerable variability in nervous system damage following exposure to TOCP probably reflects variabilities in dose and absorption. Most instances have involved oral ingestion; however, this substance is also readily absorbed through the skin and alveoli.[58] Following a single large exposure, a transient, variable cholinergic response occurs, usually diarrhea, perspiration and fasciculations, which generally lasts a day and is rarely incapacitating (in contrast to the OP esters with potent anticholinesterase properties, whose muscarinic and nicotinic properties may be instantly fatal). An asymptomatic interval of 7–21 days then ensues before clinical evidence of neuropathy appears. Should repeated low-level exposure occur, typical in industry, then cholinergic symptoms may not be appreciated.

SYMPTOMS AND SIGNS. Initial symptoms of cramping pain in the calves are followed by tingling and burning sensations in the feet and occasionally in the hands. Weakness soon appears in the legs and rapidly involves the hands as well. In severe cases, weakness may spread proximally to involve muscles acting about the knee or hips. The course is subacute, in contrast to the chronicity of most distal axonopathies, and maximum involvement usually occurs within two weeks of the first symptoms.

Weakness and flaccidity are prominent clinical signs, and despite the early paresthesias, TOCP neuropathy is predominantly motor. Sensory loss is present in every case, if carefully examined, but is usually trivial compared with the striking weakness. Foot-drop is common, and gait ataxia, disproportionate to weakness or sensory loss, occasionally occurs. The Achilles reflex is initially absent; patellar reflexes may be depressed or increased. Atrophy of the legs and intrinsic hand muscles is the rule. Cranial nerve involvement and autonomic dysfunction are not features of TOCP neuropathy.

Signs of CNS dysfunction are present in most cases. These often are obscured by PNS degeneration in the early stages; however, as the weeks pass, progressive spasticity may develop in the lower extremities, yielding a characteristic mixture of upper and lower motor-neuron involvement. A 30-year follow-up study of individuals with Jamaica Ginger poisoning revealed spastic paraparesis and distal leg atrophy in some.[61] The degree of corticospinal tract dysfunction is another feature distinguishing OP neurotoxicity from other distal axonopathies, and may be misleading.

The prognosis in mildly affected individuals, presumably with less exposure, is good. They generally make a near-complete recovery. Others with a more severe initial deficit are left with varying degrees of morbidity, including sequelae of both PNS (atrophy, claw hands, foot-drop) and CNS (spasticity, ataxia) damage. There is no specific treatment.

Laboratory Studies

CLINICAL LABORATORY. Routine laboratory studies are usually normal. Erythrocyte cholinesterase levels are only mildly depressed by TOCP and several other OP esters that produce distal axonopathy.

CEREBROSPINAL FLUID. The CSF is usually acellular and the protein level normal or mildly elevated.

ELECTRODIAGNOSTIC STUDIES. Electromyography reveals changes of denervation in every case. These are confined to distal muscles in mild instances and generally involve proximal leg muscles with severe involvement. Motor nerve conduction is usually mildly slowed in the legs and may be normal in the arms, even in distal segments of mixed nerves in atrophic limbs. Sensory nerve potentials are usually diminished in the upper extremities and may be unelicitible in the legs. This curious phenomenon is an important factor in determining an appropriate test for screening at-risk individuals for subclinical neuropathy. It is suggested that the recording of sensory-nerve-action-potential amplitude is likely to be the most sensitive measurements.[67]

Differential Diagnosis

The differential diagnosis of TOCP neuropathy is simple if there is clear evidence of its ingestion two weeks before the illness. Should such evidence be lacking, the condition becomes almost impossible to establish with certainty. In the authors' experience, several cases of organophosphorus neurotoxicity have been erroneously diagnosed as multiple sclerosis. The subacute onset of a myeloneuropathy syndrome in an otherwise healthy individual should raise the suspicion of OP intoxication.

THALLIUM

General

Thallous salts have been widely employed in rodenticides and insecticides. This use is now discouraged in North America. Rare reports of intoxication usually stem from homicidal or accidental (especially in children) ingestion.

Pathology and Pathogenesis

PATHOLOGY. Thallium salts produce a distal axonopathy in humans. Postmortem examination has clearly demonstrated axonal degeneration in the distal regions of long nerves with proximal fiber preservation.[69] Large diameter fibers of sensory nerves appear especially vulnerable. Axonal swelling is described as an early change in one case.[69] Sural nerve biopsy has yielded widely divergent findings; one recent report describes axonal vacuoles.[70] Experimental animal studies depict ultrastructural evidence of axonal damage, including swollen mitochondria, in the absence of clinical neuropathy.[71] Nervous system tissue cultures treated with thallium sulfate demonstrate similar mitochondrial swellings.[72]

PATHOGENESIS. The biochemical pathogenesis of thallium axonopathy is not known. It is suggested that thallium ions may combine with free sulfhydryl groups of proteins, or that thallium binds to mitochondrial membrane.[68] It is also proposed that some effects stem from thallium substitution for potassium,[70,73] particularly by replacing potassium in potassium-activated ATPase.

Clinical Features

GENERAL. There appear to be three distinct temporal varieties of peripheral neuropathy associated with thallium intoxication. These varieties, in order of frequency, are: an acute type beginning within one to two days of a massive (sometimes lethal) single dose,[69,70,73] a subacute type with onset within weeks of a less massive single dose,[69] and a rare chronic type occurring after prolonged continued exposure to moderate levels of thallium.[74] All three presumably are distal axonopathies. The clinical variation may reflect differences in the spatio-temporal evolution of axonal degeneration in response to different levels of intoxication.

ACUTE TYPE. Gastrointestinal symptoms usually follow within hours of poisoning; occasionally they are delayed for a day.[69,70,73] Vomiting, diarrhea and abdominal pain are common. Within two to five days, severe burning paresthesias begin in the legs and feet, often accompanied by intense joint pain. Sensory symptoms appear in the hands and sometimes the trunk. Weakness is not a prominent complaint in many instances, but is usually detectable on examination. All sensory modalities are affected. Tendon reflexes are usually present in the early stages, and may assist in differentiating thallium neuropathy from the Guillain-Barré syndrome in the rare instances with progressive severe sensorimotor neuropathy affecting both cranial and peripheral nerves. Lethargy, coma, and respiratory failure often develop, and death may occur within a week or two following ingestion. Recovery from neuropathy is gradual and may be incomplete. Sequelae of CNS anoxia (impaired mentation, seizures) may complicate rehabilitation. The diagnosis of acute thallium neuropathy is extraordinarily difficult unless there is clear evidence of homicidal, suicidal, or accidental ingestion. Alopecia, the classic indication of thallium poisoning, appears 15 to 39 days after ingestion. This reliable sign therefore is not present in the early stages of acute neuropathy. Renal damage may occur.

SUBACUTE TYPE. This polyneuropathy usually develops one or more weeks after exposure, evolves more slowly, and frequently is accompanied by scalp alopecia.[69] Less constant clinical phenomena are hyperkeratosis, Mees' lines (white striae of the nails), ataxia, chorea, and various cranial nerve palsies.

Sensory symptoms and signs are predominant in this neuropathy. Painful, distressing paresthesias of the feet and hands are initial symptoms, and individuals are often unwilling to walk because of painful feet. Weakness is rarely a prominent symptom. Signs of sensory impairment include diminished pin, touch sensation, and proprioception over the distal extremities. Mild or moderate distal weakness always occurs. Tendon reflexes are usually either normal or slightly depressed. Tachycardia and hypertension, presumably reflecting autonomic dysfunction, frequently accompany this illness. The prognosis of the subacute neuropathy is excellent. Most individuals recover completely within six months of withdrawal from exposure. Hair regrowth usually begins within 10 weeks of withdrawal. The cerebrospinal fluid is usually normal. Motor and sensory nerve conduction may be slightly slowed.

CHRONIC TYPE. Most reports of the nervous system complications of chronic thallotoxicosis focus on extrapyramidal dysfunction; the sensorimotor neuropathy is not well characterized.[74]

Diagnosis and Treatment

Diagnosis is established by analysis of urine or organs for thallium. Microgram quantitation can be achieved. Alopecia is the distinctive clinical sign of this disorder, but is not inevitable. It appears likely that instances of thallium neuropathy, especially the acute variety, go undetected. The efficacy of treatment is controversial. Various regimens combining chelating agents and potassium chloride are currently favored.

TRICHLORETHYLENE

Trichlorethylene (TCE) is used in dry cleaning, rubber production, and as a degreasing agent. It was formerly widely employed as general anesthetic. It is unlikely that chemically pure TCE is neurotoxic, and it is probable that cranial neuropathy stems from a decomposition product, dichloracetylene, resulting from interaction of TCE with alkaline materials.

Acute industrial exposure or anesthetic exposure to TCE is associated with dysfunction of the trigeminal, and to a lesser extent, the facial and impure optic nerves.[75,76] The effect of impure TCE on the trigeminal nerve is so predictable, that, for a time, victims of tic douloureux were intentionally exposed to it. These cranial nerves are affected after a period of exposure to high concentrations. Trigeminal neuropathy usually includes loss of sensory modalities in the entire distribution of the nerve, accompanied by weakness of muscles of mastication. Recovery occurs over a period of months. The pathophysiology of cranial neuropathy is obscure: it is suggested that the human clinical and electrophysiologic data are compatible with demyelinating neuropathy. One postmortem report describes extensive axon and myelin degeneration in the trigeminal nerve, sensory root, and brainstem nuclei and tracts.[76]

REFERENCES

1. SPENCER, PS AND SCHAUMBURG, HH: *A review of acrylamide neurotoxicity: I. Properties, uses and human exposure.* Can J Neurol Sci 1:143, 1974.
2. SCHAUMBURG, HH, WIŚNIEWSKI, HM, AND SPENCER, PS: *Ultrastructural studies of the dying-back process; I. Peripheral nerve terminal and axon degeneration in systemic acrylamide intoxication.* J Neuropathol Exp Neurol 33:260, 1974.
3. FULLERTON, PM: *Electrophysiological and histological observations on peripheral nerves in acrylamide poisoning in man.* J Neurol Neurosurg Psychiatry 32:186, 1969.
4. SCHAUMBURG, HH AND SPENCER, PS: *Clinical and experimental studies of distal axonopathy—a frequent form of brain and nerve damage produced by environmental chemical hazards.* Ann NY Acad Sci 329:14, 1979.
5. SUMNER, AJ AND ASBURY, AK: *Physiological studies of the dying-back phenomenon. Muscle stretch afferents in acrylamide neuropathy.* Brain 98:91, 1975.
6. EDWARDS, PM: *The distribution and metabolism of acrylamide analogues in rats.* Biochem Pharmacol 24:1277, 1975.
7. GARLAND, TO AND PATTERSON, MWH: *Six cases of acrylamide poisoning.* Br Med J 4:134, 1967.

DISORDERS OF
PERIPHERAL
NERVES

152

8. LeQuesne, PM: *Acrylamide.* In Spencer, PS and Schaumburg, HH (eds): Experimental and Clinical Neurotoxicology, Williams & Wilkins, Baltimore, 1980, p 309.

9. LeQuesne, PM: *Neurophysiological investigation of subclinical and minimal toxic neuropathies.* Muscle and Nerve 1:392, 1978.

10. Feldman, RG, et al: *Peripheral neuropathy in arsenic smelter workers.* Neurology (Minneap) 29:939, 1979.

11. LeQuesne, PM and McLeod, JG: *Peripheral neuropathy following a single exposure to arsenic.* J Neurol Sci 32:437, 1977.

12. Erlicki, A and Rybalkin: *Ueber Arseniklähmung.* Arch Psychiatr Nervenkr 23:861, 1892.

13. Politis, M, Schaumburg, HH and Spencer, PS: *Neurotoxicity of Selected Chemicals.* In Spencer, PS and Schaumburg, HH (eds): Experimental and Clinical Neurotoxicology, Williams & Wilkins, Baltimore, 1980, p 613.

14. Heyman, A, et al: *Peripheral neuropathy caused by arsenical intoxication.* N Engl J Med 254:401, 1956.

15. Jenkins, RB: *Inorganic arsenic and the nervous system.* Brain 89:479, 1966.

16. Chhuttani, PN, Chawla, LS and Sharma, TD: *Arsenical neuropathy.* Neurology (Minneap) 17:269, 1967.

17. Seppalainen, AM and Haltia, M: *Carbon Disulfide.* In Spencer, PS and Schaumburg, HH (eds): Experimental and Clinical Neurotoxicology, Williams & Wilkins, Baltimore, 1980, p 356.

18. Seppalainen, AM and Tolonen, M: *Neurotoxicity of long term exposure to carbon disulfide in the viscose rayon industry. A neurophysiological study.* Work-Environment Health 11:145, 1974.

19. Vigliani, EB: *Carbon disulphide poisoning in viscose rayon factories.* Br Med J II:235, 1954.

20. Vasilescu, C: *Motor nerve conduction velocity and electromyogram in carbon disulphide poisoning.* Revue Roumaine de Neurologie et de Psychiatri 9:63, 1972.

21. Osuntokun, BO: *An ataxic neuropathy in Nigeria.* Brain 91:215, 1968.

22. Osuntokun, BO, Aladetoyinbo, A and Adeuja, AOG: *Free cyanide levels in tropical ataxic neuropathy.* Lancet 2:372, 1970.

23. Pestronk, A, Keogh, J and Griffin, JG: *Dimethylaminopropionitrile intoxication: A new industrial neuropathy.* Neurology (Minneap) 29:540, 1979.

24. Feldman, RG, et al: *Neurotoxic dysuria due to dimethylaminopropionitrile.* Neurology (Minneap) 29:560, 1979.

25. Pestronk, A, Keogh, J and Griffin, JG: *Dimethylaminopropionitrile.* In Spencer, PS and Schaumburg, HH (eds): Experimental and Clinical Neurotoxicology, Williams & Wilkins, Baltimore, 1980, p 422.

26. Goldstein, NP, Jones, PH and Brown, JR: *Peripheral neuropathy after exposure to an ester of dichlorophenoxyacetic acid.* JAMA 171:1306, 1959.

27. Berkley, MC and Magee, KR: *Neuropathy following exposure to a dimethylamine salt of 2,4D.* Arch Int Med 111:133, 1963.

28. Fisher, CM and Adams, RD: *Diphtheritic polyneuritis: a pathological study.* J Neuropathol Exp Neurol 15:243, 1956.

29. Waxman, BH: *Experimental study of diphtheritic polyneuritis in the rabbit and guinea pig. III. The blood-nerve barrier in the rabbit.* J Neuropathol Exp Neurol 20:35, 1961.

30. Webster, H, deF et al: *Phase and electron microscopic studies of experimental demyelination. II. Schwann cell changes in guinea pig sciatic nerves during experimental diphtheritic neuritis.* J Neuropathol Exp Neurol 20:5, 1961.

31. Allt, G and Cavanagh, JB: *Ultrastructural changes in the region of the node of Ranvier in the rat caused by diphtheria toxin.* Brain 92:459, 1969.

32. Pleasure, DB, Feldman, B and Prockop, DJ: *Diphtheria toxin inhibits the synthesis of myelin proteolipid and basic proteins by peripheral nerve in vitro.* J Neurochem 20:81, 1973.

33. McDonald, WI and Kocen, RS: *Diphtheritic Neuropathy.* In Dyck, PJ, Thomas, PK and Lambert, EH (eds): Peripheral Neuropathy, Vol II, WB Saunders, Philadelphia, 1975, 1281.

34. Gross, JA, Haas, ML, Swift, TR: *Ethylene oxide neurotoxicity: Report of four cases and review of the literature.* Neurology (Minneap) 29:978, 1979.

35. Hollingsworth, RL, Rowe, UK and Oyen, F: *Toxicity or ethylene oxide determined on experimental animals.* Archives of Industrial Health 13:217, 1956.

36. DiVincenzo, GD, Hamilton, ML, Kaplan, C and Dedinas, J: *Characterization of the metabolities of methyl n-butyl ketone.* In Spencer, PS and Schaumburg, HH (eds): Experimental and Clinical Neurotoxicology, Williams & Wilkins, Baltimore, 1980, p 846.

TOXIC
NEUROPATHY:
OCCUPATIONAL,
BIOLOGICAL AND
ENVIRONMENTAL
AGENTS

153

37. SPENCER, PS, COURI, D AND SCHAUMBURG, HH: *n-Hexane and methyl n-butyl ketone.* In SPENCER, PS AND SCHAUMBURG, HH (EDS): Experimental and Clinical Neurotoxicology, Williams & Wilkins, Baltimore, 1980, p 456.

38. SPENCER, PS, ET AL: *The enlarging view of hexacarbon neurotoxicity.* CRC Crit Rev Toxicol 7:273, 1980.

39. HERSKOWITZ, A, ISHII, N AND SCHAUMBURG, HH: *n-Hexane neuropathy. A syndrome occurring as a result of industrial exposure.* N Engl J Med 285:82, 1971.

40. KOROBKIN, R, ET AL: *Glue sniffing neuropathy.* Arch Neurol 32:158, 1975.

41. ALTENKIRCH, HJ ET AL: *Toxic polyneuropathies after sniffing a glue thinner.* J Neurol 214:152, 1977.

42. ALLEN, N, ET AL: *Toxic polyneuropathy due to methyl n-butyl ketone. An industrial outbreak.* Arch Neurol 32:209, 1975.

43. SPENCER, PS AND SCHAUMBURG, HH: *Ultrastructural studies of the dying-back process. III. The evolution of experimental giant axonal degeneration.* J Neuropathol Exp Neurol 36:276, 1977.

44. SPENCER, PS AND SCHAUMBURG, HH: *Ultrastructural studies of the dying-back process. IV. Differential vulnerability of PNS and CNS fibers in experimental central-peripheral distal axonopathies.* J Neuropathol Exp Neurol 36:300, 1977.

45. POLITIS, M, PELLEGRINO, RG AND SPENCER, PS: *Ultrastructural studies of the dying-back process. V. Axonal neurofilaments accumulate at sites of 2,5-hexanedione application: evidence for nerve fibre dysfunction in experimental hexacarbon neuropathy.* J Neurocytol 9:505, 1980.

46. SEPPALAINEN, AM, RAITTA, C AND HUSKONEN, MS: *n-Hexane induced changes in visual evoked potentials and electroretinograms of industrial workers.* Electroenceph Clin Neurophysiol 47:492, 1979.

47. SCHAUMBURG, HH AND SPENCER, PS: *Environmental hydrocarbons produce degeneration in cat hypothalamus and optic tract.* Science 199:199, 1978.

48. CAVANAGH, JB AND BENNETTS, RJ: *On the pattern of change in the rat nervous system produced by 2,5-hexanediol: a topographical study by light microscopy.* Brain 104:297, 1981.

49. BUCHTHAL, F AND BEHSE, F: *Electrophysiological and nerve biopsy in men exposed to lead.* Br J Ind Med 36:135, 1979.

50. SEPPALAINEN, AM AND HERNBERG, S: *Subclinical lead neuropathy.* Am J Ind Med 1:413, 1980.

51. KRIGMAN, M, BOULDIN, T AND MUSHAK, P: *Lead.* In SPENCER, PS AND SCHAUMBURG, HH (EDS): Experimental and Clinical Neurotoxicology, Williams & Wilkins, Baltimore, 1980, p 490.

52. BOOTHBY, JA, DEJESUS, PV AND ROWLAND, LP: *Reversible forms of motor neuron disease.* Arch Neurol 31:18, 1974.

53. LAMPERT, PW AND SCHOCHET, SS: *Demyelination and remyelination in lead neuropathy— electron microscopic studies.* J Neuropathol Exp Neurol 27:527, 1968.

54. LOW, PA AND DYCK, PJ: *Increased endoneurial pressure in experimental lead neuropathy.* Nature 269:427, 1977.

55. DYCK, PJ, ET AL: *Blood nerve barrier in rat and cellular mechanisms of lead-induced segmental demyelination.* J Neuropathol Exp Neurol 39:700, 1980.

56. WINDEBANK, AJ, ET AL: *The endoneurial content of lead related to the onset and severity of segmental demyelination.* J Neuropathol Exp Neurol 38:692, 1980.

57. KANTARJIAN, AD AND SHAHEEN, AS: *Methyl bromide poisoning with nervous system manifestations resembling polyneuropathy.* Neurology (Minneap) 13:1054, 1963.

58. DAVIS, CS AND RICHARDSON, RJ: *Organophosphorus Compounds.* In SPENCER, PS AND SCHAUMBURG, HH (EDS): Experimental and Clinical Neurotoxicology, Williams & Wilkins, Baltimore, 1980, p 527.

59. SCHAUMBURG, HH AND SPENCER, PS: *Selected Outbreaks of Neurotoxic Disease.* In SPENCER, PS AND SCHAUMBURG, HH (EDS): Experimental and Clinical Neurotoxicology, Williams & Wilkins, Baltimore, 1980, p 883.

60. ABOU-DONIA, MB: *Delayed neurotoxicity of phenylphosphonothioate esters.* Science 205:713, 1979.

61. ARING, CD: *The systemic nervous affinity of triorthocresyl phosphate (Jamaican Ginger Palsy).* Brain 65:34, 1942.

62. SMITH, HV AND SPALDING, JMK: *Outbreak of paralysis in Morocco due to orthocresylphosphate poisoning.* Lancet 2:1019, 1959.

63. CAVANAGH, JB AND PATANGIA, GN: *Changes in the central nervous system of the cat as a result of tri-o-cresyl phosphate poisoning.* Brain 88:165, 1965.

64. PRINEAS, J: *The pathogenesis of dying-back polyneuropathies. Part I. An ultrastructural study of experimental tri-orthocresyl phosphate intoxication in the cat.* J Neuropathol Exp Neurol 28:571, 1969.

65. JOHNSON, MK: *Organophosphorus esters causing delayed neurotoxic effects.* Arch Toxicol (Berl) 34:259, 1975.

66. JOHNSON, MK: *The delayed neuropathy caused by some organophosphorus esters, mechanism and challenge.* CRC Crit Rev Toxicol 3:289, 1975.

67. LeQUESNE, P: *Neurophysiological investigation of subclinical and minimal toxic neuropathies.* Muscle Nerve 1:392, 1978.

68. BANK, WJ: *Thallium.* In SPENCER, PS AND SCHAUMBURG, HH (EDS): *Experimental and Clinical Neurotoxicology,* Williams & Wilkins, Baltimore, 1980, p 570.

69. CAVANAGH, JB, ET AL: *The effects of thallium salts, with particular reference to the nervous system changes.* Q J Med 43:293, 1974.

70. DAVIS, LE, ET AL: *Acute thallium poisoning: toxicological and morphological studies of the nervous system.* Ann Neurol 10:38, 1981.

71. SPENCER, PS AND SCHAUMBURG, HH: *Central-peripheral distal axonopathy—the pathology of dying-back polyneuropathies.* In ZIMMERMAN, HM (ED): *Progress in Neuropathology,* Vol 3, Grune & Stratton, New York, 1976, p 253.

72. SPENCER, PS, ET AL: *Effects of thallium salts on neuronal mitochondria in organotypic cord-ganglia-muscle combination cultures.* J Cell Biol 58:79, 1973.

73. BANK, WJ, ET AL: *Thallium poisoning.* Arch Neurol 26:456, 1972.

74. PRICK, JJG: *Thallium Poisoning.* In VINKEN, PJ AND BRUYN, GW (EDS): *Handbook of Clinical Neurology,* Vol 36, North Holland Publishing, Amsterdam, 1979, p 239.

75. FELDMAN, RG, MAYER, RM AND TAUB, A: *Evidence for peripheral neurotoxic effect of trichlorethylene.* Neurology (Minneap) 20:599, 1970.

76. BUXTON, PH AND HAYWARD, M: *Polyneuritis cranialis associated with industrial trichlorethylene poisoning.* J Neurol Neurosurg Psychiatry 30:511, 1967.

TOXIC
NEUROPATHY:
OCCUPATIONAL,
BIOLOGICAL AND
ENVIRONMENTAL
AGENTS

155

NEUROPATHIES ASSOCIATED WITH MALIGNANCY AND DYSPROTEINEMIA

CLASSIFICATION

Compression and infiltration of peripheral nerves, roots, and cranial nerves are common PNS effects of malignancy. As a remote effect of malignancy, neuropathy is probably rare. Nevertheless, occult malignancy is frequently first on the list of suspected disorders when unexplained polyneuropathies are encountered; and healthy persons with a mild peripheral neuropathy frequently undergo an elaborate, uncomfortable, expensive, and fruitless evaluation for an occult neoplasm. This practice is encouraged by earlier reports suggesting that neuropathy or 'neuromyopathy' frequently accompanies carcinoma.[1-3] It seems likely that many of the findings commonly attributed to remote effects of cancer may have reflected malnutrition, aging, neurotoxic chemotherapeutic agents, associated or coincidental metabolic and other diseases. Recent studies indicate that characteristic patterns of PNS degeneration may accompany systemic malignancy[4-6] and suggest that a classification based on the neuropathologic outline in Chapter 2 is appropriate:

Carcinoma
    Compression and Infiltration
    Sensorimotor polyneuropathy (Distal axonopathy?)
    Sensory Neuronopathy (subacute sensory neuropathy)
Lymphoma
    Compression and Endoneurial Invasion
    Demyelinating Neuropathy (Guillain-Barré Syndrome)
    Sensory Neuropathy (subacute sensory neuropathy)
    Motor Neuronopathy (subacute motor neuropathy)
Multiple Myeloma
    Compression
    Distal Axonopathy (sensorimotor neuropathy) in Typical Myeloma

Atypical Myeloma with progressive polyneuropathy
Systemic Amyloidosis
Myeloma with cryoglobulinemic neuropathy
Dysproteinemia
Cryoglobulinemic neuropathy
Macroglobulinemia—sensorimotor neuropathy with systemic amyloidosis
Paraproteinemia (benign monoclonal gammopathy)

CARCINOMA

Compression and Epineurial Invasion

Compression of peripheral nerve and roots by adjacent or epidural carcinoma is common. The clinical and pathologic features of chronic and subacute compression are discussed in Chapter 18. Compression syndromes are usually symptomatic, and frequently result in pain or dysfunction and require treatment. Epineurial invasion also frequently occurs, is usually asymptomatic, and is especially common in breast and pancreatic adenocarcinoma. The invading tumor spreads under the epineurium and surrounds individual fascicles. The perineurium is relatively resistant to invasion and usually prevents malignant cells from entering the endoneurial space. Hematogenous endoneurial metastases are extremely rare.

Sensorimotor neuropathy (Distal axonopathy?)

General

This is especially frequent in individuals with oat-cell carcinoma of the lung.[7] Primary carcinoma of the breast, stomach, colon, pancreas, uterus, cervix, thyroid, and testis are also associated with distal neuropathy.

Pathology and Pathophysiology

PATHOLOGY. Postmortem tissue and nerve biopsies in this disorder predominantly display axonal degeneration and loss of myelinated nerve fibers. These changes are most pronounced in distal limb nerves. Pallor of the dorsal columns and slight loss of anterior horn and dorsal root ganglion cells are also present. There is no systematic morphologic analysis of postmortem tissue in this disorder utilizing contemporary histopathologic techniques, and no animal model.

PATHOGENESIS. The pathogenesis of this presumed distal axonopathy is unknown. Oat-cell carcinoma originates from neural crest cells,[8] is associated with the secretion of a variety of hormone and hormone-like substances[9] and with other remote nervous system effects (Eaton-Lambert syndrome) probably mediated by circulating proteins.[10] It is suggested that a metabolic abnormality in axonal metabolism may result from a secretory product of the carcinoma, resulting in distal axonopathy[7] by mechanisms described in Chapter 2. Weight loss usually precedes the onset of this polyneuropathy, but patients are neither cachectic nor do they manifest other signs of nutritional disorder.[7] This condition clearly occurs in untreated individuals and the dysfunction cannot be attributed to chemotherapeutic axonal toxins.

Clinical Features

Symmetrical distal neuropathy may occur early or late in the course of a known carcinoma. Rarely, it may precede diagnosis of the malignancy. Most individuals experience significant weight loss before neuropathy appears.[7]

Initial symptoms are numbness and weakness of the feet. Progression is gradual, but eventually the proximal lower limbs and hands are affected. Position, vibration, and touch sense are more affected than pain, and distal tendon reflexes are absent. Weakness is present in every case, foot-drop and atrophy of intrinsic hand muscles occur in some. Autonomic and cranial nerve dysfunction are not features of this neuropathy. The previous natural history was one of slow progression;[1] however, many now experience an illness accelerated by neurotoxic chemotherapeutic agents such as vincristine. It is becoming increasingly difficult to distinguish individuals with this neuropathy from drug-induced illness.

The CSF is generally unremarkable. Electromyography usually reveals evidence of denervation in lower limb muscles. Motor and sensory conduction velocities are normal or slightly slowed. Sensory amplitudes are usually diminished.

Electrophysiologic evidence of axonal neuropathy is allegedly common in carcinomatous patients with no symptoms of nervous system dysfunction. Physical examination frequently discloses absent ankle jerks. It is claimed that such individuals have subclinical sensorimotor neuropathy.[1]

Sensory Neuronopathy (subacute sensory neuropathy)

General

This rare syndrome has been recognized since 1948 as a distinct clinico-pathologic entity, principally associated with oat-cell carcinoma.[11] Previously described as "carcinomatous sensory neuropathy," this condition is best understood as a sensory neuronopathy syndrome (see Chapter 2, Section C). Its clinical recognition is important, as it frequently produces symptoms when the underlying neoplasm is occult and potentially curable. A wide range of other tumors are occasionally associated with this condition; these include bronchial (squamous) carcinoma, breast, gastrointestinal tract, ovary, Hodgkin's disease, and reticulum cell sarcoma.[4]

Pathology and Pathogenesis

Primary degeneration of dorsal root ganglion neurons, accompanied by inflammation, is consistently demonstrated both by biopsy and postmortem examination. Salient neuropathologic findings include:[4] (1) neuronal degeneration in the dorsal root ganglia (DRG) accompanied by inflammation and phagocytosis at an early stage, with neuronal loss and fibrosis at later stages; (2) secondary degeneration in dorsal roots, sensory nerves, and dorsal columns of the spinal cord; (3) minimal change in ventral roots and muscle; and (4) occasional evidence of patchy neuronal loss in the brainstem and limbic cortex.

The etiology and pathogenesis are unknown. It appears that an inflammatory assault on the dorsal root ganglion neurons is followed by degeneration of these cells and their processes.[4] Clinical and pathologic evidence of a more diffuse encephalomyelitis is occasionally present.[12] These

NEUROPATHIES
ASSOCIATED WITH
MALIGNANCY AND
DYSPROTEINEMIA

159

features have suggested a viral etiology, perhaps accompanied by an immune-mediated cellular response. Viral particles have not been identified and culture of DRG biopsy and postmortem material has been negative.[4] There is one report of complement-fixing antibodies to brain.[13]

Clinical Features

This disorder is rare—only 29 cases were reported before 1977—and most commonly affects women in late middle age. The neurologic illness usually precedes the discovery of malignancy, often by a period as long as a year.[4]

The symptoms and signs are characteristic. The onset is subacute, with pain, paresthesias, and dysesthesias occurring in the distal extremities and spreading proximally. The trigeminal nerve is seldom involved. Unsteady gait and clumsy hands are prominent disabling complaints in nearly every case. Weakness is usually absent and wasting may evolve from disuse. Position-sense loss in the distal extremities and resulting sensory ataxia are universal signs. Loss of vibration sense parallels the loss of position sense; touch, pain, and temperature sensation are generally decreased as well. Pseudoathetoid movements appear in individuals with especially diffuse sensory loss. Autonomic neuropathy is not a feature of this condition, although urinary-bladder dysfunction is described in two individuals. Signs of more diffuse nervous system involvement—encephalomyelitis—are frequently present and impaired ocular (nystagmus, anisocoria) and higher function (memory impairment, dementia) are especially common.[4,13]

The course of the illness is subacute, worsening over a one-to-three-month interval, after which the condition remains static. In most cases, the sensory deficit is disabling. The neurologic illness appears unaffected by treatment of the underlying neoplasm. Clearly, successful treatment of the tumor prolongs survival.[4]

The cerebrospinal fluid profile is variable. Cells are not present in the majority, but occasionally a mild lymphocytosis occurs. The protein level is frequently elevated. Motor nerve conduction is usually normal. Sensory nerve action potentials are often of reduced amplitude or unelicitible in involved limbs.

Differential Diagnosis

This semiologic constellation represents a well defined, easily recognized clinical entity that should initiate a thorough search for an underlying malignancy. Individuals should be re-evaluated after six months if the initial investigations were negative. A history of an antedating febrile illness treated with antibiotics may suggest the acute sensory neuronopathy syndrome,[14] but this condition can only be diagnosed with certainty when neoplasia is eliminated.

LYMPHOMA

Compression and Endoneurial Invasion

Compression of root and plexus by epidural or retroperitoneal lymphoma is common. The clinical and pathologic features of chronic and subacute compression are discussed in Chapter 16. Endoneurial infiltration in lymphoma and leukemia can be extensive, and may present confusing clinical signs.[15] Widespread infiltrates may produce a multiple mononeuropathy or a clinical picture resembling a symmetrical distal axonopathy or the Guillain-Barré syndrome. For this reason, nerve biopsy may be necessary to dictate appropriate therapy when one of these PNS syndromes occurs in an individual with lymphoma or leukemia.

Demyelinating Neuropathy (Guillain-Barré syndrome)

Either the classic Guillain-Barré syndrome or chronic relapsing inflammatory polyneuropathy (CRIP) may occur in temporal relationship to lymphoma. The clinical and pathologic features of these conditions appear identical to those described in Chapter 3. It is suggested both that the immunosuppression that occurs in the natural course of some malignant reticuloses is a predisposition for the Guillain-Barré syndrome in these individuals,[16] and that a toxic or metabolic disorder of the Schwann cells may be associated with lymphoma.[17]

Sensory Neuropathy (subacute sensory neuropathy)

Hodgkin's disease and reticulum cell sarcoma may be associated with a subacute sensory neuropathy syndrome similar to that described for carcinoma,[4,18] but which may show considerable improvement with treatment of the underlying disease.[18]

Motor Neuronopathy (subacute motor neuronopathy)

General

This rare syndrome has been recognized since the 1960s as a distinct clinicopathologic entity associated with Hodgkin's disease. Originally described as "subacute poliomyelitis,"[19] it is best understood as a motor neuronopathy syndrome (see Chapter 2, Section 3). Its clinical recognition is important as it is a benign syndrome that usually improves, and does not require extensive evaluation or indicate further treatment of the underlying neoplasm.[5]

Pathology and Pathogenesis

Primary degeneration of anterior horn cells, accompanied by inflammation, is a consistent feature at postmortem examination. Salient neuropathologic findings include:[5] (1) degeneration of the anterior horn cells at multiple levels of the spinal cord, accompanied by inflammation and phagocytosis at an early stage and neuronal loss and gliosis at late stages; (2) lesser neuronal loss in Clarke's column, the intermediolateral cell column, and the commissural nuclei; (3) varying degrees of axonal loss in the dorsal columns and propriospinal tracts; (4) secondary axonal degeneration in ventral roots and denervation atrophy of skeletal muscle. The overall pathologic pattern suggests a mirror image of the findings in subacute sensory neuronopathy associated with carinocoma, in which DRG cells and dorsal roots are destroyed.

The etiology and pathogenesis are unknown. It appears that an inflammatory assault on the anterior horn cells and, to a lesser extent, other spinal neurons, is followed by phagocytosis of these cells and degeneration of their processes. Many features of this condition resemble poliomyelitis and it is suggested that it may represent an infection by an opportunistic virus.[5,19] Patients with Hodgkin's disease are often immunosuppressed and are susceptible to a variety of unusual infections. Radiation therapy may cause selective dysfunction of lower motor neurons and could have a role in some cases, although this syndrome has also been described in individuals who have received no radiation.[5]

Clinical Features

This disorder is uncommon, occurs equally in both sexes, at any age, and may begin at any stage in the course of the hematologic malignancy. It has not been shown to precede the discovery of malignancy, in contrast to subacute sensory neuronopathy.[4]

The illness is characterized by subacute onset of painless asymmetrical weakness of the limbs.[5,18,19] The legs are usually initially involved, although several affected individuals have first experienced weakness in the arms or in neck muscles. Involved limbs are flaccid, muscle atrophy is prominent, tendon reflexes are depressed, and fasciculation may occur. Involvement of bulbar or respiratory muscles is rare and upper motor neuron signs are not a feature of this condition. Sensation and intellect are spared.

Weakness progresses over a period of months, then stabilizes, and gradual improvement usually occurs. Rarely is this an incapacitating condition. Its course is independent of the activity of the underlying lymphoma. Individuals with this condition are stated to be unusually vulnerable to the neurotoxic effects of vincristine.[5]

The CSF protein content is sometimes increased. Electromyography reveals evidence of denervation in affected limbs. Motor and sensory conduction are normal.

Differential Diagnosis

Diagnosis of this condition is occasionally difficult despite its characteristic clinical profile. Leptomeningeal metastases, plexus compression, and the Guillain-Barré syndrome, all occur with Hodgkin's disease and may have similar clinical features. Leptomeningeal metastases frequently produce sensory complaints and cranial nerve findings; CSF cytology may be crucial in distinguishing between these conditions. Plexus compression by lymphoma is usually accompanied by pain and produces a more segmental disturbance of neurologic function. The Guillain-Barré syndrome is generally more acute and weakness is symmetrical.

MULTIPLE MYELOMA

Polyneuropathy is more common in multiple myeloma than in most other malignancies; it is suggested that subclinical neuropathy occurs frequently[20,21] and that a significant number of individuals with neuropathy of unknown cause may have a monoclonal serum protein.[22] Two common (nonamyloid) types are recognized: a sensorimotor (distal-axonopathy type) neuropathy seen with typical myeloma[23] and a predominantly motor neuropathy seen with atypical (sclerotic) myeloma.[6] Amyloidosis may coexist and the neuropathy of primary amyloidosis, described in Chapter 14, also occasionally occurs in individuals with myeloma. Both the subacute sensory neuronopathy syndrome[4] and a polyneuropathy-endocrine dysfunction syndrome may rarely occur in concert with multiple myeloma. The latter condition is seen almost exclusively in Japan.[24]

Compression

Epidural spinal-root and cranial-nerve compression syndromes produced by plasmacytomas, extending from vertebral body and skull, are common. Epineurial involvement with peripheral nerve or plexus compression syndromes are rare. Several reports demonstrate mild endoneurial infiltration with plasma cells.[15,21] The carpal tunnel syndrome in multiple myeloma suggests systemic amyloidosis.[6]

Distal Axonopathy (sensorimotor polyneuropathy)

Pathology and Pathogenesis

Postmortem and nerve biopsy studies indicate that this condition is a distal axonopathy. A thorough postmortem study has demonstrated axonal degeneration to be more pronounced in distal than in proximal segments of leg nerves.[23] Nerve biopsies consistently reveal profound loss of myelinated axons, and slight evidence of segmental demyelination.[20] Nonspecific axonal changes are described. Amyloid deposition is not a histologic feature of this condition.[20] The pathogenesis is unknown. It is widely held that this neuropathy is somehow related to the sensorimotor neuropathy occurring as a remote complication of carcinoma[6] (*vide supra*).

Clinical Features

This disorder is more common in males in late middle age. Frequently, polyneuropathy antedates discovery of the underlying malignancy. Polyneuropathy is heralded by the insidious onset of numbness and tingling in the feet accompanied by slight weakness. Symptoms intensify over a period of months and the hands are eventually involved. All sensory modalities are impaired, and distal tendon reflexes are lost. Autonomic involvement does not occur. The CSF protein may be slightly increased. Motor nerve conduction velocity is normal or minimally slowed; sensory nerve action potential amplitudes are low.

The course is variable. Some remain with a mild, nondisabling, stocking-glove sensory loss; others become profoundly weak and bedridden. There is little improvement. Treatment and improvement of the underlying malignancy does not affect the polyneuropathy. Pain is sometimes a feature in this neuropathy and *the gradual occurrence of a painful sensorimotor or sensory neuropathy in a male in middle age or later should lead to the suspicion of myeloma.*

Differential Diagnosis

There are no features of this distal axonopathy that permit distinction from the many similar conditions caused by metabolic or toxic illness. Since myeloma is usually unsuspected when the neuropathy appears, it is probably wise to perform electrophoresis and immunoelectrophoresis on serum and urine of individuals without obvious cause for neuropathy.[22]

Chronic Demyelinating Polyneuropathy

It has been suggested recently that there is a group of patients with a systemic plasma cell dyscrasia-associated neuropathy that can be distinguished from the usual myeloma polyneuropathy.[6] These patients are subject to PNS dysfunction that has clinical features of chronic inflammatory neuropathy, predominantly motor neuropathy, distinct from the usual sensorimotor neuropathy of typical myeloma. Frequently, such individuals are young, do not have anemia or renal failure, display a modestly elevated plasma monoclonal protein, and few plasma cells in bone-marrow aspirates. Many have osteosclerotic bony myelomatous lesions.[6] The neuropathy may precede the diagnosis of myeloma, sometimes by as long as two years. Simultaneous onset of weakness and sensory symptoms in the lower limbs is followed by relentless progression over months. Weakness is severe and, in general, motor loss dominates the clinical picture. Diminished position and vibration sense occurs in the feet and hands, but pain and thermal sense are spared. Tendon reflexes are depressed or absent. There is no involvement of cranial or autonomic nerves. Cerebrospinal fluid protein is usually elevated. Motor nerve conduction is profoundly slowed and sensory nerve action potentials are low or unobtainable.[6] There are no postmortem examinations in this condition; nerve biopsy tissue displays evidence of axonal degeneration and segmental demyelination. The course is steady progression and eventually stabilizes, usually at an incapacitating level. Improvement in neuropathy may occur following successful treatment of the myeloma. There is a report of improvement following myeloma treatment combined with plasma exchange.[25]

The pathology and pathogenesis of this condition are obscure. Improvement following treatment of the tumor suggests a close relationship to the primary neoplasm. It is generally held that this represents a chronic demyelinating neuropathy.[6,25] Recent reports of antibody activity, possibly directed against components of peripheral myelin in benign plasma-cell dyscrasias[25] and claims of passive transfer of human myeloma neuropathy to experimental animals[26] somewhat support this notion.

Systemic Amyloidosis

Systemic amyloidosis frequently occurs in association with multiple myeloma and may be accompanied by neuropathy.[6] Formerly it was held that myeloma neuropathy represented a variety of systemic amyloidosis. Abundant postmortem analysis has effectively contradicted this notion and most individuals with myeloma neuropathy do not have amyloid in the PNS. The peripheral neuropathy of systemic amyloidosis complicating myeloma is similar to that seen in primary amyloidosis (see Chapter 14).

DYSPROTEINEMIA

Monoclonal gammopathy

(1) Related to myeloma (vide supra)
(2) Benign gammopathy. Two varieties of polyneuropathy are described:[27–30]
    (a) A poorly characterized chronic sensorimotor neuropathy, related to a variety of benign monoclonal gammapathies.
    (b) A progressive sensorimotor demyelinating neuropathy related to IgM kappa gammapathy. There is severe slowing of nerve conduction and IgM kappa demonstrable on myelin. It is suggested both that circulating IgM proteins may have an affinity for peripheral nerve myelin and that myelin associated glycoprotein is the antigen for the monoclonal IgM[25,36]. It is possible that immunocytochemical tests could detect IgM paraproteins

with an affinity for nerve antigens and assist in the diagnosis and classification of plasma cell dyscrasia associated neuropathy[37]. This notion, and a possible role for plasmapheresis in the treatment of this demyelinative neuropathy are currently being investigated.

(3) Waldenstrom's Macroglobulinemia: This is a chronic lymphoproliferative disorder characterized by an IgM monoclonal protein. There is usually an underlying lymphoma with a wide range of clinical manifestations. An indolent distal symmetrical sensorimotor polyneuropathy is commonly seen, and may be the initial phase of the illness. The pathology and pathogenesis of polyneuropathy are poorly understood, but myelin degeneration without inflammation is described.[31] Endoneurial and endothelial deposits of amorphous IgM-containing material are described.

Cryoglobulinemia

Both essential and secondary cryoglobulinemia are associated with neuropathy in the lower limbs often precipitated by cold. One study estimates that 7 percent of all individuals with cryoglobulinemia have neuropathy.[34] The pathology, pathogenesis, and natural history of this condition are not clear. Endoneurial and intracapillary deposits of cryoglobulin are described with multiple myeloma. It is proposed that cryoglobulin thrombi render the nerves ischemic. This suggestion appears especially relevant to those cases whose neurologic deficit parallels the occurrence of purpura produced by cold. Vasculitis of the vasa nervorum, probably related to activation of the complement system by intravascular cryoglobulin deposition, has been demonstrated in cryoglobulinemic neuropathy,[35] in association with cutaneous vasculitis.

REFERENCES

1. CROFT, PB AND WILKINSON, M: *Carcinomatous neuromyopathy-its incidence in patients with carcinoma of the lung and carcinoma of the breast.* Lancet 1:184, 1963.

2. DAYAN, AD, CROFT, PB AND WILKINSON, M: *Association of carcinomatous neuromyopathy with different histological types of carcinoma of the lung.* Brain 88:435, 1965.

3. MORTON, DL ITABASHI, HH AND GRIMES, OF: *Nonmetastatic neurological complications of bronchogenic carcinoma: the carcinomatous neuromyopathies.* J Thorac Cardiovasc Surg 51:14, 1966.

4. HORWICH, MS, ET AL: *Subacute sensory neuropathy: a remote effect of carcinoma.* Ann Neurol 2:7, 1977.

5. SCHOLD, SC, ET AL: *Subacute motor neuronopathy: a remote effect of lymphoma.* Ann Neurol 5:271, 1979.

6. KELLY, JJ, ET AL: *The spectrum of peripheral neuropathy in myeloma.* Neurology (Minneap) 31:24, 1981.

7. HAWLEY, RJ, ET AL: *The carcinomatous neuromyopathy of oatcell lung cancer.* Ann Neurol 7:65, 1980.

8. BELL, EC, SEETHARAM, S AND McDANIEL, RC: *Endodermally-derived and neural crest-derived differentiation antigens expressed by a human lung tumor.* J Immunol 116:1236, 1976.

9. EAGAN, RT, ET AL: *Small cell carcinoma of the lung: staging, paraneoplastic syndromes, treatment and survival.* Cancer 33:527, 19??

10. ISHIKAWA, D, ET AL: *A neuromuscular transmission block produced by a cancer tissue extract derived from a patient with the myasthenic syndrome.* Neurology (Minneap) 27:140, 1977.

11. DENNY-BROWN, D: *Primary sensory neuropathy with muscular changes associated with carcinoma.* J Neurol Neurosurg Psychiatry 11:73, 1948.

12. HENSON, RA AND URICH, H: *Peripheral neuropathy associated with malignant disease*. In VINKEN, PJ AND BRUYN, GW (EDS): Handbook of Clinical Neurology, Vol 8, North Holland-American Elsevier, New York, 1970, p 131.

13. CROFT, PB, ET AL: *Sensory neuropathy with bronchial carcinoma: a study of four cases showing serological abnormalities*. Brain 88:501, 1965.

14. STERMAN, AB, SCHAUMBURG, HH AND ASBURY, AK: *The acute sensory neuronopathy syndrome*. Ann Neurol 7:354, 1979.

15. BARRON, KD, ROWLAND, LD AND ZIMMERMAN, HM: *Neuropathy with malignant tumor metastases*. J Nerv Ment Dis 131:10, 1960.

16. LISAK, RP, ET AL: *Guillain-Barré syndrome and Hodgkin's disease: three cases with immunological studies*. Ann Neurol 1:72, 1977.

17. WALSH, JC: *Neuropathy associated with lymphoma*. J Neurol Neurosurg Psychiatry 34:42, 1971.

18. SAGAR, HJ AND READ, DJ: *Subacute sensory neuropathy with remission: an association with lymphoma*. J Neurol Neurosurg Psychiatry 45:83, 1982.

19. WALTON, JN, TOMLINSON, BE AND PEARCE, GW: *Subacute "poliomyelitis" and Hodgkin's disease*. J Neurol Sci 6:435, 1968.

20. WALSH, JC: *The neuropathy of multiple myeloma, an electrophysiological and histological study*. Arch Neurol 25:404, 1971.

21. HESSELVICK, M: *Neuropathological studies on myelomatosis*. Acta Neurol Scand 45:95, 1969.

22. KELLY, JJ, ET AL.: *Prevalence of monoclonal protein in peripheral neuropathy*. Neurology (Minneap) 31:1480, 1981.

23. VICTOR, M, BANKER, BQ AND ADAMS, RD: *The neuropathy of multiple myeloma*. J Neurol Neurosurg Psychiatry 21:73, 1958.

24. IWASHITA, H, ET AL: *Polyneuropathy, skin hyperpigmentation, edema and hypertrichosis in localized osteosclerotic myeloma*. Neurology (Minneap) 27:675, 1977.

25. LATOV, N ET AL: *Plasma cell dyscrasia and peripheral neuropathy with a monoclonal antibody to peripheral-nerve myelin*. N Engl J Med 303:617, 1980.

26. BESINGER, UA, ET AL: *Myeloma neuropathy: passive transfer from man to mouse*. Science 213:1027, 1981.

27. CHAZOT, G, ET AL: *Manifestations neurologiques des gammopathies monoclonales*. Rev Neurol (Paris) 132:195, 1976.

28. KAHN, SN, RICHES, PG AND KOHN, J: *Paraproteinemia in neurological disease: incidence, associations and classifications of monoclonal immunoglobulins*. J Clin Pathol 33:617, 1980.

29. KYLE, RH: *Monoclonal gammopathy of undetermined significance: natural history of 241 cases*. Am J Med 64:814, 1978.

30. KYLE, RA AND GRIEPP, PR: *The diverse picture of gamma heavy chain disease (JHCD): report of seven cases and review of literature*. Mayo Clin Proc 56:439, 1981.

31. IWASHITA, H, ET AL: *Polyneuropathy in Waldenströms macroglobulinaemia*. J Neurol Sci 21:341, 1974.

32. PROPP, RP, ET AL: *Waldenstrom's macroglobulinemia and neuropathy: deposition of M-component on myelin sheaths*. Neurology (Minneap) 25:980, 1975.

33. LOGOTHETIS, J, ET AL: *Cryoglobulinemic neuropathy*. Arch Neurol 19:389, 1968.

34. VALLAT, JM, ET AL: *Cryoglobulinemic neuropathy: a pathological study*. Ann Neurol 8:179, 1980.

35. CREAM, JJ, ET AL: *Mixed or immune complex cryoglobulinemia and neuropathy*. J Neurol Neurosurg Psychiatry 37:82, 1974.

36. BRAUN, PE, LATOR, N AND FRAIL DE: *Myelin-associated glycoprotein is the antigen for a monoclonal IgM in polyneuropathy*. J Neurochem (in press).

37. ABRAMS, GM, ET AL: *Immunocytochemical studies of human peripheral nerve with serum from patients with polyneuropathy and paraproteinemia*. Neurol 32:821, 1982.

Chapter 14

AMYLOID NEUROPATHY

Extracellular deposition of the fibrous protein amyloid is associated with peripheral neuropathy in two distinct classes of neuropathic disorders, nonhereditary (immunoglobulin-derived) amyloidosis and hereditary (nonimmunoglobulin-derived) amyloidosis. Although diverse etiologies underlie the accumulation of amyloid in these conditions, they share common neuropathologic and pathophysiologic features.[1-12]

PATHOLOGY AND PATHOGENESIS

Nerve biopsy studies indicate that three patterns of amyloid deposition occur in the PNS, and all may contribute to neuropathy. One is amyloid deposition in connective tissue surrounding peripheral nerves, leading to nerve compression at potential entrapment sites.[2,4,13] The median nerve is frequently involved at the wrist, giving rise to a carpal tunnel syndrome. The second pattern is widespread endoneurial deposition of amyloid.[4,9,12] The third pattern is amyloid deposition within the walls of the vasa nervorum of both epineurium and endoneurium.[12,14] The latter two patterns of amyloid deposition are accompanied by severe depletion of unmyelinated and small diameter myelinated fibers, correlating closely with clinical findings of pain and temperature sensory loss and autonomic dysfunction. There are no detailed postmortem studies of the nervous system in systemic amyloidosis utilizing contemporary histologic techniques, and the relationship of focal amyloid deposition to fiber damage is unknown. Much of the nerve fiber degeneration in peripheral nerves could result from lesions affecting dorsal root and autonomic ganglion cells where amyloid deposits also occur.[1,3,15-17]

The pathogenesis is unknown. There are three hypotheses: one states that nerve fiber degeneration results from a generalized metabolic disorder and that amyloid deposits are an epiphenomenon;[7,8] the second hypothesis is that the peripheral nerve changes result from ischemia induced by amyloid compromising endoneurial vessels,[14] and the third holds that the amyloid deposits exert a direct mechanical effect,[9] or lead to the loss of sensory and autonomic ganglion neurons and peripheral axons by a mechanism that is not yet understood.[3,9]

CLINICAL FEATURES

Non-hereditary Amyloidosis (Primary and Dysproteinemic Types)

GENERAL. Systemic organ involvement by amyloidosis is apparent in about one half of the cases of primary amyloidosis with neuropathy, and the disorder is most common in middle-aged males.[12] The amyloid neuropathy of dysproteinemic states, especially meyloma, appears to be identical to that of primary amyloidosis, and should be distinguished from the other neuropathies associated with the dysproteinemias (Chapter 13). In both primary amyloidosis and multiple myeloma, the amyloid fibril appears homologous to the terminal region of an immunoglobulin light chain.[20-22]

Symptoms, Signs, and Course of Neuropathy

Sensory symptoms are the most prominent features in all but the few patients who present with autonomic or carpal tunnel involvement.[9,12] Symmetrical numbness of hands and feet heralds this disorder; dysesthesias and spontaneous aching pains are especially frequent. Symptoms of autonomic dysfunction (postural hypotension, bladder atony, impotence) eventually appear in most affected individuals and are often an early feature.[23-25] Distal weakness appears later.

Signs of distal limb sensory impairment are a constant feature and, characteristically, pain and temperature sensation are more affected than position and vibration sense. Distal weakness and atrophy are present, usually mild at first. Signs of autonomic dysfunction include orthostatic hypotension, hypoactive pupils, diminished sweating and abnormal cystometrograms.[23-25] The peripheral nerves may be enlarged.

The course is one of gradual incapacity by sensory, motor and autonomic dysfunction.[9-12] Sensorimotor impairment progressively moves proximally and the distal limbs become numb and atrophic. Most patients eventually require orthopedic appliances or become unable to walk. Primary amyloidosis is fatal, usually secondary to cardiac or renal decompensation. Survival of individuals with neuropathy range from 2 to 10 years following the initial sensory symptoms. Patients exhibiting dysproteinemia with amyloid neuropathy usually die because of the underlying disorder, but occasionally succumb from systemic amyloidosis. There is no specific treatment for systemic amyloidosis.

Laboratory Studies

CLINICAL LABORATORY. Abnormal routine laboratory values are common in primary amyloidosis, often reflecting renal and cardiac involvement. Serum protein electrophoretic patterns are abnormal in half the patients and urine patterns in 70 percent. Monoclonal proteins are present in 90 percent when both urine and blood are studied. Amyloid may be demonstrated by histologic examination of gingival or rectal biopsy tissue. Myeloma patients display additional abnormalities including many plasma cells in the bone marrow, large amounts of monoclonal protein in urine and serum, lytic bone lesions, and severe anemia.[13,18,19]

CEREBROSPINAL FLUID. Protein levels are usually moderately elevated, and electrophoresis may reveal elevation of the IgG fraction.

ELECTRODIAGNOSTIC STUDIES. Motor conduction velocities are usually normal or slightly slowed, while sensory nerve action potentials, certainly in the later stages, are either markedly reduced or unobtainable. Electromyography reveals evidence of denervation in distal limb muscles.

NERVE BIOPSY. Amyloid deposits are usually present in sural nerve biopsy specimens on light microscope examination of sections stained with Congo red or thioflavin T.

Differential Diagnosis

Sensorimotor-autonomic neuropathy appearing in a nondiabetic middle-aged male should strongly suggest the diagnosis of amyloid neuropathy. Demonstration of amyloid on nerve, rectal, or gingival biopsy confirms its presence. Diabetic autonomic and sensorimotor neuropathy resembles this disorder, although distal motor involvement is less severe and dissociated pain and temperature sensory loss less apparent. Tabes dorsalis is also featured by pupillary abnormalities, bladder dysfunction and pains in the extremities; abnormal proprioception and preservation of strength help distinguish tabes from amyloid neuropathy.

Case History* and Comment

At age 61, the patient developed a feeling of coldness in his fingers and feet which slowly spread proximally as far as the wrists and knees. About two years later, he became aware that he was unable to appreciate the temperature of bath water with his feet. At about the same time, he began to experience occasional stabbing pains in the legs and, a little later, a persistent aching in both lower legs. He became impotent and constipated and on a few occasions had felt faint on standing up abruptly. He had no definite urinary symptoms. He also slowly became aware of wasting of his legs and of unsteadiness in walking. Apart from a myocardial infarct at age 53, his previous health had been good, and there was no family history of similar disorder.

He was admitted for investigation in the following year. Examination showed small, unequal pupils; the response to light was absent on the left and reduced on the right; they constricted normally on convergence. There was slight, generalized wasting in the arms, with focal wasting of the small hand muscles. The small hand muscles were weak bilaterally, as were the finger and wrist extensors. There was generalized wasting and weakness in the legs, maximal distally. The right triceps and both ankle jerks were absent; the other tendon reflexes were obtainable only on reinforcement. The plantar responses were absent. The appreciation of light touch was lost in the hands and below both knees. Pain and temperature sensation was lost over a similar distribution. Joint position sense was impaired in the

AMYLOID
NEUROPATHY

*Case 4. From Thomas and King,[9] with permission

toes but preserved in the fingers. Vibration sense was lost in the feet but remained in the hands. The peripheral nerves were not thickened. A sweating test showed absent sweating over the trunk and limbs except in the axillae. Intradermal histamine failed to produce a flare in the legs, but did so on the forearm and on the abdominal wall. His blood pressure decreased from 140/90 when lying to 90/70 on standing. The liver and spleen were not enlarged.

A full blood count was normal and the ESR was 8 mm at one hour. A bone-marrow biopsy was normal, as was a glucose tolerance test. The blood urea concentration was 23 mg per dl and the creatinine clearance was 109 ml per min. A three-day fecal fat collection yielded 3 to 5 gm per day. Chest X-ray was normal. The CSF showed no pleocytosis but the protein content was 240 mg per dl.

Motor nerve conduction velocity in the right median and peroneal nerves was 46 and 31 m per sec, respectively. No sensory action potentials were detectable on percutaneous recording at the wrist on stimulation of the digital nerves of the index and fifth fingers.

Sural nerve biopsy revealed gross depletion of myelinated nerve fibers; remaining fibers showed evidence both of degeneration and regeneration. The number of unmyelinated axons was grossly reduced. Congo red staining revealed the presence of amyloid deposits around endoneurial blood vessels and free in the endoneurium.

COMMENT. This case clearly illustrates the cardinal clinical features of primary amyloid neuropathy: autonomic involvement, onset in late middle age, insidious progression, and distal limb loss of pain, temperature and tactile sense. No evidence of multiple myeloma was found and nerve biopsy was diagnostic.

Hereditary Amyloidosis

Clinical patterns form the sole basis for differentiating one type of hereditary amyloidosis from another, since there are no specific biochemical, hematologic or immunologic tests in these disorders. All four varieties featured by prominent PNS involvement are inherited in an autosomal dominant manner. The pathologic features of peripheral nerve involvement appear identical to those of the nonhereditary types (vide supra). Abnormal immunoglobulins are not present in individuals with hereditary amyloidosis and the pathogenesis of these disorders is unknown.

TYPE I (LOWER-LIMB ONSET). Three similar variants of this fatal disorder have been described in Portuguese,[1] Japanese[26] and Swedish kinships.[27] The onset is usually in the third decade, with initial symptoms of numb paresthetic feet or gastrointestinal or other evidence of autonomic dysfunction. The disorder progresses slowly, leading to the development of a severe sensory and autonomic neuropathy, featured by dissociated sensory loss with pain and temperature sense most affected. Attacks of stabbing pain, trophic changes, and ulcerated skin are common. Signs of autonomic dysfunction include impotence, constipation, diarrhea, postural hypotension, and pupillary inequality. Distal limb weakness later appears with muscle atrophy and sometimes fasciculation. Amyloid deposits in the heart, kidneys, and liver commonly occur in this disorder. Clinical signs of dysfunction of these organs are not prominent features of this condition, nor is nerve compression (carpal tunnel syndrome) by extraneural deposits of amyloid. The diagnosis may be established by skin or nerve biopsy. Death usually occurs before the age of 50.

TYPE II (UPPER-LIMB ONSET). Two similar variants of a milder disorder featured by the carpal tunnel syndrome and vitreous opacities have been described in families of Swiss origin in Indiana[2] and German origin in Maryland, USA.[5] This condition begins in middle age with progressive bilateral median nerve compression at the wrist, sometimes accompanied by vitreous opacities. In time, there is more widespread sensory loss, but peripheral neuropathy is rarely disabling and autonomic involvement is not a prominent feature of the disorder. The carpal tunnel syndrome is usually relieved by decompression of the flexor retinaculum. Individuals may survive as long as 35 years with little disability, although vitreous opacities may lead to serious impairment of vision. Postmortem examination in several instances has revealed widespared, clinically inapparent, systemic amyloid deposition.

TYPE III (GENERALIZED). This disorder is described in an Iowa, USA, family whose ancestors originated in Britain.[6] Both upper and lower extremities are severely affected but the carpal tunnel syndrome does not appear. The onset is in the fourth decade and death from renal involvement occurs within twenty years. Initial symptoms of pain, dysesthesias, and weakness of the distal lower limbs are followed by progressive proximal and upper limb involvement. Autonomic dysfunction is not prominent. Most individuals are disabled by the peripheral neuropathy within ten years. Hypertension and uremia are additional debilitating features of the illness. Postmortem examination has revealed abundant amyloid deposition in the kidneys, liver, adrenal, testes, and peripheral nerve.

TYPE IV (CRANIAL NERVE). A further distinctive form has been described in Finland and is characterized by the combination of a lattice corneal dystrophy and multiple cranial nerve involvement.[28]

REFERENCES

1. ANDRADE, C: *A peculiar form of peripheral neuropathy: familial atypical generalized amyloidosis with special involvement of the peripheral nerves.* Brain 75:408, 1952.

2. RUKAVINA, JG, ET AL: *Primary systemic amyloidosis: a review and an experimental, genetic and clinical study of 29 cases with particular emphasis on the familial form.* Medicine 35:239, 1956.

3. KRÜCKE, W: *Zür pathologischen Anatomie der Paramyloidose.* Acta Neuropathol, Suppl 11:74, 1963.

4. DYCK, PJ AND LAMBERT, EH: *Dissociated sensation in amyloidosis: compound action potential, quantitative histologic and teased-fiber, and electron microscopic studies of sural nerve biopsies.* Arch Neurol 20:490, 1969.

5. MAHLOUDJI, M, ET AL: *The genetic amyloidoses with particular reference to hereditary neuropathic amyloidosis, type II (Indiana or Rukavina type).* Medicine 48:1, 1969.

6. VAN ALLEN, MW, FROHLICH, JA AND DAVIS, JR: *Inherited predisposition to generalized amyloidosis. Clinical and pathological study of a family with neuropathy, nephropathy and peptic ulcer.* Neurology (Minneap) 19:10, 1969.

7. COIMBRA, A AND ANDRADE, C: *Familial amyloid polyneuropathy: an electron microscope study of the peripheral nerve in five cases. I. Interstitial changes.* Brain 94:199, 1971.

8. COIMBRA, A AND ANDRADE, C: *Familial amyloid polyneuropathy: an electron microscope study of the peripheral nerve in five cases. II. Nerve fibre changes.* Brain 94:207, 1971.

9. THOMAS, PK AND KING, RHM: *Peripheral nerve changes in amyloid neuropathy.* Brain 97:395, 1974.

10. KYLE, RA AND BAYRD, ED: *Amyloidosis: review of 236 cases.* Medicine 54:271, 1975.

11. NEUNDORFER, B, MEYER, JG AND VOLK, B: *Amyloid neuropathy due to monoclonal gammopathy: A case report.* J Neurol 216:207, 1977.

12. KELLEY, JJ ET AL: *The natural history of peripheral neuropathy in primary systemic amyloidosis.* Ann Neurol 6:1, 1979.

13. DAYAN, AD, URICH, H AND GARDNER-THORPE, C: *Peripheral neuropathy and myeloma.* J Neurol Sci 14:2, 1971.

14. KERNOHAN, JW AND WOLTMAN, HW: *Amyloid neuritis.* Arch Neurol Psychiatry 47:132, 1942.

15. DE NAVASQUEZ, S AND TREBLE, HA: *A case of primary generalized amyloid disease with involvement of the nerves.* Brain 61:116, 1938.

16. GOTZE, W AND KRUCKE, W: *Uber Paramyloidose mit besondener Beteiligung der peripheren Nerven und granular Atrophie des Gehirns, und uber ihre Beziehungen zu den intracerbralen Gefassverkalkungen.* Arch Psychiat Nerv Krank 114:182, 1941.

17. JEDRZEJOWSKA, H: *Some historic aspects of amyloid polyneuropathy.* Acta Neuropathol 37:119, 1977.

18. DAVIES-JONES, GAB AND ESIRI, MM: *Neuropathy due to amyloid in myelomatosis.* Br Med J 2:444, 1971.

19. KELLY, JJ, ET AL: *The spectrum of peripheral neuropathy in myeloma.* Neurology (Minneap) 31:24, 1981.

20. GLENNER, GG, EIN, D AND TERRY, WD: *The immunoglobulin origin of amyloid.* Am J Med 52:141, 1972.

21. BENSON, MD: *Partial amino acid sequence homology between an heredofamilial amyloid protein and human plasma prealbumin.* J Clin Invest 67:1035, 1981.

22. SOJI, S, ET AL: *Immunologic and immunohistochemical study of familial amyloid polyneuropathy.* Neurology (Minneap) 31:1493, 1981.

23. FRENCH, JM, ET AL: *Peripheral and autonomic nerve involvement in primary amyloidosis associated with uncontrollable diarrhea and steatorrhea.* Am J Med 39:277, 1965.

24. GANN, D, ET AL: *Postural hypotension in amyloid disease.* Am Heart J 84:395, 1972.

25. NORDBERG, C, ET AL: *Involvement of the autonomous nervous system in primary and secondary amyloidosis.* Acta Neurol Scand 49:31, 1973.

26. ARAKI, S, ET AL: *Polyneuritic amyloidosis in a Japanese family.* Arch Neurol 18:593, 1968.

27. ANDERSSON, R: *Hereditary amyloidosis with polyneuropathy.* Acta Med Scand 188:85, 1970.

28. MERETOJA, J: *Familial systemic paramyloidosis with lattice dystrophy of the cornea, progressive cranial neuropathy, skin changes, and various internal symptoms.* Ann Clin Res 1:314, 1969.

CHAPTER 15

ISCHEMIC NEUROPATHY (PERIPHERAL-VASCULAR OCCLUSIVE DISEASE AND VASCULITIS)

Clinicians most commonly equate ischemic disease of the PNS with diabetic mononeuropathy or with nerve compassion or trauma (see Chapters 4, 17 and 18). Peripheral neuropathy associated with chronic peripheral vascular occlusive disease is probably frequent but has been little studied, whereas that associated with necrotizing angiopathy is rare but well described.

NEUROPATHY OF PERIPHERAL VASCULAR DISEASE

It is generally held that peripheral nerve is relatively resistant to large-vessel occlusive disease, and only widespread, severe involvement of small blood vessels produces ischemic nerve damage. Experimental studies that failed to produce ischemic lesions in leg nerves by ligating single large limb vessels have supported this notion,[1] and emphasize the abundant collateral sources of blood flow in peripheral nerve. It is usually necessary to ligate multiple limb vessels[2] or the aorta[3] to produce limb nerve ischemia in an experimental animal. Nevertheless, several clinical reports have documented neurologic abnormalities in the extremities of individuals with chronic severe peripheral vascular disease. Studies of individuals with chronic obliterative arterial disease of the lower limbs describe evidence of sensory peripheral neuropathy in 50[4] to 88 percent.[5] The extent of the deficit appeared proportional to the degree of ischemia. One half were weak and many had no tendon reflexes. Nerve biopsy revealed loss of myelinated fibers with evidence of segmental demyelination, Wallerian degeneration, and abundant occlusion of small epineurial vessels. The latter finding suggests the possibility that the arteriosclerotic process extended into many of the arterioles of nerve, resulting in a "diffuse-small-vessel" neuropathy. It appears likely that neuropathy is a common feature of chronic vascular insufficiency, and goes unrecognized, since the more obvious effects of ischemia on skin and muscle dominate the clinical picture.

NEUROPATHY DUE TO NECROTIZING ANGIITIS

No fewer than nine disorders are clearly associated with vasculitis and ischemic neuropathy:[6]

Polyarteritis nodosa
Rheumatoid arthritis
Systemic lupus erythematosus (SLE)
Hypersensitivity angiitis
Allergic granulomatosis (Churg-Strauss)
Systemic sclerosis
Sjögrens' syndrome
Wegener's granulomatosis
Cranial arteritis (temporal arteritis)
Spanish oil syndrome

Although there is considerable variety among these conditions, they present similar clinical and pathologic profiles of peripheral nerve involvement. Only polyarteritis nodosa, rheumatoid arthritis, and lupus erythematosus are encountered with any frequency in clinical practice and these conditions are discussed individually, in addition to the recently described "Spanish oil syndrome." Angiitis characteristically gives rise to a focal or multifocal neuropathy.[7] A symmetrical sensory polyneuropathy may be encountered in relation to SLE, rheumatoid arthritis, and Sjögren's syndrome, and a subacute motor polyneuropathy in SLE.[6] They possibly have a differing pathogenesis.

Polyarteritis Nodosa

PATHOLOGY AND PATHOGENESIS. Spinal or cranial nerves display vascular lesions in 75 percent of cases.[9] Nerves may be focally swollen and hemorrhagic. In polyarteritis the necrotizing inflammation involves medium-sized and small arteries and, occasionally, veins. Capillaries and venules are spared. Thus, the epineurial vessels are heavily involved while endoneurial capillaries are preserved. Segments of vessels are affected and there appears to be a predilection for bifurcation points where small, fragile aneurysms occur. Acute lesions are featured by fibrinoid necrosis of the vessel wall accompanied by focal accumulations of polymorphonuclear leucocytes; chronic (or healed) lesions by modest numbers of mononuclear cells, granulation tissue, and collagen.[5]

The pathogenesis of nerve fiber destruction presumably is related to focal ischemia resulting from arteriolar occlusion. Nerve biopsy usually reveals abundant vascular change and teased nerve fiber preparations a combination of axonal degeneration and segmental demyelination.[6] Postmortem sampling of nerves clearly demonstrates distally accentuated loss of nerve fibers. Focal infarcts of nerve have not been convincingly demonstrated in polyarteritis.

CLINICAL FEATURES. Polyarteritis nodosa is rare, but clinically detectable neuropathy occurs in almost two thirds of cases at some stage in the illness and may be the presenting feature.[8] Neuropathy usually occurs subsequent to other manifestation of generalized disease, such as fever, pericarditis, hypertension, renal failure, abdominal pain. Occasionally, peripheral neuropathy may be the first clear indication of specific organ involvement in an individual with puzzling nonspecific debilitating illness. Polyarteritic neuropathy is usually heralded by dysfunction of one or more scattered peripheral nerves (multiple mononeuropathy). Branches of the radial, median, and sciatic nerves are especially frequent early sites for mononeuropathy in this condition. The onset of dysfunction is abrupt, accompanied by pain and numbness in the distribution of the affected nerve and may be followed in days by near-total motor and sensory loss. In time, other nerves often become involved, eventuating in a severe, symmetrical, predominantly distal polyneuropathy affecting arms as well as legs. This profile is so well recognized that the occurrence of a multiple mononeuropathy in a nondiabetic, chronically ill elderly person immediately suggests a polyarteritic basis. Occasional cases of polyarteritic neuropathy display a distal symmetrical pattern from the outset, clinically indistinguishable from the toxic-metabolic neuropathies. This probably is secondary to an especially widespread and fulminant vasculitic involvement of many peripheral nerves.

The prognosis is poor for polyarteritis nodosa with multiple organ involvement. Treatment with high doses of corticosteroids (60 mg prednisone on alternate days) is customary and may produce rapid, albeit temporary, improvement. Higher dosages may be necessary. Occasional cases may have vasculitis that predominantly affects the nervous system and spares the heart, abdominal viscera, and kidney. In our experience, such individuals tend to have more prolonged survival, and occasionally display a remarkable recovery from severe generalized polyneuropathy following prolonged corticosteroid therapy.

RHEUMATOID ARTHRITIS

Compression Syndromes

Pressure palsy and entrapment mononeuropathies are common in rheumatoid arthritis, reflecting prolonged immobilized postures and compression of nerve by articular deformity.[10] The carpal tunnel syndrome is especially frequent in advanced cases. The pathology, pathogenesis, and clinical features of these conditions are discussed in Chapter 18.

Chronic Symmetrical Sensory Neuropathy

A few individuals with long-standing, moderately severe rheumatoid arthritis develop a mild, distally symmetrical sensory neuropathy. All modalities of sensation are equally affected. It is likely that some weakness accompanies this predominantly sensory neuropathy, and electrodiagnostic studies support this view;[11] however, strength is difficult to evaluate in patients with prolonged immobilization and severe joint deformity. This symmetrical polyneuropathy is generally a benign condition, spontaneous improvement is the rule, and corticosteroid treatment is not indicated. Occasionally, severe pain may accompany this condition, even in its mild form. The symmetrical sensory neuropathy, in itself, is rarely debilitating. A careful histologic study of nerve biopsies from three individuals with mild sensory neuropathy demonstrated epineurial vessels occluded by nonspecific thickening, large-fiber loss, and axonal degeneration.[12]

Subacute Multiple Mononeuropathy Due to Necrotizing Angiitis

This rare condition is the most severe peripheral nervous system complication of rheumatoid arthritis. The clinico-pathological profile closely resembles that of polyarteritis nodosa.[10,13] Most cases occur after many years of chronic arthritis with destructive joint change and rheumatoid nodules, but may be encouraged in comparatively mild cases. Mononeuritis is usually part of an overall changing clinical picture reflecting systemic vasculitis (Raynaud's phenomenon, nail bed infarctions, skin ulcers, coronary and mesenteric artery occlusions). The clinical profile is an acute onset of painful paresthesias within the distribution of one peripheral nerve, followed within days by appropriate motor and sensory dysfunction. Usually, multiple nerves in several limbs become involved within a few months and the prognosis is poor. There is a high incidence of life-threatening complications from coronary artery disease, mesenteric artery occlusion, and septicemia. The pathophysiology of this condition clearly is related to ischemia secondary to necrotizing vasculitis. High-dose corticosteroid treatment, possibly in combination with azathioprine or cyclophosphamide, is merited, but the response is often disappointing. A meticulous postmortem study of this condition has highlighted several features of the PNS pathology including focal areas of nerve fiber degeneration. Changes appear mostly in the center of fascicles, and focal lesions in major limb nerves which begin at mid-humeral and mid-femoral levels, suggesting these areas are watersheds of poor perfusion.[14] Endoneurial infarction is not described in this study. A recent experimental study suggests that unmyelinated fibers are most vulnerable following acute small-vessel occlusion of peripheral nerve,[15] but this is not reflected in the pattern of sensory loss observed in humans.

SYSTEMIC LUPUS ERYTHEMATOSUS (SLE)

Approximately 10 percent of SLE develop peripheral neuropathy in one of three varieties: a subacute illness of Guillain-Barré type, a diffuse distal sensory or sensorimotor neuropathy, and multiple mononeuropathy.[6,16] None of these conditions has been thoroughly characterized morphologically. Presumably the Guillain-Barré picture results from immune-mediated demyelination and resembles the condition discussed in Chapter 3. It is generally held that both diffuse sensorimotor neuropathy and multiple mononeuropathy somehow result from ischemia secondary to vasculitis, since arteritis is clearly associated with other manifestations of SLE. Severe multifocal neuropathy carries a bad prognosis and is best treated with high-dose corticosteroids. Whether the cases of symmetrical sensory neuropathy that may occur also have a vascular basis is still uncertain. The symmetrical sensorimotor neuropathy may be mild and is not inevitably an ominous prognostic sign. A postmortem study of one such case demonstrated widespread endoneurial deposition of amorphous material regarded as similar to the hematoxylin bodies characteristic of arteriolar deposits in SLE.[17]

SPANISH OIL SYNDROME

Consumption of adulterated rapeseed oil has been held responsible for the 1981 epidemic of pneumonitis, vasculitis, and myalgia involving approximately 20,000 people living in central and north-central Spain. A few months after the initial outbreak, a small proportion (10 to 15 percent) of affected individuals developed sensory-motor polyneuropathy which eventuated in profound, sometimes global, muscle atrophy, fibrosis and scleroderma, accompanied by severe body-weight loss.[18] In the initial phases of the illness, pathologic studies reveal a global, non-necrotizing vasculitis mainly affecting the initima and accompanied by inflammatory edema of lungs and affected muscles. Subsequently, peripheral nerves display epineurial inflammation, perineural fibrosis, and variable patterns of intrafascicular necrosis, possibly related to infarcts in the vasa nervorum; affected muscles commonly show extensive neuromuscular atrophy and interstitial fibrosis.[19] The causative agent of this devastating, multisystem disease is unknown; the pathology suggests an immune-mediated condition, and experimental animal studies fail to demonstrate a direct-acting neurotoxin.[20]

REFERENCES

1. ADAMS, WE: *The blood supply of nerves. II. The effects of exclusion of its regional sources of supply on the sciatic nerve of the rabbit.* J Anat 77:243, 1943.
2. HESS, K, ET AL: *Acute ischemic neuropathy in rabbit.* J Neurol Sci 44:19, 1979.
3. KORTHALS, JK AND WISNIEWSKI, HM: *Peripheral nerve ischemia. Part I. Experimental model.* J Neurol Sci 24:65, 1975.
4. HUTCHINSON, EC AND LIVERSEDGE, LA: *Neuropathy in peripheral vascular disease.* Quart J Med 25:267, 1956.
5. EAMES, RA AND LANGE, LS: *Clinical and pathological study of ischemic neuropathy.* J Neurol Neurosurg Psychiatry 30:215, 1967.
6. ASBURY, AK AND JOHNSON, PC: *Pathology of Peripheral Nerve.* WB Saunders, Philadelphia, 1978, p 110.
7. DYCK, PJ, ET AL: *Necrotizing angiopathic neuropathy: three dimensional morphology of fiber degeneration related to sites of occluded vessels.* Mayo Clin Proc 47:461, 1972.
8. KERNOHAN, JW AND WOLTMAN, HW: *Periarteritis nodosa: a clinico-pathologic study with special reference to the nervous system.* Arch Neurol 39:655, 1938.
9. LOVSHIN, LL AND KERNOHAN, JW: *Peripheral neuritis in periarteritis nodosa. A clinicopathologic study.* Arch Int Med 82:321, 1948.
10. PALLIS, CA AND SCOTT, JT: *Peripheral neuropathy in rheumatoid arthritis.* Br Med J 1:1141, 1965.
11. CHAMBERLAIN, MA AND BRUCKNER, FE: *Clinical and electrophysiological features of rheumatoid neuropathy.* Ann Rheum Dis 29:609, 1970.
12. WELLER, RO, BRUCKNER, FE AND CHAMBERLAIN, MA: *Rheumatoid neuropathy: a histological and electrophysiology study.* J Neurol Neurosurg Psychiatry 33:592, 1970.
13. CONN, DL AND DYCK, PJ: *Angiopathic neuropathy in connective tissue diseases.* In DYCK, PJ, THOMAS, PK AND LAMBERT, EH (EDS): Peripheral Neuropathy, Vol II, WB Saunders, Philadelphia, 1975, p 1149.
14. DYCK, PJ, CONN, DL AND OKAZAKI, H: *Necrotizing angiopathic neuropathy.* Mayo Clin Proc 47:461–475, 1972.
15. PARRY, GJ AND BROWN, MJ: *Selective fiber vulnerability in acute ischemic neuropathy.* Ann Neurol 11:147, 1982.
16. JOHNSON, RT AND RICHARDSON, EP: *The neurologic manifestations of lupus erythematosis: a clinical-pathological study of 24 cases and review of the literature.* Medicine 47:337, 1968.
17. SCHEINBERG, LC: *Polyneuritis in systemic lupus erythematosus. Review of the literature and report of a case.* N Engl J Med 255:416, 1956.
18. TABUENCA, JM: *Toxic-allergic syndrome caused by ingestion of rapeseed oil denatured with aniline.* Lancet 11:567, 1981.
19. MARTINEZ-TELLO, FJ, ET AL: *Pathology of a new toxic syndrome caused by ingestion of adultered oil in Spain.* Virch Arch (Path Anat), in press.
20. BEAUBERNARD, C, ET AL: *Spanish Oil Syndrome: experimental neurotoxicological study with rats.* Lancet, in press.

Chapter 16

INFECTIOUS AND GRANULOMATOUS NEUROPATHY (HERPES ZOSTER, LEPROSY, SARCOIDOSIS)

HERPES ZOSTER

Definition and Etiology

This condition results from infection of the nervous system with varicella-zoster virus. Peripheral nerve dysfunction stems from involvement of the sensory ganglia, peripheral nerves, and segments of the spinal cord.

Pathology and Pathogenesis

PATHOLOGY. Inflammation and hemorrhagic necrosis of sensory ganglion neurons is the hallmark of varicella-zoster. Distribution of lesions in any case is usually confined to one or two adjacent dorsal root ganglia, but the trigeminal ganglia and geniculate ganglia of the facial nerve may also be affected. Varicella-zoster virus particles can be seen in the appropriate ganglion neurons, and virus can be recovered from these loci during the active inflammatory phase.[1] Inflammatory changes, usually confined to the dorsal root ganglia and adjacent dorsal roots, occasionally involve the corresponding segments of the spinal cord. Necrotizing myelitis is present in the adjacent dorsal root entry zone and extends into the ventral horns.[2] The segmental nerves and dorsal columns display varying amounts of secondary axonal degeneration.

PATHOGENESIS. The pathogenesis of herpes zoster is poorly understood. It is generally held that, following a generalized varicella-zoster infection, virus lies dormant in sensory ganglia and becomes activated during various provocative situations (altered immune states, and so forth).[3] There is no direct proof of this notion, and in contrast with herpes simplex, the virus has never been recovered from the ganglia of asymptomatic individuals.

Clinical Features

Herpes zoster can occur at any age, may recur, is more frequent in older individuals and has an annual incidence of 0.1 to 4.8 per thousand. Malignancy, especially lymphoma, is the most common predisposing factor.[4]

Pain and paresthesias in one sensory dermatome often precede the appearance of vesicles by one to three weeks, and persist throughout the illness.[5] The vesicular rash is usually confined to one spinal segment, most commonly a thoracic dermatome. Vesicles become encrusted by 5 to 10 days and then disappear, leaving small scars. Rapidly developing segmental paralysis may follow the cutaneous eruption, especially in lumbosacral and cervical zoster.[6]

The CSF displays a variable pleocytosis and moderate increase in protein. Electromyographic evidence of denervation is present in cases with segmental weakness.

The prognosis for recovery is good in most cases. The most disabling feature of herpes zoster ganglionitis is persistent pain (postherpetic neuralgia). This syndrome of intense segmental pain occurs in about 10 to 20 percent of cases and may last for months or years.[7] Suggested treatments include local cold, local anesthesia, local counter irritation, vibration, and amitriptyline.[3] None is completely effective.

LEPROSY

General

At present there are estimated to be 10 to 20 million persons with leprosy.[8] Although unusual in Western medicine, apart from nerve injury and diabetes, leprosy is the most common treatable neuropathy in the world.

Definition and Etiology

Leprosy represents a chronic granulomatous infection by *Mycobacterium leprae* (Hansen's bacillus) which primarily affects cutaneous nerve, skin, and nasal mucosa. The two major clinical types are *lepromatous* and *tuberculoid*; a third type, *boderline* or dimorphous, has features of both major varieties.

Pathology and Pathogenesis

PATHOLOGY. The *lepromatous* and *tuberculoid* forms represent the polar extremes of immunologic response to *M. leprae*. The widespread neuropathy of *lepromatous* leprosy is thought to result from a poor immune response.[9] It is an extensive, diffuse, symmetrical neuropathy, featured by many organisms in Schwann cells and macrophages, and in the early stages, by well preserved nerve architecture and little focal granulomatous inflammatory reaction. PNS involvement extends well beyond the patchy skin lesions. Early stages are characterized by predominant infestation of Schwann cells of unmyelinated fibers by clusters of organisms, occasional foamy macrophages, and little inflammatory response. Eventually there is diffuse, near-total fiber loss; many cutaneous nerves are converted to swollen bundles of connective tissue.[10]

Tuberculoid leprosy, in contrast, is a focal or multifocal condition, and the superficial nerve involvement is often localized near the immediate zone of the skin lesions.[2] The nerve architecture is totally destroyed, even in early stages, by an intense inflammatory-granulomatous reaction. Few organisms are present. The focal nature and severe inflammatory cell reaction of *tuberculoid* leprosy are thought to result from a strong immunological response.

PATHOGENESIS. *M. leprae* probably enters the body through the skin or nasal mucosa. In *lepromatous* leprosy, bacillemia follows local infection[11] and organisms settle in stereotyped cool locations (distal extremities, exposed areas of the face, ears, scrotum) that are all several degrees lower than 37°C. This tendency probably explains the initial involvement of superficial cutaneous nerves.[12] Some focal nerve lesions may be related to entrapment secondary to enlargement of nerve trunks. Bloodstream dissemination probably has a much less important role in tuberculoid leprosy, and the initial lesions may be sited close to the portal of entry. It is suggested that there is both local spread from Schwann cell to Schwann cell[10,13] and along the axon.[2]

The eventual distribution of destructive nervous system lesions in leprosy thus appears to be dictated by the immune response of the host; for example, persons who develop diffuse PNS involvement (*lepromatous*) probably have poor specific cellular immunity, while individuals with *tuberculoid* leprosy, whose lesions may be restricted to patchy skin areas with adjacent nerve destruction, are immunologically competent.

Clinical Features

Sensory loss is the cardinal feature of leprosy, regardless of type. Initial sensory loss is due to intracutaneous nerve damage and not in the pattern of individual peripheral nerves or nerve roots. Generally, pain and temperature are the first modalities affected, perhaps reflecting early involvement of Schwann cells of unmyelinated fibers in superficial nerves.[14] Loss of sweating in anesthetic areas is also an early feature. Position and vibration sense and tendon reflexes are preserved because they are carried by fibers in deeply placed (i.e., warm) nerve branches. The overall spatio-temporal pattern of peripheral nervous system involvement is determined by the type of leprosy.

Tuberculoid Leprosy

Skin lesions (hypopigmentation) are anesthetic, reflecting concurrence of skin and nerve involvement. Anesthesia rarely extends far beyond the edge of the affected skin.[15] Generally, only one or two lesions are present over the entire body. The most commonly involved sensory nerves are the digital, sural, radial, and posterior auricular. Motor involvement may occur in the distribution of ulnar, median, or peroneal nerves. Affected nerves often are swollen, can be palpated, and usually display slowed nerve conduction from the earliest stages. Autonomic dysfunction of affected nerves is the rule, probably reflecting unmyelinated fiber involvement, so that the cutaneous lesions are anhidrotic.

Lepromatous Leprosy

Skin lesions are multiple and often not anesthetic, in contrast to *tuberculoid* leprosy. The stereotyped pattern and widespread nature of PNS involvement reflect respectively the tendency of *M. leprae* to localize in cool areas and the diffuse hematogeneous spread in low-resistance lepromatous leprosy.[16] Cutaneous thermal and pin sensory loss first appears over the ears, the dorsal surface of hands, forearms, feet, and lateral legs. In time (usually years) sensory loss extends to yield a stocking-and-glove distribution with palmar sparing, as well as nasal, malar, eyebrow region, and ear involvement.[15] At this stage, paralysis of the hands appears, secondary to ulnar nerve involvement above the elbow. Other motor nerves are spared at this stage, save for the deep peroneal branch at the ankle. Untreated cases then gradually develop sensory loss over the face and palms, paralysis of selected facial muscles and involvement of median and common peroneal nerves. Widespread anhidrosis is a pronounced feature of this illness. The tendon reflexes are relatively spared. In contrast to tuberculoid leprosy, the enlarged nerves of *lepromatous* leprosy may function well in the initial stages of the disease.[17]

Prognosis and Treatment

The prognosis for recovery from individual peripheral nerve lesions in *tuberculoid* leprosy is poor because of the extensive destruction of nerve architecture that characterizes even the early lesions. Early peripheral nerve lesions in *lepromatous* leprosy may be stabilized by antibacterial treatment and considerable function preserved. Later stages of *lepromatous* leprosy neuropathy carry a poor prognosis.[15]

The treatment of leprosy is best left to specialists. Specific chemotherapy with sulfones forms the cornerstone of therapy and diamino-diphenylsulfone (dapsone, DDS) is the drug of choice.[18] The daily dose is 50 to 100 mg, and in tuberculoid leprosy is continued for two years after the disease has become inactive. Therapy for lepromatous leprosy is continued for 6 to 10 years after bacilli can no longer be detected in skin smears, or perhaps for life. Multiple drug therapy is often used because of drug resistance, and the most common additional drugs are clufazimine[19] (B663) and rifampicin (rifampin).[15]

A most important aspect in the management of leprous neuropathy is the prevention of damage to anesthetic areas by accidental injury in burns, ill-fitting footwear, and so forth. Careful instruction must be given to patients at risk.

Reconstructive plastic and orthopedic surgery is helpful in individuals with severe neuropathy. Facial surgery and tendon transplants are among the most common procedures. In many parts of the world, the psychologic trauma that formerly resulted from prolonged hospitalization is now prevented by home treatment.

SARCOID NEUROPATHY

Definition and Etiology

Sarcoidosis is a multisystem granulomatous disorder of unknown etiology, most commonly affecting young adults and presenting most frequently with bilateral hilar lymphadenopathy, pulmonary infiltration, skin, or eye lesions.[20] Peripheral neuropathy of uncertain pathogenesis develops in 5 percent of cases; both multiple mononeuropathy, involving cranial and limb nerves, and symmetrical polyneuropathy occur.[21]

Pathology and Pathogenesis

It is likely that a mixture of localized granulomatous infiltration and vascular compromise play predominant roles in all forms of sarcoid polyneuropathy.[22,23] There are surprisingly few careful postmortem or nerve-biopsy studies of sarcoid polyneuropathy. Noncaseating granulomas develop within the endoneurium or perineurium of cranial nerve roots, spinal nerve roots, and peripheral nerves. Presumably they displace and compress adjacent fibers with resultant axonal degeneration. Granulomas may also infiltrate perineurial arterioles. A recent nerve-biopsy report from a case of symmetrical polyneuropathy describes near-occlusion of arterioles by granulomata, in addition to perivascular inflammation.[22] Necrotizing vasculitis and focal areas of ischemic nerve have not been described. There is no explanation for the frequent involvement of the seventh cranial nerve. Although the pathologic descriptions are sketchy, there now seems little support for the previous notions that facial neuropathy stems from parotid involvement or basal meningitis.

Clinical Features

MULTIPLE MONONEUROPATHY. There are two distinct types of multifocal neuropathy, one affecting cranial nerves (cranial polyneuritis) and the other, spinal nerves. Each may occur alone, or both patterns may coexist in the same individual.

CRANIAL MONONEUROPATHY. Cranial mononeuropathy in sarcoidosis is almost synonomous with facial palsy.[24] The clinical profile of an episode of facial nerve palsy in sarcoidosis is indistinguishable from severe idiopathic Bell's palsy. Pain behind the ear, sudden onset, and loss of taste are all characteristic. Hyperacusis is rare. Paralysis is usually complete, denervation is common, and incomplete recovery the rule. Although bilateral involvement is frequent, *simultaneous* bilateral involvement is rare; generally one side of the face becomes paralyzed and recovers before the other side is affected. Facial palsy may be the initial sign of sarcoidosis, or may appear after systemic disease is obvious. Other lower cranial nerves (8, 9, 10) are less commonly involved.[25,26]

SPINAL MONONEUROPATHIES. The spinal-nerve mononeuropathies of sarcoidosis have an acute or subacute onset and are generally indistinguishable from other mononeuritides (diabetes, necrotizing vasculitis). Patchy sensory loss over the trunk or abdomen accompanied by pain is particularly characteristic.[27] Rarely, there is predominant involvement of ventral roots, producing a syndrome of diffuse weakness resembling the Guillain-Barré syndrome,[28] but with a more insidious onset.

SYMMETRICAL POLYNEUROPATHY. This is a rare complication of sarcoidosis and few cases have been described.[22,23] The condition is a progressive, distal sensorimotor polyneuropathy, clinically indistinguishable from symmetrical polyneuropathies caused by toxic or metabolic diseases. Progression is either subacute or chronic, and the lower limbs are principally involved. Bilateral facial weakness may coexist. There may be little in the clinical profile to suggest multifocal destruction of nerves, and nerve biopsies have often failed to demonstrate the presence of sarcoid granulomata. Nevertheless, it is still possible that this disorder stems from widespread granulomatous infiltration. Paradoxically, this form of neuropathy is not usually accompanied by obtrusive evidence of systemic disease.

Diagnosis and Prognosis

The diagnosis of sarcoid mononeuropathy is not difficult when accompanied by signs of widespread systemic involvement (pulmonary, skin, ocular). Sural nerve biopsy is usually less helpful than muscle biopsy in mononeuropathy, unless there is clear evidence of sural nerve involvement. The differential diagnosis of the symmetrical polyneuropathy is difficult, since most patients do not display overt signs of systemic disease. The presence of facial nerve involvement would heighten suspicion of this disorder, and muscle or nerve biopsy is merited in such cases.

Little is known about the prognosis or natural history of symmetrical sarcoid polyneuropathy. Since some cases respond to corticosteroids,[28] a course of treatment is justified, the duration depending upon response. The mononeuropathies generally have a benign prognosis and gradual recovery appears to be the rule. Again, corticosteroid therapy may hasten and improve the degree of recovery. The usual regimen is prednisone 60 mg per day, tapered to 15 mg daily, and continued for the duration of the mononeuropathy.

REFERENCES

1. BASTIAN, FO, ET AL: *Herpes virus varicellae.* Arch Pathol 97:331, 1974.
2. HOGAN, EL AND KRIGMAN, MR: *Herpes zoster myelitis: evidence for viral invasion of spinal cord.* Arch Neurol 29:309, 1973.
3. BARINGER JR AND TOWNSEND, JJ: *Herpes virus infection of the peripheral nervous system.* In DYCK, PJ, THOMAS, PK AND LAMBERT, EH (EDS): Peripheral Neuropathy, Vol II, WB Saunders, Philadelphia, 1975, p 1092.
4. MULLER, SA: *Association of zoster and malignant disorders in children.* Arch Dermatol 96:657, 1967.
5. JUEL-JENSEN, BE AND MCCALLUM, BO: *Herpes Simplex Varicella and Zoster.* JB Lippincott, Philadelphia, 1972.
6. THOMAS, JE AND HOWARD, FM: *Segmental zoster paresis—a disease profile.* Neurology (Minneap) 22:459, 1972.
7. HOPE-SIMPSON, RE: *The nature of herpes zoster: A long term study and a new hypothesis.* Proc R Soc Med 58:9, 1965.
8. TRAUTMAN, JR AND ENNA, CD: *Leprosy.* In Tice's *Practice of Medicine,* Vol III, Harper and Row, New York 1970, p 1.
9. ASBURY, AK AND JOHNSON, PC: *Pathology of Peripheral Nerve.* WB Saunders, Philadelphia, 1978, p 184.
10. JOB, CK: *Pathology of peripheral nerve lesions in lepromatous leprosy: a light and electron microscopic study.* Int J Lepr 39:251, 1971.
11. DRUTZ, DJ, ET AL: *The continuous bacteremia of lepromatous leprosy.* N Engl J Med 287:159, 1972.
12. SABIN, TD, ET AL: *Temperature along the course of certain nerves affected in leprosy.* Int J Lepr 42:33 1974.
13. DASTUR, DK, ET AL: *Ultrastructure of lepromatous nerves: neural pathogenesis in leprosy.* Int J Lepr 41:47, 1973.
14. SABIN, TD: *Temperature-linked sensory loss: a unique pattern in leprosy.* Arch Neurol 20:257, 1969.
15. SABIN, TD AND SWIFT, TR: *Leprosy.* In DYCK, PJ, THOMAS, PK AND LAMBERT, EH (EDS): Peripheral Neuropathy, Vol II, WB Saunders, Philadelphia, 1975, p 1166.
16. HASTINGS, RC, ET AL: *Bacterial density in the skin in lepromatous leprosy as related to temperature.* Lepr Rev 39:71, 1968.

17. DASTUR, DK: *Cutaneous nerve in leprosy: the relationship between histopathology and cutaneous sensibility.* Brain 78:615, 1955.

18. JACOBSON, RR AND TRAUTMAN, JR: *The treatment of leprosy with the sulfones. I. Faget's original 22 patients: a thirty year follow-up on sulfone therapy for leprosy.* Int J Lepr 39:726, 1971.

19. HASTINGS, RC AND TRAUTMAN, JR: *B663 in lepromatous leprosy: Effect in erythema nodusum leprosum.* Lepr Rev 39:3, 1968.

20. SILTZBACH, LE, ET AL: *Course and prognosis of sarcoidosis around the world.* Am J Med 57:847, 1974.

21. DELANEY, P: *Neurological manifestations of sarcoidosis: review of the literature, with a report of 23 cases.* Ann Int Med 87:336, 1977.

22. OH, SJ: *Sarcoid polyneuropathy: A histologically proved case.* Ann Neurol 7:178, 1980.

23. NEMMI, R, ET AL: *Symmetric sarcoid polyneuropathy: analysis of a sural nerve biopsy.* Neurology (Minneap) 31:1217, 1981.

24. SUCHENWIRTH, R: *Die Sarkoidose des Nervensystems.* Münch Med Wochenschr 110:580, 1968.

25. MATTHEWS, WB: *Sarcoidosis of the nervous system.* J Neurol Neurosurg Psychiatry 28:23, 1965.

26. THARP, BR AND PFEIFFER, JB: *Sarcoidosis and the acoustic nerve.* Arch Otolaryngol 90:360, 1969.

27. COLOREX, J: *Sarcoidosis with involvement of the nervous system.* Brain 71:451, 1948.

28. STRICKLAND, GT AND MOSER, KM: *Sarcoidosis with a Landry-Guillain-Barré syndrome and clinical response to corticosteroids.* Am J Med 43:131, 1967.

Chapter 17

ACUTE TRAUMATIC LESIONS OF NERVE

DEFINITION AND ETIOLOGY

Acute nerve injury refers to damage resulting from sudden compression, transection, or stretching.

Classification

Classification of acute nerve injury continues to be a source of controversy.[1-5] Experimental studies indicate three basic types: mild injury where axonal integrity is maintained but myelin may be damaged;[6] more severe, where axonal continuity is lost but the connective tissue framework of the nerve is maintained;[7] and most severe injuries in which nerve fibers and connective tissue are damaged to varying degrees.[8-11] Table 6 shows the anatomic classification of acute nerve injury.

Pathology and Pathogenesis

CLASS 1 (NEURAPRAXIA[1]). This lesion is a blockade of nerve conduction commonly associated with mild or moderate focal compression of nerve.

TABLE 6. Anatomic Classification of Acute Nerve Injury

SUGGESTED NOMENCLATURE	PREVIOUS NOMENCLATURE	ANATOMIC LESION
Class 1	Neurapraxia transient delayed reversible	Conduction block due to ischemia demyelination
Class 2	Axonotmesis	Axonal interruption
Class 3	Neurotmesis partial	Nerve fiber interruption with connective tissue damage
	complete	with nerve severance

There are two types: one is a mild, rapidly reversible type of block, most commonly resulting from transient *ischemia* of nerve (sitting with legs crossed); there is no anatomic lesion.[12] The other type results in more persistent conduction block and is assumed to result from paranodal demyelination (although direct pathologic confirmation in man is not available). This type of conduction block has been reproduced experimentally by inflating a pneumatic tourniquet around limbs of cats[13] and baboons.[6] Myelin sheaths are displaced away from the site of compression, causing overriding and damage of adjacent myelin segments, which results in localized demyelination (see Figure 12, Chapter 2). Large-diameter fibers are affected more than smaller. Recovery is associated with paranodal remyelination.

CLASS 2 (AXONOTMESIS[1]). This lesion is associated with closed-crush and percussion injuries. Axonal interruption occurs, but the Schwann cell basal lamina around each fiber remains intact, as does the endoneurial connective tissue[14] (see Figure 13, Chapter 2). Although Wallerian degeneration occurs distal to the lesion site, regeneration is usually effective. All functions are restored since regenerating axons are guided back to their former terminations at the periphery by the continuous columns of Schwann cells which develop distally during the degenerative process.[7] Class 2 nerve injury is readily produced in experimental animals by crushing a surgically exposed peripheral nerve with smooth-tipped forceps.

CLASS 3 (NEUROTMESIS[1]). Severe nerve injuries of this type result from stab wounds, the close passage of a high-velocity bullet, or nerve stretching sufficient to rupture the connective tissue components of the nerve (see Figure 14, Chapter 2). As in Class 2 injuries, nerve fibers undergo degeneration distal to the injury, and regenerating sprouts grow from the proximal ends.[8-12] Some axons may traverse the lesion site and successfully grow along distal Schwann cell columns, but misrouting of axons commonly occurs and inappropriate end-organ connection may be established. Many regenerating fibers will grow in random fashion at the injury site because their basal laminae and connective tissue framework have been disrupted and collagen production is profuse. Continued growth and sprouting of these aberrantly regenerating axons results in the formation of a neuroma at the site of injury.[15] Neuromata may be intrafascicular if the perineurium has not been breached, lateral, or, in the case of total neurotmesis with wide separation of the nerve stumps, a bulbous terminal neuroma may develop. Such structures display a characteristic resilient texture and must be surgically removed if reunion of the cut ends is to be attempted. Surgical repair of individual fascicles is now preferred over simple anastomosis of the entire nerve, although the issue remains controversial.[4]

ACUTE COMPRESSION

TYPE OF INJURY. Focal compression of nerve commonly follows habitual adoption of certain postures (leaning on elbows), prolonged abnormal posture (drug overdose), moderate constrictive lesion (tourniquet paralysis), or a sudden crushing blow.[16] It is widely held that subclinically diseased nerves are more susceptible to the effects of pressure, while compression syndromes are allegedly more common in individuals with uremia, diabetes, malnutrition, and alcoholism.[17-19] Genetic factors may predispose to pressure neuropathy; for example, there is a rare hereditary form of multiple mononeuropathy that becomes symptomatic when individuals have minor trauma.[20,21]

ANATOMICAL CLASSIFICATION. Mild or moderate acute compression injuries, such as sleeping with an arm draped over a bedrail, usually produce Class 1 lesions. Severe compression (closed-crush) injury, such as being struck by a moving object, frequently results in a Class 2 lesion. Prolonged compression injuries, such as following drug overdose, may result in a mixed Class 1—Class 2 lesion. Both closed-crush injuries and severe prolonged compression may be associated with disruption of subcutaneous tissue, causing a connective tissue proliferation that impedes nerve repair,[5] and prolonged compression may result in bulbous cutaneous lesions.

Clinical Features

Class 1 Injury

GENERAL. Strength usually is severely impaired and tendon reflexes absent below the compression site in a Class 1 lesion, while sensory loss is less obvious and confined to large-fiber modalities. Sympathetic function is spared. This constellation of findings probably reflects the low vulnerability of unmyelinated sympathetic and small myelinated sensory fibers, and dependence of motor and tendon-reflex function upon larger myelinated axons which undergo focal demyelination.[5]

Careful nerve conduction studies will usually demonstrate a block and preserved response to nerve stimulation below the lesion. Nerve conduction studies are not helpful in distinguishing Class 1 (demyelinative) injuries from Class 2 (axon interruption) unless performed after an interval of five days, since distal portions of transected axons may continue to conduct for four days.[22]

RECOVERY AND TREATMENT. Recovery from Class 1 injuries usually occurs spontaneously within three months.[4] Recovery is simultaneous throughout the distribution of the affected nerve. Denervation atrophy of muscle does not develop because axonal continuity is maintained.

There is no specific treatment of Class 1 lesions other than appropriate orthotic devices (wrist splint for radial nerve palsy, etc.) and behavioral advice aimed at preventing recurrences.

Case History and Comment: Class 1 Compression Injury

An 18-year-old narcotics addict became unconscious following an accidental overdose. For six hours he lay on the right side with his elbow pressed against a table leg. When aroused, he discovered that his right hand was weak and numb, and came to the hospital. Examination revealed paralysis of all muscles of ulnar innervation, and diminished touch sensation over the hand in the ulnar distribution, with splitting of the ring finger. Pin and thermal sense was normal. A simple hand-wrist splint was applied to prevent claw-hand deformity. Three days later sensory recovery began. Motor nerve conduction studies on the sixth day revealed normal conduction in the ulnar nerve below the elbow and total conduction block across the elbow. On the tenth day, motor recovery commenced in the interosseous muscles and flexor carpi ulnaris, and, two days later, in the flexor digitorum profundus and adductor pollicis. Two months following the injury, motor and sensory function was almost normal.

COMMENT. Preservation of pin and thermal sense supported the clinical impression that the ulnar nerve was in continuity and unmyelinated axons were spared. Normal motor nerve conduction below the lesion of total blockade after six days suggested that most axons were not affected and the prognosis for full recovery excellent. Recovery began almost simultaneously in muscles innervated at multiple levels of the ulnar nerve, typical for this class of injury.

Class 2 Injury

GENERAL. Variable loss of sensory, motor, and sympathetic function occurs from interruption of unmyelinated and myelinated axons. Muscle atrophy is apparent after one month and may become extreme if all motor axons are transected. Areflexia is the rule. It is unusual in closed-crush injuries for all axons to be severed. Should this occur, anesthesia and total sympathetic dysfunction appear distal to the site of injury.[5]

Motor and sensory conduction studies performed after five days are useful both to document conduction failure and determine if any fibers have survived the injury. Electromyography performed after 14 days may demonstrate denervation potentials (fibrillation, positive sharp waves), although these are not constantly present.

RECOVERY AND TREATMENT. Although recovery is slow, the prognosis in closed-crush injuries is usually excellent since regenerating axons grow along their original Schwann cell tubes, ensuring that the pattern of motor and sensory restoration is appropriate. Recovery varies from a few months in a distal lesion, to over a year with proximal lesions since regenerating axons elongate slowly (1 to 2 mm each day). The pattern of slow recovery is proximal to distal, reflecting rate and course of axonal regeneration. Recovery occurs first in muscles closest to the site of injury. Electromyography will detect recovery earlier than clinical observation. During regeneration, light percussion over advancing tips of the axons may elicit a tingling sensation (Tinel's sign) referred to the area of distal innervation of that nerve. With time, this sign can be elicited in more distal sites, indicating continuing advance of regenerating axons. Reinnervation of denervated skin frequently is accompanied by distorted sensations, and a slight stimulus may produce unpleasant sensations. This state usually abates when reinnervation is complete.[4]

Treatment of Class 2 lesions is similar to that previously described for Class 1. Simple orthotic devices, physical therapy, and reassurance are all that is required. Surgical exploration and neurolysis (clearing of excess connective tissue to free nerve fascicles) are not indicated, except in cases where there has been severe trauma to adjacent subcutaneous tissues. Electrical stimulation of denervated muscles is of no benefit.

STRETCH INJURIES

TYPES OF INJURY. Stretch injuries are more often encountered with closed injury to the brachial plexus or roots.[23,24] They are seen following birth injuries, motorcycle accidents, heavy blows with downward displacement of shoulder, traction during falls when an individual hangs with an outstretched arm (straphanger's palsy), and so forth. Roots may be torn from the spinal cord with especially severe trauma, (nerve root avulsion), such as falling from a great height or from a moving vehicle. It is less well appreciated that stretch injuries of nerve may also be related to bony fracture dislocations. The site of nerve injury is sometimes remote from the bony injury (for example, common peroneal nerve at neck of fibula with displaced fractures at ankle). In addition, nerve injury from gunshot wounds is usually in part related to nerve displacement and stretch because of sudden expansion of tissues in the path of the bullet.[5,25]

ANATOMIC CLASSIFICATION. Stretch injuries commonly involve neurotmesis. The injury to axons and connective tissue is often diffuse, may be initially accompanied by hemorrhage, and eventually, intraneural fibrosis. Severe head or shoulder displacement may cause one more or cervical nerve roots to be torn from their attachment to the spinal cord.

Clinical Features

GENERAL. Traction injuries are characterized by complete loss of motor, sensory, and autonomic function in the distribution of the involved nerve.[4] There is considerable variation in the clinical pattern of traction injuries as exemplified by the following description of various brachial plexus lesions.

Severe traction lesions, commonly encountered in current medical practice as a result of motorcycle accidents, often damage the whole of the brachial plexus. With forcible downward displacement of the shoulder, as when someone is thrown forward and the shoulder strikes against an obstacle, only the *upper part* of the plexus, involving the contribution from the fifth and sixth cervical nerve roots, may be damaged. This pattern may also be encountered as a birth injury from traction on the head, or on the trunk in a breech presentation (*Erb's palsy*), and rarely in anesthetized patients during operation, or in individuals carrying heavy backpacks. Selective injury to the *lower part* of the plexus, involving the contributions from the eighth cervical and first thoracic nerve roots, occurs as a result of traction with the arm extended, as when an individual falls from a height and tries to save himself by hanging on to a ledge. It may also occur as a birth injury following traction with the arm extended (*Klumpke's paralysis*), but is less common than upper plexus damage.

The clinical profile of traction injury is sometimes complicated by neuroma formation or causalgia, or both. Since both entities are more frequent with penetrating wounds, they are described in the next section.

Electrodiagnostic procedures may help to localize the lesion following traction injury of the arm.[5] If the roots are avulsed, all muscles innervated by those roots will show denervation changes, including proximal paraspinal muscles. Sensory nerve action potentials will be preserved despite complete sensory loss (if additional damage in the plexus is not present), since the transection is proximal to the ganglion neurons. Myelography can also be used to confirm root avulsion by demonstrating empty root sheaths and, occasionally, meningoceles.

RECOVERY AND TREATMENT. Recovery from traction injuries is limited owing to the severe axonal and connective tissue disruption and the diffuse nature of the lesion. When the spinal roots are avulsed from the cord, efficacious regeneration is impossible. With total brachial plexus lesions, amputation of the limb may be advisable. Where the injury is distal to the dorsal root ganglia, lesions of the upper portion of the brachial plexus recover more satisfactorily than lower plexus lesions. Early recognition and the application of measures to reduce the risk of joint contractures are important in all traction injuries. Surgical treatment appears of little value in closed traction injuries, but is sometimes undertaken. Electrical stimulation of atrophic muscles or distal nerves is of no use, and drug therapy (e.g., carbamazepine) for pain, which may be severe and persistent, has little effect. Secondary depression is often a complicating feature and may sometimes be helped by antidepressants.

Spontaneous recovery is generally satisfactory in some birth injury cases. In the proximal (Erb's) form of brachial plexus damage from birth injury, weakness of abduction at the shoulder and flexion at the elbow often persist, although there may be little residual sensory loss. Full recovery takes place in about a third of these cases.

Case History and Comment: Traction Injury of Brachial Plexus

A 41-year-old policeman fell from his motorcycle at high speed, striking his head and the point of the right shoulder. He was unconscious for two hours, and on awakening in the emergency room, was unable to move his right arm. Examination revealed paralysis of all muscles of the right arm and shoulder and anesthesia of the entire arm below the axilla. Horner's syndrome was not present. X-rays of the chest and shoulder revealed no fractures, and he was discharged after one week in the hospital. Evaluation six and twelve months later revealed paralysis and atrophy of right upper extremity and shoulder muscles, descent of the head of the humerus, and total sensory loss below the axillary line. Electrodiagnostic studies demonstrated no motor or sensory conduction in nerves of the right upper limb and complete denervation of limb and scapular muscles. The patient declined myelography.

COMMENT. This case represents a severe traction injury to the entire brachial plexus, with an unusual degree of proximal damage as evidenced by scapular weakness. A myelogram might have helped to determine if root avulsion had also occurred. There was little to be gained by surgical exploration of the plexus in the absence of fracture, bony dislocation, or massive subcutaneous tissue damage. Failure of proximal muscles to recover after a one-year interval implies considerable endoneurial disruption in this case, accompanying nerve-root avulsion, and a poor prognosis.

PENETRATING WOUNDS OF NERVE

TYPE OF INJURY. Injuries that penetrate nerves are commonly associated with high velocity missiles, broken glass, and motor vehicle and industrial accidents. Rarely, nerves may be severely lacerated by fractures.

ANATOMIC CLASSIFICATION. Penetrating wounds generally produce partial or complete Class 3 lesions and are characterized by considerable disruption of connective tissue.[4]

Stretch injury to nerve often occurs together with penetrating wounds, additionally disrupting neural architecture over considerable lengths (see previous section). High-velocity missile wounds may cause all degrees of nerve damage.[2,4,25]

Clinical Features

GENERAL. Injuries associated with partial or complete nerve transection produce clearly defined areas of total motor, sensory, and autonomic dysfunction. Muscle atrophy proceeds rapidly for about three months, at which time about 80 percent of bulk is lost. Muscle can still recover function if reinnervated up to three years following nerve transection. Thereafter, there is a progressive loss of muscle fibers, and the prognosis for recovery becomes increasingly less satisfactory.

Shrinkage of the autonomous sensory zone of a nerve, its area of superficial cutaneous sensation, follows within days of complete transection. Presumably, this phenomenon reflects overlap in normal innervation. Clinically, it is important to recognize that shrinkage of an injured nerve's autonomous zone does not reflect regeneration. Pain, of a superficial "pins and needles" type, is commonly present in the autonomous zone of a transected nerve and abates within several months. Persistent deep pain or a dysesthetic over-response to touch may indicate neuroma formation. Both neuromas, in continuity with partial injury or stump neuromas, may be associated with spontaneous severe pain. Neuroma pain may also be generated by cold or pressure.[5]

With partial or complete lesions of median and tibial nerves, or the lower part of the brachial plexus, *causalgic* pain may be a troublesome consequence.[2,4] Although well described after missile wounds, causalgia may appear after a variety of nerve injuries. Causalgic pain may begin immediately or after an interval of up to 60 days or longer. The pain of causalgia is severe, intractable, and has a burning or smarting quality. Upon this may be superimposed severe paroxysms of pain provoked by touching or jarring the hand or foot, or by emotional factors. Vasomotor and sudomotor changes may be associated: the skin usually becomes dry and scaly, but excessive sweating may also be a feature. The patient adopts a protective attitude towards the limb, so that fixation of the joints of the fingers and wrist may develop, together with atrophic changes in skin and subcutaneous tissue. About 80 percent of cases are relieved by sympathectomy. Untreated, the pain gradually subsides over months or years. The pathogenesis of causalgia is unknown.

Transection of autonomic fibers causes diminished sweating and impaired vasomotor repsonses. Diminished sweating usually corresponds to the zone of autonomous cutaneous sensory loss, and it may be helpful to perform repeated sweat tests in detecting signs of recovery from nerve injury. Vasodilatation develops and persists for several weeks following injury. Moderate vasoconstriction then appears, resulting in a cold, pale extremity. Numerous "trophic" disturbances commonly affect denervated extremities, such as thickened fingertips and shiny, atrophic keratotic skin.[4] Minor trauma, acting in conjunction with vasomotor malfunction in anesthetic fingers and toes, probably accounts for most of these phenomena.

RECOVERY AND TREATMENT. The prognosis for recovery, even with optimal surgical care, is usually only fair because axons often fail to reach their original end-organs. The treatment of penetrating nerve injuries is by reconstructive surgery and is best carried out by expert teams. Its discussion is beyond the scope of this book.

A decision to operate on a functionless injured nerve is facilitated by knowledge that the nerve has been severed. The initial clinical examination cannot disclose whether the loss of function is due to nerve severance or whether the nerve remains in total or partial continuity. This information is crucial in deciding the course of management. Loss of function following injury from sharp objects usually indicates complete or partial nerve severance. However, it is remarkable how often a nerve remains in continuity following lacerating missile wounds, probably reflecting the tensile strength of its connective tissue.

The following general rules are helpful in managing suspected penetrating wounds of nerve:

(1) In any instance where the nerve is known to be transected, surgical intervention (at the appropriate time) is mandatory.

(2) In a *distal* wound, such as the ulnar nerve at the wrist, where the nerve is not known to be transected, approximately three months should be allowed for the earliest signs of reinnervation before surgical intervention.

(3) In a *proximal* lesion, such as a missile wound of the buttock or axilla, surgery is almost always indicated, since the patient may have to wait 200 days for the first signs of spontaneous recovery.

CLINICAL FEATURES OF ACUTE AND SUBACUTE INJURIES OF SPECIFIC NERVES

Brachial Plexus

UPPER. Selective acute damage to the upper portion of the plexus (C_5 and C_6 roots or upper trunk) results in paralysis of deltoid, biceps, brachialis, brachioradialis and, sometimes, supraspinatus, infraspinatus, and subscapularis (see Figure 17). If the roots are avulsed from the cord, the rhomboids, serratus anterior, levator scapulae, and the scalene muscles will be affected. The arms hangs at the side, internally rotated at the shoulder, with the elbow extended and the forearm pronated in the 'waiter's tip' position. Abduction at the shoulder and flexion at the elbow are not possible. The biceps and brachioradialis jerks are lost. Sensory loss affects the lateral aspect of the shoulder and upper arm and the radial border of the forearm.

LOWER. Selective paralysis of the lower brachial plexus (C_8, T_1) results in paralysis of all the intrinsic hand muscles and a consequent claw-hand deformity, weakness of the medial finger and wrist flexors, and sensory loss along the medial border of the forearm and hand and over the medial two fingers. Cervical sympathetic paralysis, giving rise to Horner's syndrome, is frequently associated. Subacutely, the lower plexus may be invaded by tumors. Most commonly, this occurs from carcinoma of the lung (Pancoast syndrome), which gives rise to wasting and weakness of the small hand muscles and of the medial-forearm wrist and finger flexors, pain and sensory loss affecting the medial border of the forearm and hand, and cervical sympathetic paralysis. Other tumors that may invade the lower brachial plexus include carcinoma of the breast and malignant lymphomas affecting the lymph glands in the root of the neck. Subacute upper-plexus damage may also occur months or years after radiotherapy for breast carcinoma. It can be difficult to distinguish from tumor recurrence but is less likely to be painful.

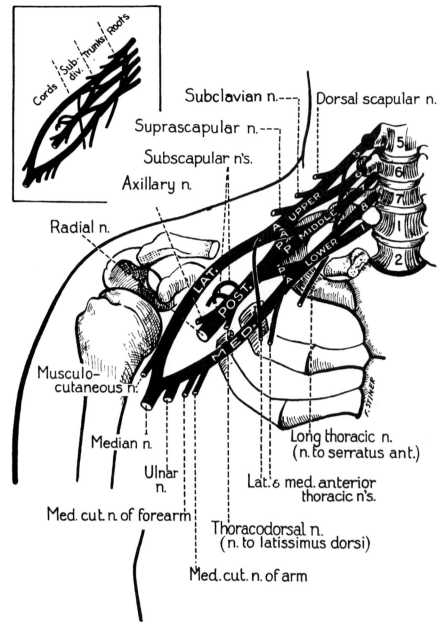

FIGURE 17. Diagram of the brachial plexus. The components of the plexus are depicted (out of scale) in the upper left. (From Haymaker, W and Woodhall, B: *Peripheral Nerve Injuries,* WB Saunders, Philadelphia, 1953, with permission.)

Radial Nerve (C$_5$-C$_8$)

The long course of the radial nerve and its position in relation to the humerus make this nerve unusually susceptible to external compression. It is a continuation of the posterior cord of the brachial plexus (Figure 18). In the upper arm, it supplies triceps and anconeus and the skin on the back of the arm through the posterior brachial cutaneous nerve. The lateral aspect of the lower part of the upper arm is supplied by the lower lateral brachial

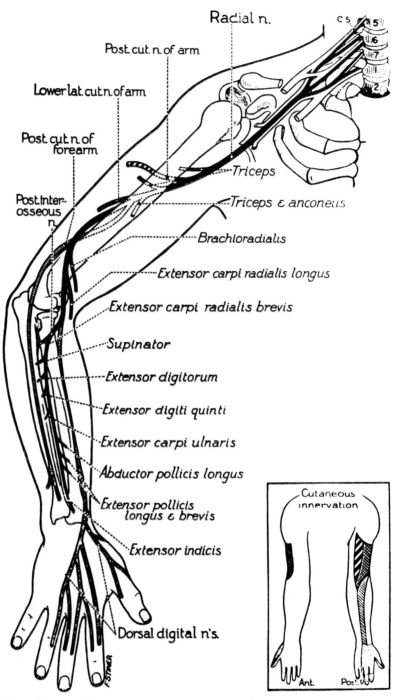

Radial n.

Post. cut. n. of arm

Lower lat. cut. n. of arm

Post. cut. n. of forearm

Post. inter-osseous n.

C 5 5
6
7
2

Triceps

Triceps & anconeus

Brachioradialis

Extensor carpi radialis longus

Extensor carpi radialis brevis

Supinator

Extensor digitorum

Extensor digiti quinti

Extensor carpi ulnaris

Abductor pollicis longus

Extensor pollicis longus & brevis

Extensor indicis

Dorsal digital n's.

Cutaneous innervation

Ant. Post.

FIGURE 18. The course and distribution of the radial nerve. (From Haymaker, W and Wood-hall, B: *Peripheral Nerve Injuries*, WB Saunders, Philadelphia, 1953, with permission.)

cutaneous branch and the dorsal aspect of the forearm by the posterior anterbrachial cutaneous nerve. Muscular branches of the radial nerve innervate brachioradialis and extensor carpi radialis longus and brevis. The superficial branch of the nerve is its continuation. It descends along the radial border of the forearm and supplies the skin over the dorsum of the hand and the thumb, index, and middle fingers. The deep branch winds around the lateral aspect of the radius, passes through the supinator, which it supplies, and innervates the extensor digitorum, extensor digiti minimi, extensor carpi ulnaris, and often extensor carpi radialis brevis. Its continuation is the posterior interosseus nerve which supplies the abductor pollicis longus, extensor pollicis longus and brevis and extensor indicis.

The nerve may be injured in wounds of the axilla so that paralysis includes triceps, resulting in loss of extension at the elbow. The most frequent type of injury is compression of the nerve in the middle third of the arm against the humerus. This is encountered as 'Saturday night paralysis', in which an individual falls asleep when intoxicated with his upper arm over the arm of a chair. In this injury triceps is spared, but brachioradialis, supinator, and all the forearm extensor muscles are paralyzed. Sensory impairment is limited to the dorsum of the hand. Commonly, the lesion consists of a localized conduction block (Class 1 lesion) so that muscle wasting does not occur and a muscle response can be obtained on stimulation of the nerve below the level of the lesion. Recovery is complete within a matter of weeks. A cock-up wrist splint may be helpful while recovery is awaited. At times, there is some associated axonal degeneration, so that electromyographic evidence of denervation is detectable and full recovery is correspondingly delayed.

Many muscles not supplied by the radial nerve work at a disadvantage when the wrist and finger extensors are paralyzed. These defects must not be mistaken for signs of injury to other nerves. Owing to the flexed position of the wrist, gripping is impaired, but if the power of the wrist and finger flexors is tested with the wrist extended, it can be shown to be normal. The action of the interossei in abducting and adducting the fingers is also feeble when the wrist is flexed, but full power is demonstrable if these muscles are tested with the hand resting flat on a table.

The deep branch of the nerve may be injured distal to the supinator muscle. The muscle is, of course, spared, together with the brachioradialis and the radial wrist extensors, and there is no sensory loss. A lesion of the posterior interosseus nerve gives rise to weakness confined to abduction and extension of the thumb and extension of the index finger.

Axillary Nerve

This is a branch of the posterior cord of the brachial plexus. It supplies deltoid and teres minor and the skin over the deltoid through the upper lateral brachial cutaneous nerve. It may be damaged in injuries to the shoulder, and the chief sign is an almost complete inability to raise the arm at the shoulder. In the past, the axillary nerve was sometimes injured by pressure from a crutch ('crutch palsy').

Musculocutaneous Nerve (C_5-C_6)

This nerve is rarely damaged alone, but may be involved in injuries to the brachial plexus. It supplies coracobrachialis, biceps, and brachialis and the skin over the lateral aspect of the forearm through the lateral antebrachial cutaneous nerve. Flexion at the elbow is still possible by brachioradialis, but is weak, and sensation may be impaired along the radial border of the forearm.

Median Nerve (C₆-C₈, T₁)

The median nerve arises from the medial and lateral cords of the brachial plexus and descends with the brachial artery through the upper arm, entering the forearm deep to the bicipital aponeurosis (Figure 19). It has no muscular branches above the elbow. It supplies all the muscles in the anterior apsect of the forearm, except flexor carpi ulnaris and the medial half of flexor digitorum profundus. The main trunk of the nerve supplies pronator teres, flexor carpi radialis, palmaris longus, and flexor digitorum superficialis. Through the anterior interosseous branch, it also supplies flexor pollicis longus, the lateral aspect of flexor digitorum profundus, and pronator quadratus. The main trunk passes deep to the flexor retinaculum of the wrist, and its recurrent muscular branch supplies abductor pollicis brevis, opponens pollicis, and contributes to the innervation of flexor pollicis brevis. It also supplies the lateral two lumbrical muscles and the skin of the lateral aspect of the palm, and the lateral three and a half digits over their palmar aspects and terminal parts of their dorsal aspects.

Lesions in the Forearm

The median nerve may be injured in the region of the elbow or compressed at the level of the pronator teres muscle. Occasionally, the anterior interosseus branch is involved in isolation.

Complete lesions of the median nerve at the elbow cause paralysis of pronator teres, the radial flexor of the wrist, the long finger flexors (except the ulnar half of the deep flexor), most of the muscles of the thenar eminence, and the two radial lumbricals. In brief, there is an inability to flex the index finger and the distal phalanx of the thumb, flexion of the middle finger is weak, and opposition of the thumb is defective. The appearance of the hand has been described as simian; it shows ulnar deviation, the index and middle fingers are more extended than normal, and the thumb lies in the same plane as the fingers.

Sensory loss is evident over the lateral three and a half digits and the lateral aspect of the palm, although individual variations occur. There is almost complete anesthesia over the two terminal phalanges of the index and middle fingers. This degree of sensory loss, combined with the motor deficit, renders the thumb and index finger almost useless and *makes paralysis of the median the most serious single nerve lesion in the upper limb.*

Lesions at the Wrist

The superficial situation of the median nerve at the wrist renders it liable to injury in lacerations sustained by falling against a window with the hand outstretched or in sucidal attempts. The clinical profile of injury at this level described in Chapter 18 under Carpal Tunnel Syndrome.

Ulnar Nerve (C₇, C₈, T₁)

This nerve arises from the medial cord of the plexus, usually with a contribution from the lateral cord (Figure 20). It descends in the medial side of

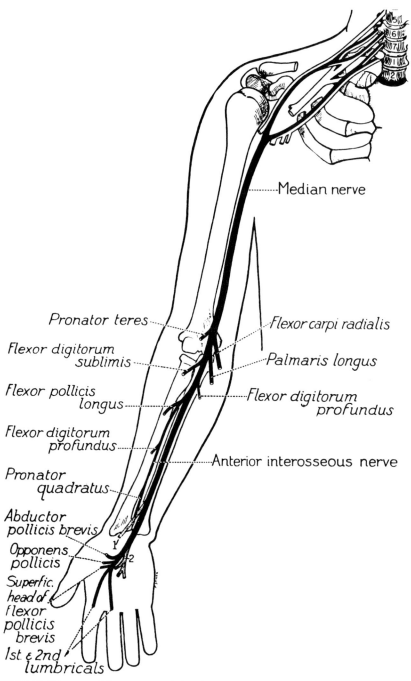

Median nerve

Pronator teres

Flexor digitorum sublimis

Flexor pollicis longus

Flexor digitorum profundus

Pronator quadratus

Abductor pollicis brevis

Opponens pollicis

Superfic. head of flexor pollicis brevis

1st. & 2nd lumbricals

Flexor carpi radialis

Palmaris longus

Flexor digitorum profundus

Anterior interosseous nerve

FIGURE 19. Diagram of the course and distribution of the median nerve. Number 1 indicates the palmar cutaneous branch, number 2 the palmar digital nerves. (From Haymaker, W and Woodhall, B: *Peripheral Nerve Injuries*, WB Saunders, Philadelphia, 1953, with permission.)

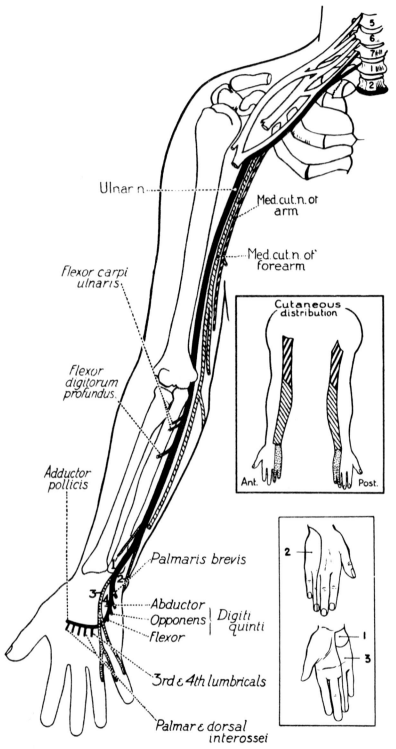

Ulnar n
Med. cut. n. of arm
Med. cut. n. of forearm
Flexor carpi ulnaris
Flexor digitorum profundus
Adductor pollicis

Cutaneous distribution
Ant.   Post.

Palmaris brevis

Abductor
Opponens } Digiti quinti
flexor

3rd & 4th lumbricals

Palmar & dorsal interossei

FIGURE 20. The origin and distribution of the ulnar nerve, the medial cutaneous nerve of the forearm and medial cutaneous nerve of the arm. The numbered nerves are the following: 1, palmar branch; 2, dorsal branch; 3, superficial terminal branch; 4, deep terminal branch. The fields of innervation of 1, 2, and 3 are depicted in the inset. (From Haymaker, W and Woodhall, B: *Peripheral Nerve Injuries*, WB Saunders, Philadelphia, 1953, with permission.)

the upper arm, passes around the elbow in the ulnar groove and enters the forearm under an aponeurotic band between the humeral and ulnar heads of flexor carpi ulnaris. It then runs superficial to flexor digitorum profundus to the wrist and enters the hand between the pisiform bone and the hook of the hamate, superficial to the flexor retinaculum. After penetrating the hypothenar muscles, its deep branch crosses the palm and ends in the flexor pollicis brevis.

In the upper arm, branches arise that supply flexor carpi ulnaris and the medial part of flexor digitorum profundus. In the forearm, the dorsal branch arises and winds around the ulnar and supplies the skin over the dorsal aspect of the hand and the medial one and a half fingers. In the hand, a superficial branch supplies palmaris brevis and the skin over the medial aspect of the palm and the medial one and a half fingers. The deep branch, after supplying the hypothenar muscles, innervates the interossei, the third and fourth lumbricals, the adductor pollicis, and part of flexor pollicis brevis.

Lesions of the ulnar nerve in the arm and forearm are common with penetrating wounds and at the wrist in suicide attempts. The specific clinical pattern in ulnar nerve lesions at various levels is described in Chapter 18.

Lumbosacral Plexus

Acute lesions of the lumbosacral plexus are uncommon. It may be compressed by a hematoma in patients receiving anticoagulant therapy or suffering from hemophilia, or be involved in fractures of the pelvis. The lumbosacral cord may be compressed against the rim of the pelvis during parturition by the fetal head, with consequent weakness of the anterior tibial and peroneal muscles, and sensory impairment in the distribution of the fourth and fifth lumbar dermatomes. The superior gluteal nerve may also be affected. Recovery is initially good but may not be complete. Subacute injury to the plexus may stem from pelvic malignancy, such as from carcinoma of the cervix, bladder, prostate or rectum, or be the site of a local neural tumor.

Femoral Nerve (L_2-L_4)

This nerve arises from the lumbar plexus, crosses the iliac fossa between the psoas and iliacus muscles, and enters the thigh deep to the middle of the inguinal ligament (Figure 21). In the iliac fossa it supplies the iliacus, and in the thigh, pectineus, sartorius, and quadriceps femoris, and anterior cutaneous branches to the front of the thigh. The continuation of the femo-

Damage to the femoral nerve causes weakness of knee extension, wasting of the quadriceps, loss of the knee jerk, and sensory impairment over the front of the thigh and in the distribution of the saphenous nerve. With a proximal lesion, there may also be weakness of hip flexion from paralysis of iliacus.

The femoral nerve may be injured in fractures of the pelvis or femur, in dislocations of the hip, and at times during operations on the hip. Subacutely, it may be involved by psoas abscesses, tumors, or implicated in wounds of the thigh. Owing to the rapid dispersion of the branches of the thigh, partial lesions are common from wounds at the site. The nerve to quadriceps is most often injured. The resulting paralysis causes consider-

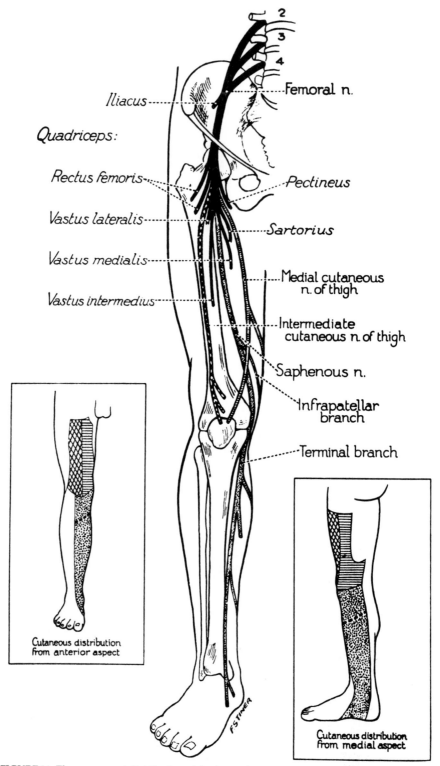

Figure labels:

2
3
4

Iliacus

Quadriceps:

Rectus femoris

Vastus lateralis

Vastus medialis

Vastus intermedius

Femoral n.

Pectineus

Sartorius

Medial cutaneous n. of thigh

Intermediate cutaneous n. of thigh

Saphenous n.

Infrapatellar branch

Terminal branch

Cutaneous distribution from anterior aspect

Cutaneous distribution from medial aspect

F STINER

FIGURE 21. The course and distribution of the femoral nerve. The broken line in the cutaneous field of the saphenous nerve represents the boundry between the infrapatellar and terminal branches. (From Haymaker, W and Woodhall, B: *Peripheral Nerve Injuries*, WB Saunders, Philadelphia, 1953, with permission.)

able difficulty in walking, as the knee cannot be locked in extension and gives way, especially when descending stairs. The saphenous nerve is sometimes damaged in operations for the treatment of varicose veins.

Obturator Nerve (L$_2$-L$_4$)

The nerve emerges from the lateral border of psoas, crosses the lateral wall of the pelvis, and enters the thigh through the obturator foramen where it supplies gracilis, adductor longus and brevis, adductor magnus, obturator externus, and sometimes also pectineus, and the skin over the lower medial aspect of the thigh.

Damage to the obturator nerve results in weakness of adduction and internal rotation at the hip, pain in the groin, and sensory impairment on the medial part of the thigh. Subacutely, the nerve may be involved in neoplastic infiltration in the pelvis and can be acutely damaged by the fetal head or by forceps during parturition.

Sciatic Nerve (L$_4$, L$_5$, S$_{1-3}$)

The sciatic nerve enters the thigh through the sciatic notch. It is composed of the tibial and peroneal divisions, which are usually bound together within a common sheath (Figure 22) . It descends the posterior aspect of the thigh, initially deep to gluteus maximus and supplies semitendinosus, semimembranosus, and the long head of biceps femoris and adductor magnus through the tibial division, and the short head of biceps femoris through its peroneal division. It separates into the tibial and common peroneal nerves in the lower thigh, which supply all muscles below the knee, and both nerves contribute to the formation of the sural nerve.

Total interruption of the sciatic nerve gives rise to foot-drop. Walking is possible, but the patient cannot stand on the toes or the heel of the affected foot and the ankle is unstable. All muscles below the knee are paralyzed. If the injury is in the upper thigh, flexion of the knee is also weak. The skin is completely anesthetic over the entire foot, except for the medial border, which is supplied by the saphenous nerve. Pressure sores may develop. Anesthesia extends upwards on the posterolateral aspect of the calf in its lower two-thirds. Joint-position sense is abolished in the foot and toes. Beyond this area of complete anesthesia, there is a wide zone in which sensibility may be diminished. Sweating is absent on the sole and dorsum of the foot, but is preserved on the medial side. The ankle jerk is lost but the knee jerk is retained.

The sciatic nerve may be injured during misdirected intramuscular injections and fractures of the pelvis or femur. After the radial and ulnar, it is implicated in gunshot wounds more frequently than any other nerve. Partial injury of the tibial division may be followed by causalgia. Incomplete lesions of the nerve may be caused by pressure of the nerve against the hard edge of a chair in individuals who fall asleep while intoxicated. Similar lesions may occur in diabetic subjects, in whom the peripheral nerves are more susceptible to pressure neuropathy.

Tibial Nerve (L$_4$, L$_5$-S$_{1-3}$)

After separating from the peroneal division of the sciatic nerve in the lower thigh, this nerve passes through the popliteal fossa and enters the calf deep to gastrocnemius through the fibrous arch of soleus. It descends through the calf to the medial side of the ankle, passes beneath the flexor retinacu-

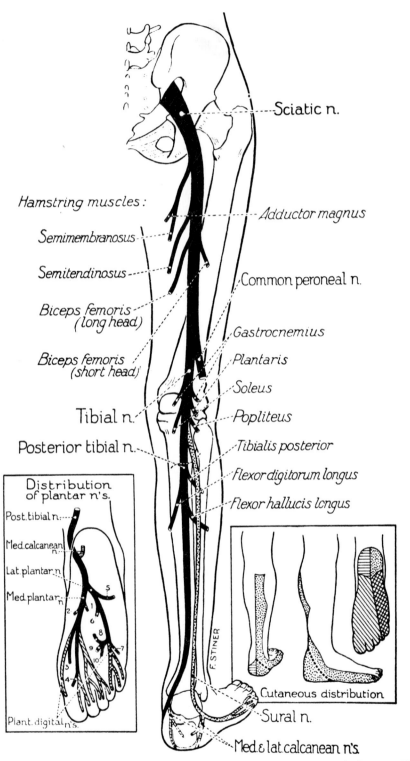

Sciatic n.

Hamstring muscles:

Semimembranosus

Semitendinosus

Biceps femoris
(long head)

Biceps femoris
(short head)

Tibial n.

Posterior tibial n.

Adductor magnus

Common peroneal n.

Gastrocnemius

Plantaris

Soleus

Popliteus

Tibialis posterior

Flexor digitorum longus

Flexor hallucis longus

Distribution
of plantar n's.

Post. tibial n.

Med. calcanean
n.

Lat. plantar. n.

Med. plantar.
n.

Plant. digital n's.

F. STINER

Cutaneous distribution

Sural n.

Med. & lat. calcanean n's.

FIGURE 22. The course and distribution of the sciatic, tibial and posterior tibial nerves. The cutaneous fields of the medial calcaneal and medial plantar nerves are indicated in the inset by lines, the sural nerve by dots, and the lateral plantar nerve by crosshatching. The numbered branches of the plantar nerves supply intrinsic foot muscles. (From Haymaker, W and Woodhall, B: *Peripheral Nerve Injuries*, WB Saunders, Philadelphia, 1953, with permission.)

lum, and divides into the medial and lateral plantar nerves (see Fig. 22). It supplies the popliteus, all the muscles of the calf, and through the plantar nerves, the small muscles of the sole of the foot and sensation to the sole.

When the nerve is interrupted, usually by a gunshot or stab wound, the patient is unable to plantarflex or invert the foot, or flex the toes. The calf muscles eventually atrophy. He cannot stand on the ball of the foot. Paralysis of the interossei leads to a claw-like deformity of the toes. Sensation is lost over the sole. Causalgia may arise after partial lesions. Injury to the distal portion is followed by atrophy of the intrinsic muscles of the medial sole.

The "tarsal-tunnel syndrome" associated with entrapment to the terminal portion of the nerve beneath the tarsal tunnel is considered in Chapter 18.

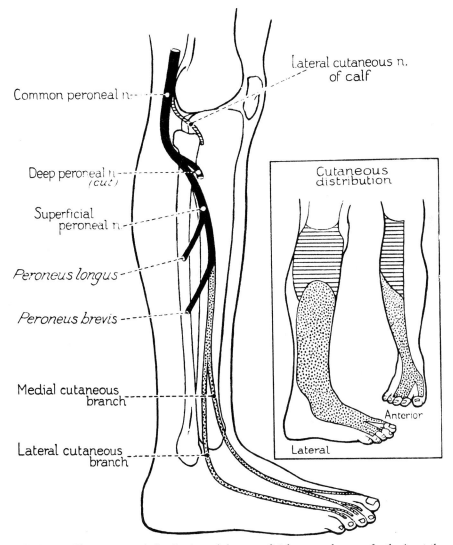

FIGURE 23. The course and distribution of the superficial peroneal nerve. In the inset the dotted pattern is the cutaneous field of the superficial peroneal nerve, the lined pattern that of the lateral cutaneous nerve of the calf. (From Haymaker, W and Woodhall, B: *Peripheral Nerve Injuries*, WB Saunders, Philadelphia, 1953, with permission.)

Sural Nerve (L_5, $S_{1,2}$)

This arises from the sciatic nerve and descends to the back of the calf, winds around to the lateral side of the ankle and reaches the lateral border of the foot (see Fig. 22). It supplies the skin in this distribution and has no motor fibers except for an aberrant innervation of extensor digitorum brevis in some individuals. Sensory impairment occasionally results from pressure on the nerve as it lies in a superficial situation in the back of the calf, but most commonly is seen following diagnostic nerve biopsy if the whole nerve is removed at the ankle.

Common Peroneal Nerve (L_4, L_5 $S_{1,2}$)

After separating from the tibial division of the sciatic nerve in the lower part of the thigh, this nerve descends through the popliteal fossa, winds

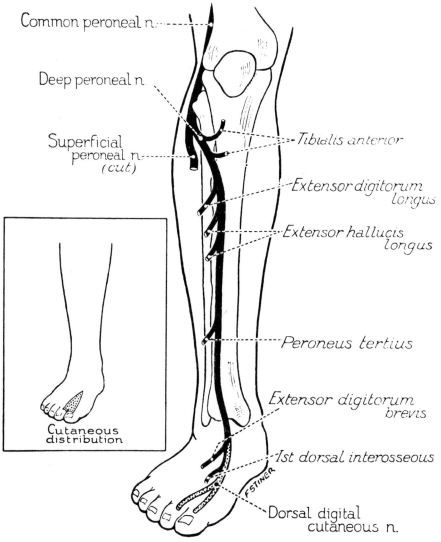

FIGURE 24. The course and distribution of the deep peroneal nerve. (From Haymaker, W and Woodhall, B: *Peripheral Nerve Injuries*, WB Saunders, Philadelphia, 1953, with permission.)

around the neck of the fibula, and divides into its superficial and deep branches. The superficial peroneal nerve passes down in front of the fibula, supplies peroneus longus and brevis, and emerges in the lower leg (Figure 23). It crosses the extensor retinaculum and supplies the skin on the dorsum of the foot and the second to the fifth toes. The deep peroneal branch continues to wind around the fibula, pierces the anterior intermuscular septum, and then descends on the anterior interosseous membrane (Figure 24) . It innervates tibialis anterior, extensor hallucis longus, extensor digitorum longus, and peroneus tertius. It passes deep to the extensor retinaculum where it supplies the extensor digitorum brevis and the skin of the adjacent sides of the first and second toes.

Damage to the common peroneal nerve is more frequent than injury to its two branches because of its vulnerable superficial position at the neck of the fibula. Trivial trauma, sometimes unnoticed by the patient, may cause dysfunction of the common peroneal nerve. Injury gives rise to footdrop with paralysis of dorsiflexion and eversion at the ankle and of toe extension. Cutaneous sensation is impaired over the lateral aspect of the lower leg and ankle and on the dorsum of the foot.

The common peroneal nerve may be compressed at the neck of the fibula by habitual sitting with the legs crossed, prolonged squatting, pressure during sleep or while anesthetized, and various other events. It can be damaged by traction caused by fractures of the tibia and fibula and is sometimes damaged by ischemia in the anterior tibial syndrome. Paralysis caused by external pressure frequently gives rise to a local conduction block (Class 1 injury) with satisfactory recovery within a few weeks. If electromyography indicates that nerve degeneration has taken place, a foot-drop support should be provided while axonal regeneration is awaited.

REFERENCES

1. SEDDON, HJ: *Three types of nerve injury.* Brain 66:327, 1943.

2. SEDDON, HJ: *Surgical Disorders of Peripheral Nerves.* Churchill Livingstone, London and Edinburgh, 1972.

3. THOMAS, PK: *Nerve Injury.* In BELLAIRS, R AND GRAY, EG (EDS): *Essays on the Nervous System—A Festschrift for Professor J. Z. Young.* Clarendon Press, Oxford, 1974, p 44.

4. SUNDERLAND, S: *Nerves and Nerve Injuries.* 2e, Churchill Livingstone, Edinburgh and London, 1978.

5. GILLIATT, RW: *Physical injury to peripheral nerves: physiologic and electrodiagnostic aspects.* Mayo Clin Proc 56:361, 1981.

6. OCHOA, J, ET AL: *Anatomical changes in peripheral nerves compressed by a pneumatic tourniquet.* J Anat 113:433, 1972.

7. HAFTEK, J AND THOMAS, PK: *Electron-microscope observations on the effects of localized crush injuries on the connective tissues of peripheral nerve.* J Anat 103:233, 1968.

8. MORRIS, JH, ET AL: *A study of degeneration and regeneration in the divided rat sciatic nerve based on electron microscopy. I. The traumatic degeneration of myelin in the proximal stump of the divided nerve.* Z Zellforsch Mikrosk Anat 124:76, 1972.

9. MORRIS, JH, ET AL: *A study of degeneration and regeneration in the divided rat sciatic nerve based on electron microscopy. II. The development of the 'regenerating unit'.* Z Zellforsch Mikrosk Anat 124:103, 1972.

10. MORRIS, JH, ET AL: *A study of degeneration and regeneration in the divided rat sciatic nerve based on electron microscopy. III. Changes in the axons in the proximal stump.* Z Zellforsch Mikrosk Anat 124:131, 1972.

11. MORRIS, JH, ET AL: *A study of degeneration and regeneration in the divided rat sciatic nerve based on electron microscopy. IV. Changes in fascicular microtopography, perineurium and endoneurial fibroblasts.* Z Zellforsch Mikrosk Anat 124:165, 1972.

12. LEWIS, T, ET AL: *Centripetal paralysis arising out of arrested bloodflow to the limb, including notes on a form of tingling.* Heart 16:1, 1931.

13. Mayer, RF and Denny-Brown, D: *Conduction velocity in peripheral nerve during experimental demyelination in the cat.* Neurology (Minneap) 14:714, 1970.

14. Thomas, PK: *Changes in the endoneurial sheaths of peripheral myelinated nerve fibers during Wallerian degeneration.* J Anat 98:175, 1964.

15. Spencer, PS: *The traumatic neuroma and proximal stump.* Bull Hosp Joint Dis 35:85, 1974.

16. Gilliatt, RW: *Peripheral nerve compression and entrapment.* In Lant, AF (ed): Eleventh Symposium on Advanced Medicine: Proceedings of a Conference held at the Royal College of Physicians of London, 17-21 February, 1975. Pitman Medical, London p 144, 1975.

17. Denny-Brown, D: *Neurological conditions resulting from prolonged and severe dietary restriction.* Medicine 26:41, 1947.

18. Gilliatt, RW and Willison, RG: *Peripheral nerve conduction in diabetic neuropathies.* J Neurol Neurosurg Psychiatry 25:11, 1962.

19. Preswick, G and Jeremy, D: *Subclinical polyneuropathy in renal insufficiency.* Lancet 2:731, 1964.

20. Earl, CJ, et al: *Hereditary neuropathy with liability to pressure palsies.* Q J Med 33:481, 1967.

21. Behse, F, et al: *Hereditary neuropathy with liability to pressure palsies: electrophysiological and histopathological aspects.* Brain 95:777, 1972.

22. Landau, WM: *The duration of neuromuscular function after nerve section in man.* J Neurosurg 10:64, 1953.

23. Bonney, G: *Prognosis in traction lesions of the brachial plexus.* J Bone Joint Surg 41:4, 1959.

24. Bonney, G: *Some lesions of the brachial plexus.* Am R Cell Surg 59:298, 1977.

25. Puckett, WO, et al: *Damage to peripheral nerves by high velocity missiles without a direct hit.* J Neurosurg 3:294, 1946.

Chapter 18

CHRONIC NERVE ENTRAPMENT AND COMPRESSION SYNDROMES

DEFINITION AND ETIOLOGY

At least three types of injury are associated with chronic trauma to peripheral nerve:

(1) Compression in a fibro-osseous tunnel (carpal, cubital, tarsal tunnels)
(2) Angulation and stretch (over arthritic joints, cervical rib, under ligaments)
(3) Recurrent compression (occupational trauma to hands and feet).

Pathology, Pathogenesis and Animal Models

There is considerable variation among the three types of injury listed above. The histopathology of the tunnel syndromes has been extensively studied in man and in experimental animals; little is known about types 2 and 3.

In the human carpal tunnel syndrome the nerve appears enlarged immediately above the site and constricted in the compressed zone. Demyelination is prominent at the site of compression.[1,2] The morphologic features of demyelination in chronic entrapment differ sharply from the picture of invaginated nodes of Ranvier described in acute compression (see Figure 12, Chapter 2). Studies of the naturally occurring carpal tunnel syndrome in the guinea pig reveal that myelin segments are deformed in a tadpole-like manner, being bulbous at one end and tapered at the other.[3] The bulbous ends point away from the site of compression, indicating the direction of mechanical force. In time, myelin slips away and bare axons become remyelinated with thin sheaths. Eventually, in older animals, there is axonal destruction and Wallerian degeneration.[4] Unmyelinated fibers resist until late. Examination of human median nerves at the wrist, ulnar nerves at the elbow, and lateral femoral cutaneous nerves under the inguinal ligament has confirmed the observations in the guinea pig. It appears that mechanical factors are dominant in the demyelination of chronic compression. The role of ischemia is less certain. It is probably responsible for the acute attacks of pain in the carpal tunnel syndrome, and short periods of ischemia can reversibly block conduction in damaged fibers.[5] It is possible that ischemia has a role in the pathogenesis of long-standing chronic entrapment.

Experimental chronic nerve constrictions have been less adequately studied than acute constrictions. They have been examined by applying snug ligatures around the nerves in immature animals leading to constriction developing *pari passu* with growth,[6] and also by the application of contricting devices around nerves in adult animals.[7]

Clinical Features of Individual Conditions

Carpal Tunnel Syndrome

The median nerve (see Figure 19, Chapter 17) is compressed at the wrist as it passes deep to the flexor retinaculum. The usual presentation is with acroparesthesias.[8] These consist of numbness, tingling, and burning sensations felt in the hand and fingers, the pain sometimes radiating up the forearm as far as the elbow or even as high as the shoulder or root of the neck. The paresthesias are occasionally restricted to the radial fingers, but may affect all the digits, as some fibers from the median nerve are distributed to the fifth finger through a communication with the ulnar nerve in the palm.[9] The attacks of pain and paresthesias are most common at night and often wake the patient from sleep. They are then relieved by shaking the hand. The hand tends to feel numb and useless on waking in the morning but recovers after it has been used for some minutes. The symptoms may recur during the day following use, or at times when sitting with the hands immobile. Such symptoms of acroparesthesia may persist for many years without the appearance of symptoms of median nerve damage. In other patients, weakness of the thenar muscles develops, particularly of abduction of the thumb, and is associated with atrophy of the lateral aspect of the thenar eminence. Sensory loss may appear over the tips of the median-innervated fingers. Occasionally, patients present with symptoms of median nerve deficit (Figure 25) in the hand without acroparesthesias having occurred, or motor and sensory signs may be discovered incidentally in the absence of symptoms, particularly in older individuals.

The symptoms are usually characteristic. If confirmation is required in atypical cases, this can generally be obtained by nerve conduction studies.[10,11] In patients who are experiencing frequent acroparesthetic attacks, the symptoms may be reproduced by inflating a sphygmomanometer cuff around the arm above arterial pressure for two minutes.[12] At times, percussion over the carpal tunnel may elicit a Tinel's sign, or symptoms may be provoked by hyperextension of the wrist.[10]

The majority of cases occur in middle-aged and often obese housewives.[10] In younger women it is commonly associated with excessive use of the hands, and it may develop in males after unaccustomed use of the hands, such as in house-painting. In these instances, tenosynovitis of the flexor tendons is responsible. It may also be caused by tuberculous tenosynovitis at the wrist or involvement of the wrist joint in rheumatoid arthritis. It may develop as a consequence of osteoarthritis of the carpus, perhaps related to an old fracture. Other predisposing causes are pregnancy, myxedema, acromegaly, and infiltration of the transverse carpal ligament in

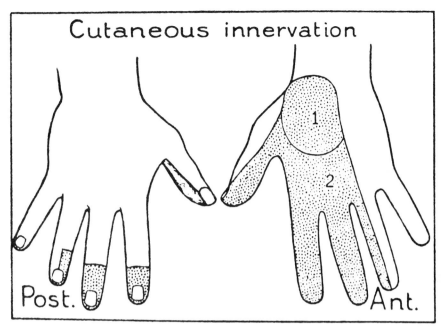

FIGURE 25. Cutaneous innervation of the hand by the median nerve. (From Haymaker, W and Woodhall, B: *Peripheral Nerve Injuries*, WB Saunders, Philadelphia, 1953, with permission.)

primary amyloidosis.[13] It is a frequent occurrence in patients who have been treated by hemodialysis for several years.

Individuals who present with muscle weakness and wasting, or sensory loss, should undergo decompression of the nerve by section of the transverse carpal ligament. In patients with acroparesthesia alone, and in which the cause is probably tenosynovitis at the wrist, reduction in the amount of activity engaged in with the hands may be sufficient to allow the symptoms to subside. Injection of the carpal tunnel with a long-acting hydrocortisone preparation may give temporary relief. Splinting of the wrist to reduce movement during the day may also be useful. If symptoms persist despite conservative measures, decompression is then advisable.

Most patients with acroparesthesia are relieved by decompression. In patients with sensory impairment and cutaneous hyperesthesia, such symptoms may persist for prolonged periods, and if denervation of the thenar muscles has been present for any length of time, recovery may not occur.[14]

Case History and Comment

A 60-year-old woman developed numbness and tingling over the palmar tips of the thumb, index, and middle fingers of the right hand. These sensations, initially most pronounced during vigorous house cleaning, in the course of a year became especially severe at night and were accompanied by an aching sensation of the right forearm. The sensation of numbness spread over the entire medial palm, accompanied both by a "pins-and-needles sensation" and a "tight, bursting" feeling. These sensations were temporarily relieved by exercising the fingers or swinging the arm. She tolerated this condition until handwriting became difficult because of palmar dysesthesias and weakness of the thumb. On physical examination, there was diminished sensation to pin, touch, and thermal stimuli over the palmar surface of the thumb, index, and middle fingers, with splitting of the ring finger. Sensation was normal above the wrist and over the dorsal hand. The right thenar eminence was less prominent than the left, and strength in the right opponens pollicis and abductor pollicis brevis muscle was 4/5. Tapping the wrist at the palmar junction elicited a tingling sensation that radiated into the tips of the affected fingers (Tinel's sign). Flexing the hands at the wrist for one minute aggravated the paresthesias in the right hand (Phalen's sign) and had no effect on the left. The remainder of the physical examination was unremarkable. Radiologic and laboratory investigations disclosed no evidence of rheumatoid arthritis, dysproteinemia, or thyroid dysfunction. Electromyography revealed fibrillation potentials and positive sharp waves at rest in the right opponens pollicis and abductor pollicis brevis muscles. Motor nerve conduction velocities, measured from elbow to wrist in both right and left median nerves were normal (48 m per sec). The wrist-muscle in the median nerve was 2 m per sec (normal) on the left and 9.3 m per sec on the right (prolonged). Sensory nerve action potentials elicited by digital nerve stimulation in the first digit and recorded from the median nerve at the wrist were of normal amplitude and latency (3 m per sec) on the left; none could be detected on the right. The patient refused surgery and was treated for two months with immobilization of the wrist with only moderate relief. An injection of prednisone into the carpal tunnel was followed by rapid amelioration of paresthesias which persisted for three months. However, the abnormal sensations gradually returned, were not helped by a second local corticosteroid injection, and the patient consented to surgery. The day following operative transection of the flexor retinaculum there was a dramatic lessening of the abnormal sensations. Nine months following surgery, sensation and strength were normal in the right hand, the right wrist-muscle median-nerve motor latency was 5 m per sec, and the sensory latency 4 m per sec.

COMMENT. This individual displayed many common features of the carpal tunnel syndrome. The condition frequently occurs in housewives, who presumably aggravate the entrapment by vigorous motions of the wrist. Nocturnal worsening, pain in the forearm, and distressing acroparesthesias promptly relieved by surgery are typical. Muscle wasting was definitive clinical evidence of axonal destruction and mandated surgery in this case.

Ulnar Compression

The ulnar nerve (see Figure 20, Chapter 17) may be damaged by dislocations or fracture dislocations at the elbow and is sometimes compressed in individuals who habitually lean on their elbows.[13] Entrapment may occur in the cubital tunnel where the nerve underlies the aponeurotic band between the two heads of the flexor carpi ulnaris.[15] This is most likely to occur in heavy manual workers, or if there is an excessive carrying angle at the elbow, or may occur years following a previous malunited supracondylar fracture of the humerus with bony overgrowth ('tardy ulnar palsy'). The medial wall of the cubital tunnel is formed by the elbow joint: osteoarthritis of the elbow can lead to osteophytic encroachment on the tunnel and compression of the ulnar nerve. In the cubital tunnel syndrome, the ulnar nerve is often palpably enlarged in the ulnar groove and for a short distance proximally. Ulnar nerve lesions are not infrequent in leprosy, where the enlargement of the nerve may result in compression. Here the enlargement of the nerve tends to be maximal just above the elbow.

Total paralysis from lesions at this level involves muscles innervated by the branches to flexor carpi ulnaris and flexor digitorum profundus, and gives rise to wasting along the medial side of the forearm flexor mass. Paralysis of the hypothenar muscles abolishes abduction of the fifth finger. Paralysis of the interossei and the medial two lumbricals gives rise to the 'claw-hand' deformity. Sensory loss affects the dorsal and palmar aspects of the medial side of the hand and the medial one and a half fingers.[13]

When it is suspected that the nerve has been subjected to repeated compression at the elbow, surgical transposition to the front of the medial epicondyle should be considered.[16] If the nerve is compressed in the cubital tunnel, decompression by slitting the aponeurosis may suffice. Damage to the nerve at the wrist will spare the dorsal branch, so that cutaneous sensation over the dorsum of the hand and fingers is spared.[17]

Lesions at the wrist or in the hand are usually the result of compression by ganglia or by repeated occupational trauma.[18] Damage to the deep palmar branch, for example, may be caused by firm pressure from a screwdriver or drill. If occupational injury is the problem, recovery follows cessation of the precipitating cause. Should improvement fail to occur after an appropriate interval, surgical exploration to establish whether a ganglion is present is merited.

It is not always easy on clinical grounds to decide whether the lesion is at the elbow or the wrist. Compression of the nerve in the cubital tunnel, for example, may spare the branches to the flexor carpi ulnaris and flexor digitorum profundus. In these circumstances, nerve conduction studies may be helpful, as they may in distinguishing between lesions of the ulnar nerve and damage to the eighth cervical and first thoracic spinal roots.[19]

Cervical Rib

The branches of the eighth cervical and first thoracic roots to the brachial plexus may be damaged by angulation over an abnormal rib or fibrous band arising from the seventh cervical vertebra and attached to the first rib. Although local structures such as the tendon of scalenus anterior may be involved in the production of symptoms, the isolation of a separate 'scalenus anterior syndrome' or of 'costo-clavicular compression' is not justified. The subclavian artery may be affected by cervical ribs, giving rise to aneurysmal dilatation and vascular symptoms such as Raynaud's syndrome and embolic events, but the simultaneous occurrence of both neural and vascular phenomena is rare.

Damage to the lower part of the brachial plexus by a cervical rib leads to weakness and wasting of the small hand muscles, and of the medial forearm wrist and finger flexors.[19] Occasionally, there is selective wasting of the thenar pad in the hand, mimicking to some extent the appearances of the carpal tunnel syndrome. Numbness, pain, and paresthesias occur along the inner border of the forearm and hand, extending into the medial two fingers. The pain tends to be provoked by carrying heavy articles in the hand on the affected side. Horner's syndrome may be a feature. Nerve conduction studies are helpful when there are difficulties in distinguishing a cervical rib syndrome from a lesion of the ulnar or median nerves on clinical grounds between.[19,22] Surgical removal of the rib or fibrous band often leads to abolition of the pain and paresthesias, but recovery of power in the small hand muscles is frequently disappointing.[23]

Lateral Cutaneous Nerve of the Thigh

This nerve arises from the lumbar plexus, passes obliquely across the iliacus muscle and enters the thigh under the lateral part of the inguinal ligament. It supplies the skin over the anterolateral aspect of the thigh.

Meralgia paresthetica is an entrapment neuropathy resulting from compression of this nerve as it passes under the inguinal ligament.[20] It is more common in obese men, and may be unilateral or bilateral. The symptoms consist of numbness in the territory of the nerve combined with tingling or burning paresthesias provoked by prolonged standing, or following excessive walking. Weight reduction may be helpful and in many instances the condition subsides spontaneously. Decompression of the nerve is rarely necessary.[21]

Tibial Nerve

The tibial nerve (see Figure 22, Chapter 17) is occasionally compressed under the flexor retinaculum at the ankle (*tarsal tunnel syndrome*), usually precipitated by osteoarthritis, post-traumatic deformities at the ankle or by tenosynovitis.[24,25] Burning pain and tingling paresthesias occur in the sole, usually following prolonged standing or walking. The condition is generally unilateral. Careful examination may demonstrate wasting of the intrinsic muscles in the medial aspect of the foot, and sensory impairment over the sole. Nerve conduction studies may be diagnostically helpful. Treatment is by surgical section of the flexor retinaculum.

Painful neuromas sometimes develop on the digital branches of the plantar nerves.[26] These give rise to the syndrome of 'Morton's metatarsalgia' in which pain occurs in the anterior part of the foot on standing. A localized area of tenderness is detectable on palpation. The condition is relieved by excision of the neuroma.

REFERENCES

1. NEARY, D AND EAMES, RA: *The pathology of ulnar nerve compression in man.* Neuropathology and Applied Neurobiology 1:69, 1975.
2. NEARY, D, ET AL: *Sub-clinical entrapment neuropathy in man.* J Neurol Sci 24:283, 1975.
3. OCHOA, J AND MAROTTE, L: *The nature of the nerve lesion caused by chronic entrapment in the guinea-pig.* J Neurol Sci 19:491, 1973.
4. FULLERTON, PM AND GILLIATT, RW: *Median and ulnar neuropathy in the guinea-pig.* J Neurol Neurosurg Psychiatry 30:393, 1967.
5. FULLERTON, PM: *The effect of ischaemia on nerve conduction in the carpal tunnel syndrome.* J Neurol Neurosurg Psychiatry 26:385, 1963.
6. AGUAYO, A, ET AL: *Experimental progressive compression neuropathy in the rabbit.* Arch Neurol 24:358, 1971.
7. SPENCER, PS: *Reappraisal of the model for "bulk axoplasmic flow."* Nature 240:283, 1972.
8. HEATHFIELD, KWG: *Acroparesthesiae and the carpal tunnel syndrome.* Lancet 11:663, 1957.
9. KENDALL, D: *Aetiology, diagnosis and treatment of paresthesiae in the hands.* Br Med J 2:1633, 1960.
10. KAESER, HE: *Diagnostische Problem beim Carpal-tunnel syndrome.* Dtsch Z Nervenheilk 185:453, 1963.
11. FULLERTON, PM AND GILLIATT, RW: *The carpal tunnel syndrome.* Lancet II:241, 1965.
12. GILLIATT, RW AND WILSON, TG: *A pneumatic tourniquet test in the carpal tunnel syndrome.* Lancet II:595, 1953.
13. STAAL, A: *General discussion on pressure neuropathies.* In VINKEN, PJ AND BRUYN, GW (EDS): Handbook of Clinical Neurology, Vol 7, North Holland-American Elsevier, Amsterdam and New York, 1970, p 276.

14. SEMPLE, JC AND CARGILL, AO: *Carpal-tunnel syndrome.* Lancet I:918, 1969.

15. EBELING, P, ET AL: *A clinical and electrical study of ulnar nerve lesions in the hand.* J Neurol Neurosurg Psychiatry 23:1, 1960.

16. HARRISON, MJG AND NURICK, S: *Results of anterior transposition of the ulnar nerve for ulnar neuritis.* Br Med J 1:27, 1970.

17. FEINDEL, W AND STRATFORD, J: *The role of the cubital tunnel in tardy ulnar palsy.* Can J Surg 1:287, 1958.

18. MUMENTHALER, M: *Die Ulnarisparesen.* Thieme Verlag, Stuttgart, 1961.

19. GILLIATT, RW, ET AL: *Wasting of the hand associated with a cervical rib or band.* J Neurol Neurosurg Psychiatry 33:615, 1970.

20. KEEGAN, JJ AND HOLYOKE, EA: *Meralgia paresthetica.* J Neurosurg 19:341, 1962.

21. ECKER, AD AND WOLTMAN, HW: *Meralgia paresthetica: a report of one hundred and fifty cases.* JAMA 110:1650, 1938.

22. URSCHEL, HG, ET AL: *Objective diagnosis (ulnar) nerve conduction velocity and current therapy of the thoracic outlet syndrome.* Ann Thorac Surg 12:608, 1971.

23. ROOS, DB: *Experience with first rib resection for thoracic outlet syndrome.* Ann Surg 173:429, 1971.

24. LAM, SJS: *Tarsal tunnel syndrome.* J Bone Joint Surg 49B:87, 1967.

25. LINSCHEID, RL, ET AL: *The tarsal tunnel syndrome.* South Med J 63:1313, 1970.

26. SCOTTI, TM: *The lesion of Morton's metatarsalgia (Morton's toe).* Arch Pathol 63:91, 1952.

CHRONIC NERVE
ENTRAPMENT AND
COMPRESSION
SYNDROMES

215

Chapter 19

CRYPTOGENIC NEUROPATHIES

These neuropathies comprise a group of common and uncommon disorders whose cause is either unknown or uncertain. Their importance lies mainly in their frequency.

SYMMETRICAL POLYNEUROPATHY

Acute and Subacute Polyneuropathy

These cases usually involve diffuse weakness, areflexia, sometimes cranial nerve involvement, and often an elevated CSF protein content. Most represent acute idiopathic inflammatory polyneuropathies without obvious antecedent viral illness, obscuring a ready diagnosis of postinfectious polyneuropathy of the Guillain-Barré type. This syndrome, when accompanied by mental changes, should suggest acute intermittent porphyria or thallium intoxication. Heavy metal intoxication, in particular arsenic and pharmaceutical agents (nitrofurantoin, vincristine), may also cause subacute polyneuropathy. These now are rarely cryptogenic conditions, since heavy-metal analysis has become part of a routine neuropathy evaluation and a history of drug ingestion, apart from alcohol, which may be denied, is customarily elicited. Acute and subacute polyneuropathies tend to prove diagnostically insoluble less often than chronic polyneuropathies.

Chronic Progressive Polyneuropathy

This group includes a mixture of adult-onset motor, sensory, and sensorimotor neuropathies.

Routine clinical evaluation yields a correct diagnosis in about one-half of individuals with symmetrical polyneuropathy. A recent report of 207 cases of symmetrical polyneuropathy, undiagnosed by initial evaluation and subsequently referred to a special center, claims that further intensive study can categorize about three quarters of the remaining "cryptogenic" cases.[1] Of the cryptogenic cases, about 42 percent were inherited disorders, 21 percent were chronic inflammatory demyelinating neuropathies, 13 percent were a mixture of diabetic, toxic, paraneoplastic, dysproteinemic and leprous neuropathies, and 24 percent remained undiagnosed.

Assessment of the individual with cryptogenic chronic symmetrical polyneuropathy is time consuming, expensive, entails considerable effort and inconvenience, and often requires hospitalization. Clinical laboratory studies will rapidly identify renal failure, diabetes, pernicious anemia, thyroid disease, dysproteinemia, malabsorption, and heavy-metal intoxication. A meticulous history, including interviews with siblings and parents, is crucial in detecting occupational and pharmaceutical neuropathies and hereditary conditions. It may prove necessary to examine and perform nerve conduction tests on family members with unsuspected, subclinical hereditary neuropathy. Nerve biopsy and sophisticated electrophysiologic testing will usually indicate whether the process is demyelinating or axonal in nature. Nerve biopsy is frequently diagnostic in multifocal neuropathies (leprosy, vasculitis) masquerading as diffuse symmetrical conditions.

Mononeuropathy Syndromes

Cases of chronic and slowly progressive multiple mononeuropathy, for which no explanation can be obtained, constitute an important category of cryptogenic neuropathy. There is no involvement of other systems and investigations reveal no evidence of arteritis, dysproteinemia, diabetes, leprosy, sarcoidosis, amyloidosis, hereditary liability to pressure neuropathy, or other conditions that may present in this way. Follow-up occasionally yields the explanation, but many remain undiagnosed.

Focal Cranial Neuropathy

Idiopathic Isolated Trigeminal Neuropathy

Rare cases are encountered of slowly progressive, bilateral sensory loss confined to the territory of the trigeminal nerve.[2] This may lead to tissue destruction, particularly around the nostrils, as a result of repeated picking and scratching. Sjögren's syndrome[3] and systemic sclerosis[4] require to be excluded, and some cases have been found at autopsy to show infiltration of the trigeminal ganglion with amyloid. The explanation in others is obscure.

Idiopathic Facial Paralysis

Bell's palsy is common: the incidence in the United States is 20 per 100,000 each year[5]. Although the condition was initially described over 150 years ago and has been thoroughly investigated, its pathology and pathogenesis are unknown and treatment is empirical.[6]

PATHOLOGY AND PATHOGENESIS. It is widely held that swelling of the facial nerve within the tight confines of the facial canal occurs in most cases; however, this notion stems from operative descriptions by enthusiastic surgeons and is not supported by morphologic data. Similarly, none of the postmortem studies has used modern neuropathologic techniques, and most reports appear to describe Wallerian degeneration.[7,8] It is likely that mild cases with rapid recovery reflect conduction block with segmental demyelination, and axonal degeneration occurs in instances with severe paralysis and prolonged or poor recovery. Hypotheses about the etiology of facial nerve dysfunction in Bell's palsy include injury from vasospasm, cold, viral, or immunologic inflammation, and venous thrombosis.[6,9-11]

CLINICAL FEATURES. Unilateral facial paralysis usually develops rapidly within a few hours or evolves over one or two days and is often accompanied by pain behind the ear and excess tearing. Numbness of the face is a common complaint, but inevitably refers to the sensation that accompanies weakness. Rarely are hyperacusis and diminished taste significant to the patient. Global facial muscle weakness is the hallmark of this condition, and is partial in 30 percent of cases. Hyperacusis, diminished lacrimation, and abnormal taste sensation are present to variable degrees. Figure 26 delineates the putative levels of involvement of the facial nerve in the common Bell's palsy syndromes.

Untreated, 80 to 85 percent of all patients with Bell's palsy recover completely or virtually completely. This applies to those in which the lesion is wholly or mainly a conduction block. In the smaller proportion, in which all or most of the fibers undergo Wallerian degeneration, recovery, which has to take place by axonal regeneration, is generally unsatisfactory and leads to persistent facial weakness. In occasional cases, motor recovery fails completely. Aberrant regeneration is frequently observed. There may be embarrassing synkinetic movements (Fig. 27) or excessive lacrimation, sometimes related to gustatory stimuli ('crocodile tears'). Patients who are going to recover completely usually begin to improve during the first two weeks, while those with permanent residual disability remain unchanged for approximately three months. Except in cases where paralysis is incomplete (Type I), there is little in the acute clinical profile that indicates prognosis. In patients with complete paralysis from the onset (Type II), reliance must be placed on careful observation and electrodiagnostic tests of nerve excitability (performed at about one week after the onset). Direct stimulation of the facial nerve trunk at the stylomastoid foramen reveals a normal

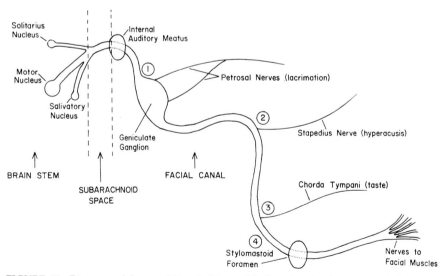

FIGURE 26. Diagram of four putative facial-canal lesion sites in the various Bell's palsy syndromes. Site 1—impaired lacrimation, hyperacusis, impaired taste, facial paralysis. Site 2—hyperacusis, impaired taste, facial paralysis. Site 3—impaired taste, facial paralysis. Site 4—facial paralysis.

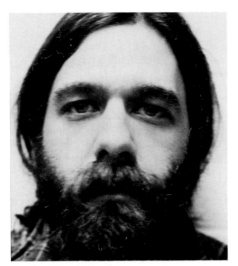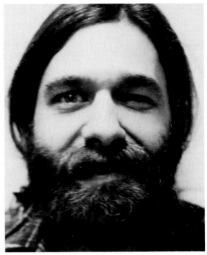

FIGURE 27. *Left,* Young man with residua of left Bell's palsy obscured by abundant beard. *Right,* Smiling results in synkinetic eye closure on the side of the old Bell's palsy. Residual left facial paralysis is also evident on smiling (an asymmetry of nasolabial fold and uneven lip spread).

evoked muscle response in cases of conduction block; these patients have a good prognosis. No response is obtained in cases where axonal degeneration has occurred.[6]

Treatment is with 1 mg per kg prednisone daily (in two divided doses) for four days, and tapered to 5 mg per day within 10 days.[10,12] It is claimed that prednisone should be instituted as soon as possible if it is to have an effect, that is, to prevent a mild lesion with only conduction block developing into axon degeneration—and it should be continued an additional 5 days if the paralysis remains complete.[10] Prompt treatment may result in dramatic lessening of pain. Steroid administration is also alleged to decrease residual paralysis and synkinetic movements, although these notions are controversial.[13] Male patients frequently choose to grow a beard to lessen the cosmetic impact if there is persistent facial paralysis (see Figure 27). The cosmetic effect is more embarrassing in women. Hypoglossal facial nerve anastomosis will restore facial tone and is the operation of choice. Facial slings from the temporalis fascia to the angle of the mouth are generally unsatisfactory. Radical facial plastic surgery ("face lifts") has produced considerable improvement in facial symmetry and reduced lacrimation in persistent cases of bilateral facial palsy following the Guillain-Barré syndrome. Even if the facial paralysis is recoverable, elderly subjects may develop exposure conjunctivitis or keratitis from lagophthalmos, and a lateral tarsorrhaphy may be necessary. There is no treatment for synkinetic movements (see Fig 26).

Other Cranial Mononeuropathies

Isolated lesions of other cranial nerves for which no explanation can be found are occasionally encountered. These are usually of acute onset. Among these, lesions of the recurrent laryngeal and spinal accessory nerves are the most frequent. The onset in the latter may be painful, and recovery usually occurs within three months. The occasional involvement of both of these nerves in patients with idiopathic brachial plexus neuropathy suggests that these isolated lesions may share the same pathogenesis. The term "cranial polyneuritis" is often used to describe simultaneous dysfunction of several lower cranial nerves, in the absence of extramedullary compression or meningeal lesions. This syndrome may recur.[14]

Plexus Neuropathies

Idiopathic Brachial Plexus Neuropathy

DEFINITION. This condition is best defined as an idiopathic acute, painful, and usually monophasic illness characterized by brachial plexus (see Figure 14, Chapter 17) dysfunction.[15] Synonyms for this disorder include *neuralgic amyotrophy*,[16] *acute brachial radiculitis*,[17] and *acute shoulder-girdle neuritis*.[18] The relationship of this condition to the syndromes of post-vaccinial,[19] toxic,[20] and hereditary brachial plexopathies[21] is uncertain.

PATHOLOGY AND PATHOGENESIS. There is no postmortem examination of this condition and no animal model. Biopsy of cutaneous nerves has revealed nonspecific axonal degeneration.

The pathogenesis is unknown. Most cases have no common antecedent illness, immunization, or toxic exposure; some follow surgical procedures. The clinical profile is usually identical to the serum vaccine (presumably allergic) syndrome,[19] and a common immunologic basis has therefore been proposed, although not substantiated.[15]

CLINICAL FEATURES. This condition can occur at any age; in our experience it is especially common in males aged 18 to 40. A cardinal feature is severe shoulder girdle-scapular pain, occasionally extending into the arm or hand. The pain persists for a few days to a week, and then subsides coincident with the appearance of weakness, although it sometimes persists for several weeks. It is often made worse by neck or arm movements. Proximal weakness, either partial or total paralysis, is usually in the distribution of subscapular and axillary nerves. The serratus anterior is the single most commonly affected muscle. Distal weakness less frequently occurs and, rarely, the entire arm and ipsilateral diaphragm are affected. Weakness may also appear in the other arm. Tendon reflexes are diminished in the involved extremity, but sensory loss is slight or negligible. Involvement is usually restricted to muscles innervated by the brachial plexus, although, as already stated, the diaphragm may become paralyzed, and accompanying laryngeal paralysis has been observed. Some cases of isolated and unexplained unilateral or bilateral diaphragmatic paralysis may be from this cause.

Routine clinical laboratory tests are normal. The CSF is acellular and protein content is not elevated.

COURSE, PROGNOSIS AND TREATMENT. Persistent weakness and atrophy of involved muscles develops in many cases. The prognosis is excellent; total recovery occurs in 90 percent of cases within two or three years.[15] Individuals with lower brachial plexus lesions have a worse prognosis. Treatment consists of physical therapy and orthotic devices to prevent joint damage. There is no evidence that corticosteroid therapy is of value. Recurrences, sometimes multiple, occasionally occur.

DIFFERENTIAL DIAGNOSIS. Brachial plexus neuropathies following serum or vaccine injections,[19] heroin abuse,[20] and of the hereditary type[21] are nearly identical clinical entities and can only be differentiated by careful history. Cervical spondylosis at the C_4-C_6 interspaces can cause severe shoulder pain and local weakness; myelography may be necessary to eliminate this possibility in an older patient. Thoracic outlet syndromes and carcinoma of lung and breast each may produce a painful brachial plexopathy, but seldom appear suddenly, and usually involve the lower plexus.[22] Anterior or posterior interosseous nerve-entrapment neuropathies in which the symptoms begin following unaccustomed exercise and are associated with pain sometimes give rise to diagnositic difficulty.

Case History and Comment

A 60-year-old man developed severe pain in the left shoulder that required opiates for relief. This persisted for two days, and because of some minor abnormalities on an electrocardiogram, he was admitted to a coronary care unit. Shortly following admission, the pain abated, and his left arm became weak. On examination, there was 2/5 weakness of the left supraspinatus, infraspinatus, deltoid, and biceps muscles. The triceps and wrist extensors were slightly weak. The remaining muscles of the arm were strong, and there was no weakness in the other limbs. All modalities of sensation were impaired in a band extending from the tip of the right shoulder down over the outer surface of the arm and forearm. The biceps tendon reflex was absent. The remainder of the neurologic examination was normal. A myelogram revealed no significant evidence of cervical intervertebral-disc disease and the CSF was normal. He was discharged.

One month later, he was re-examined and there was striking atrophy and fasciculation of the left infraspinatus, supraspinatus deltoid, and biceps muscles. The left biceps tendon reflex remained absent, but sensation was now normal over the left shoulder. An electromyogram disclosed fibrillation potentials in the atrophic muscles. Motor and sensory conduction studies of the ulnar and median nerves were normal.

Four months later, there was slight return of strength, and after one year the upper limb could be moved through a full range of notion against moderate resistance.

COMMENT. The signs and symptoms were largely confined to structures innervated by C_5-C_6 roots. Suspected cervical disc disease is a common diagnostic problem in older individuals with this condition. Typical for brachial plexus neuropathy were the predominance of motor over sensory signs, severe pain, and the satisfactory outcome.

Idiopathic Lumbar Plexopathy

This disorder is rare and has only recently been recognized.[23,24] Except for location, it is similar to cryptogenic brachial plexopathy. Lumbar plexopathy may also accompany hereditary brachial plexopathy and can occur as a result of heroin abuse.

The clinical features of cryptogenic lumbar plexopathy include a painful prodome, unilateral weakness in the distribution of several nerves, no underlying illness, and a gradual satisfactory recovery. As in brachial plexopathy, weakness is the predominant finding and sensory loss is trivial. The CSF is normal.

Differential diagnosis includes herniated lumbar intervertebral disc, proximal diabetic neuropathy, poliomyelitis, and tumor.

REFERENCES

1. DYCK, PJ, ET AL: *Intensive evaluation of referred unclassified neuropathies yields improved diagnosis.* Ann Neurol 10:222, 1981.
2. SPILLANE, JD AND WELLS, CEC: *Isolated trigeminal neuropathy. A report of 16 cases.* Brain 82:391, 1959.
3. KALTREIDER, HB AND TALAL, N: *The neuropathy of Sjögren's syndrome: trigeminal nerve involvement.* Ann Int Med 70:751, 1969.
4. ASHWORTH, B AND TAIT, GBW: *Trigeminal neuropathy in connective tissue disease.* Neurology (Minneap) 21:609, 1971.
5. HAUSER, WA, ET AL: *Incidence and prognosis of Bell's palsy in the population of Rochester, Minnesota.* Mayo Clin Proc 46:258, 1971.
6. MOLDAVER, J AND CONLEY, J: The Facial Palsies. Charles C Thomas, Springfield, Ill, 1979.
7. REDDY, JB, ET AL: *Histopathology of Bell's palsy.* Eye, Ear, Nose and Throat Mon 45:62, 1966.
8. FOWLER, EP: *The pathologic findings in a case of facial paralysis.* Acta Otolaryngol 68:1655, 1958.
9. BLUNT, MJ: *The possible role of vascular changes in the etiology of Bell's palsy.* J Laryngol Otol 70:701, 1956.
10. ADOUR, KK, ET AL: *The diagnosis and management of facial paralysis.* New Engl J Med 307:347, 1982.
11. ROWLAND, LP: *Treatment of Bell's palsy.* N Engl J Med 287:1298, 1972.
12. ADOUR, K, ET AL: *Prednisone treatment for idiopathic facial paralysis.* N Engl J Med 287:1268, 1972.
13. WOLF, SM: *Treatment of Bell's palsy with prednisone: a prospective, randomized study.* Neurology (Minneap) 28:158, 1978.
14. HOKKÄNEN, E, HALTIA, T AND MYLLYLA, VV: *Recurrent multiple cranial neuropathies.* Eur Neurol 17:32, 1978.
15. TSAIRIS, P, DYCK, PJ AND MULDER, DW: *Natural history of brachial plexus neuropathy: report on 99 patients.* Arch Neurol 27:109, 1972.
16. PARSONAGE, JM AND TURNER, JWA: *Neuralgic amyotrophy: the shoulder girdle syndrome.* Lancet I:973, 1948.
17. TURNER, JWA: *Acute brachial radiculitis.* Br Med J 2:592, 1944.
18. SPILLANE, JD: *Localized neuritis of the shoulder girdle: a report of 46 cases in the MEF.* Lancet 2:532, 1943.
19. SPILLANE, JD AND WELLS, CEC: *The neurology of Jennerian vaccination.* Brain 87:1, 1964.
20. CHALLENOR, YB, ET AL: *Nontraumatic plexitis and heroin addiction.* JAMA 225:958, 1973.
21. SMITH, BH, TAMARKVISNA, T AND SCHLAGENHAUF, RE: *Familial brachial neuropathy: Two case reports with discussion.* Neurology (Minneap) 21:941, 1971.
22. KORI, SH, FOLEY, KM AND POSNER, JB: *Brachial plexus lesions in patients with cancer: 100 cases.* Neurology (Minneap) 31:45, 1981.
23. SANDER, JE AND SHARP, FR: *Lumbosacral plexus neuritis.* Neurology (Minneap) 31:470, 1981.
24. EVANS, BA, STEVENS, JC AND DYCK, PJ: *Lumbosacral plexus neuropathy.* Neurology (Minneap) 31:1327, 1981.

Chapter 20

LABORATORY INVESTIGATION OF PERIPHERAL NERVE DISEASE: CLINICAL ELECTROPHYSIOLOGY AND NERVE BIOPSY

CLINICAL ELECTROPHYSIOLOGY*

EMG and motor and sensory nerve conduction studies, including the recording of "late responses," receive most emphasis because they are widely employed and simple to perform and considerable experience has established their value in the investigation and management of peripheral nerve disease.[1,2] Somatosensory evoked response (SER) recording techniques, useful in the evaluation of many polyneuropathies, are now widely available.

Electromyography

Indications and Usefulness

(1) In the differential diagnosis of weakness, that is, neurogenic, myopathic, volitional. Some neuropathies with pronounced proximal weakness, such as porphyria or the Guillain-Barré syndrome, may mimic myopathies.

(2) In confirmation (or refutation) of distribution of denervation changes predicted by clinical findings; for example, radicular versus peripheral nerve distribution.

(3) In detecting early recovery after peripheral nerve injury. The results of EMG examination may help decide whether surgical exploration is indicated.

(4) Special circumstances; for example, detection of neuromyotonia.

Techniques Employed and Significance of Findings

(1) Needle EMG technique is useful for assessment of:

*Prepared with the assistance of Jerry Kaplan, M.D.

(a) Presence of fibrillation and positive monophasic potentials. If present, these indicate denervation, or isolation of portions of muscle fibers from endplates in certain myopathies.

(b) Presence of fasciculation. These potentials are seen especially in anterior-horn-cell disease, but also may occur in axonopathies and demyelinating neuropathies and in benign conditions.

(c) Parameters of motor unit potentials. Amplitude and duration are reduced in myopathies because of loss of muscle fibers from motor units; increased in chronic partial denervation from expansion of the motor unit by collateral reinnervation.

(d) Motor unit recruitment pattern. Recruitment pattern remains normal in myopathies; is reduced in denervation, with normal firing rates on maximal volition; and is reduced in volitional weakness or upper motor neuron lesions with reduced firing rate on volition.

(2) Surface EMG technique, with large-plate electrodes placed anteriorly and posteriorly on proximal and distal segments of the limbs, is useful for detection of fasciculations.

Nerve Conduction Studies (Table 7)

Indications and usefulness

(1) A cardinal use is in *determining the presence of neuropathy,* either by establishing a neuropathic basis for clinically detected abnormalities, or in detecting subclinical neuropathy. Nerve conduction studies may be essential in establishing the location of focal peripheral nerve lesions, for example, compression of the ulnar nerve at the elbow.

TABLE 7. Normal Values for Nerve Conduction*

NERVE	STIMULUS SITE	RECORDING SITE	CONDUCTION VELOCITY (METERS PER SECOND)	AMPLITUDE
Motor			Range†	Lower limit of normal range (in mV)†
median	elbow	abductor pollicis brevis	50–70	4.5
ulnar	elbow	abductor digiti minimi	50–70	4.5
peroneal	ankle	extensor digitorum brevis	40–60	2.5
Sensory				(in μV)
sural	lateral malleolus	mid calf	50–70	5
median	second digit	wrist	50–70	8
ulnar	fifth digit	wrist	50–70	8
radial	wrist	mid-forearm	50–70	

*These are approximate values for adults below the age of 60. Conduction velocity and sensory-nerve action-potential amplitude decline in later life.

†It is advisable that precise ranges of normal be established for individual laboratories, as some of the values will be altered by variations in technique.

(2) Nerve conduction studies may suggest whether a symmetrical polyneuropathy is *axonal* or *demyelinating*. Differentiating between axonal and demyelinative change is also important in classifying nerve injuries (see Chapters 17 and 18) and certain other focal nerve lesions, for example, Bell's Palsy (see Chapter 19).

(3) Nerve conduction studies are not particularly useful in *following the progress* of distal symmetrical axonopathies, since nerve conduction alters slowly, but may aid in assessing recovery from focal conduction block or an acute demyelinating neuropathy.

Techniques employed

MOTOR CONDUCTION. As illustrated in Figure 28, measurements of motor nerve conduction velocity (or latency) and evoked muscle potential amplitude (MAP) are simple, but require scrupulous attention to the details of the technique, especially temperature control and measurement of conduction distance. Surface recording electrodes are over a distal muscle whose nerve has been stimulated at two proximal sites. The generated MAP is only an *indirect* measure of nerve function, in contrast to sensory nerve conduction studies (*vida infra*) where recording electrodes are over the nerve itself (Figure 29).

Motor conduction techniques are especially useful for:

(a) The detection of generalized neuropathies and prediction of the type of pathology. Slight or moderate reductions in conduction velocity characterize neuronopathies and axonopathies; for example, median nerve conduction velocity of 40 m per sec in alcoholic-nutritional neuropathy; moderate or severe reductions often occur in demyelinating neuropathies;

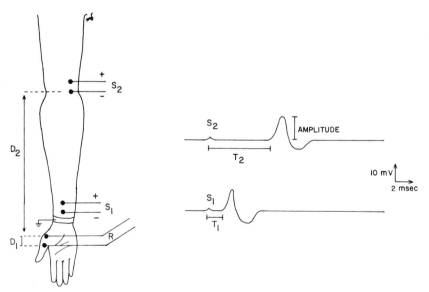

FIGURE 28. The examination of motor nerve conduction is illustrated for the median nerve or recording from the abductor policis brevis muscle (R). The median nerve is supra-maximally stimulated at the two sites (S_1 & S_2) and compound muscle action potentials are recorded. Latencies (T_1 & T_2) and distances (D_1 & D_2) are measured and conduction velocity between the stimulation sites is calculated as $\dfrac{D_2}{T_1 - T_2}$. The amplitude is measured from the baseline to the peak of negative (upward) deflection, as shown.

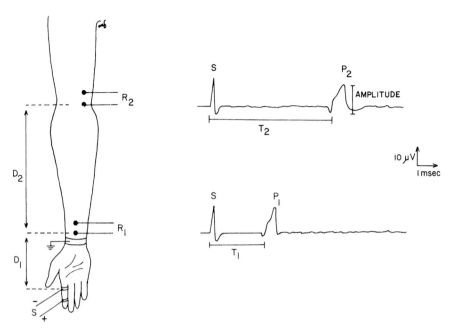

FIGURE 29. The technique for recording sensory nerve action potentials is illustrated, using the median nerve as an example. The digital nerves are stimulated (S) with the cathode at the proximal interphalangeal joint and potentials (P_1, P_2) are recorded at two proximal sites (R_1 & R_2). Latencies (T_1 & T_2) and distances (D_1 & D_2) are measured. Conduction velocity between the two recording sites is calculated as $\dfrac{D_2}{T_2\text{-}T_1}$. The amplitude is measured from peak to peak as shown.

for example, median nerve conduction velocity of 25 m per sec in the Guillain-Barré syndrome.

(b) The detection of traumatic and compression lesions; for example, focal slowing of conduction in the cubital tunnel syndrome. The existence of conduction block is further established by demonstrating preservation of conduction and evoked muscle action potential below the compressive lesion.

SENSORY CONDUCTION. Measurement of sensory and mixed-nerve action-potential velocity (or latency) and amplitude are simple, reliable means of *directly* studying peripheral nerves, but as for motor nerve conduction studies, require careful attention to the details of the recording technique. As illustrated in Figure 29, the nerve is stimulated at a distal site and action potentials are usually recorded over the nerve at one or more proximal sites in the limbs. The technique of distal stimulation and recording, for example, when both stimulus and recording are confined to one digit, is an especially sensitive means of detecting distal sensory polyneuropathy. Surface electrodes are sufficient for most clinical situations, although occasionally, subcutaneous needle electrodes are necessary. Reduction in amplitude may be related to fiber loss or, particularly in demyelinating neuropathies, to temporal dispersion.

Sensory nerve conduction techniques are especially useful for:

(a) The detection of sensory and sensorimotor neuropathy, where it is probably the single most helpful procedure.

(b) The detection of focal lesions; for example, carpal tunnel syndrome, by demonstrating differential involvement of digits or slowing of conduction across the wrist.

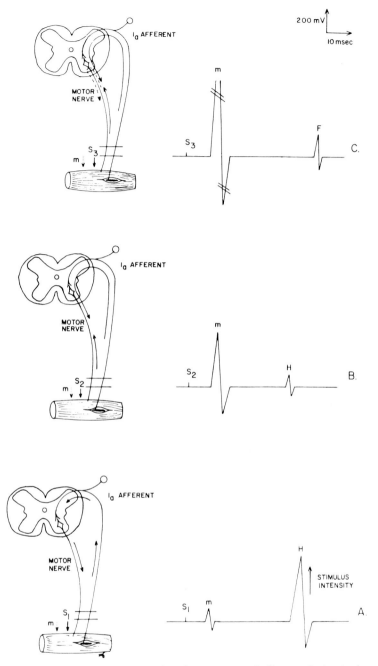

FIGURE 30. (A) The technique for recording late responses is illustrated. A mixed nerve is stimulated with a small current causing excitation of the low-threshold 1a fibers with minimal stimulation of motor fibers. A long-latency potential (H reflex) is indirectly evoked following motor neuron synaptic stimulation by 1a afferents, at a time when the short-latency directly evoked compound muscle action potential is of minimal amplitude. (B) With larger stimulus currents, more motor axons are excited; the larger antidromic potential collides with and reduces the reflexedly-generated H response, while the orthodromically-induced M response is larger. (C) With supramaximal stimulation of the motor nerve, the H reflex is completely blocked and the M response is maximal. Under these circumstances, the antidromic volley in the motor axons leads to retrograde firing of anterior horn cells, which generates descending impulses that give rise to low-amplitude long-latency muscle action potentials (F waves).

LABORATORY
INVESTIGATION
OF PERIPHERAL
NERVE
DISEASE

229

(c) Establishing whether lesions causing sensory loss are proximal or distal to dorsal root ganglia, for example, in deciding between avulsion of spinal roots and a brachial plexus lesion, or between a cauda equina and lumbosacral plexus lesion.

LATE-RESPONSE TECHNIQUES. Late responses are long-latency potentials encountered in nerve conduction studies. They are sensitive indicators of *proximal peripheral nerve* dysfunction. Figure 30 is a diagram of the two types of late responses, F waves and H reflexes.

F waves are centrifugal potentials in motor axons induced by firing of anterior horn cells by motor nerve stimulation. This technique is useful for assessing conduction in proximal portions of diffuse lesions of motor fibers in both axonopathies and demyelinating neuropathies, especially when pathologic changes are concentrated in plexus and roots, as in the Guillain-Barré syndrome. It is also useful in detecting focal proximal lesions in limb nerves, plexuses, or roots.

The H reflex is a monosynaptic reflex usually elicited from triceps surae (calf muscle) on stimulation of the tibial nerve in the popliteal fossa. Starting with a subthreshold stimulus and gradually increasing the amplitude, the H response appears before the direct or M response (i.e., with a weaker stimulus), as the afferent fibers of this reflex are large muscle-spindle afferent axons with a lower threshold than motor axons. The H reflex is useful for assessing conduction in proximal fibers in both axonopathies and demyelinating neuropathies, particularly if the pathology is predominantly radicular. In neuropathies with selective loss of large sensory fibers (e.g., Friedreich's ataxia), H reflexes may be lost while F waves are preserved.

RECORDING OF CONDUCTION IN SMALL FIBERS. Specialized procedures are available for recording from small myelinated and unmyelinated fibers, either employing collision techniques, which are applicable both to motor and sensory fibers, or computer-assisted averaging of large numbers of responses. These techniques are usually reserved for those unusual instances where clinical signs of small fiber dysfunction dominate the clinical profile, for example, amyloid neuropathy.

Potentials from small myelinated sensory and unmyelinated C fibers can be detected.

INTRANEURAL RECORDING. Intraneural microelectrode recordings and *in vitro* recordings of compound action potentials from excised nerve usually are only performed in centers dedicated to research activities.

Spinal and cortical somatosensory evoked response (SER)

Indications and usefulness

These techniques are useful for assessment of dysfunction in conditions where the centrally-directed axons of the primary sensory neurons are affected; for example, central axonopathies and distal axonopathies.[3,4] Unfortunately, the SER is unobtainable in some instances because of destruction of sensory axons in the peripheral nerves.

NERVE BIOPSY

Indications

The indications for nerve biopsy are now moderately well defined.[5] Biopsy is most helpful in identifying certain systemic illnesses that produce multiple mononeuropathy syndromes, for example, amyloidosis, sarcoidosis, leprosy, and vasculitis. Inherited metabolic illness such as metachromatic leukodystrophy, Krabbe disease, adreno-leukodystrophy, and Fabry disease are associated with specific changes in peripheral nerve, but are now more readily identified by biochemical analysis of peripheral blood samples. Demyelinating neuropathies may be readily identified on biopsy if the specimen is examined by careful teased fiber techniques. Biopsy appears justified in cases of diffuse cryptogenic neuropathy whose investigation, as outlined in Chapter 19, has failed to suggest an etiology. Conditions masquerading atypically as distal axonopathies (chronic demyelinating neuropathy, vasculitis, sarcoidosis) are occasionally revealed only at biopsy.

Individuals whose diagnosis is relatively secure on clinical grounds (diabetes, alcoholic-malnutrition, porphyria, uremia, Guillain-Barré syndrome, and those metabolic-toxic disorders whose etiology is clearly established) do not require biopsy. Distal symmetrical axonal neuropathies, of the type associated with most metabolic or toxic conditions, show similar nonspecific morphologic features, and biopsy is rarely as informative as meticulous medical evaluation.

Technical Considerations

Surgery

The sural nerve at the ankle is favored for nerve biopsy; however, the radial nerve at the wrist is sometimes used. Both are sensory nerves and a suitable length may be excised under local anesthesia as an outpatient procedure. Following biopsy at these sites, cutaneous sensory loss appears in the distribution of the nerve, and may be accompanied by dysesthesias for several weeks. Removal of the whole nerve is customary in many centers; allegedly this procedure has a greater diagnostic yield than fascicular biopsy.[5] Advocates of fascicular biopsy maintain that it is usually adequate for diagnosis and is followed by less sensory loss.[6] In any event, it is helpful if a single individual in an institution becomes thoroughly familiar with the technique and performs all the diagnostic biopsies. Although this seems a simple and trivial procedure, even an experienced surgeon can easily biopsy a vein or rough handle a specimen of nerve.

Histologic Technique

Three preparations should be available for every nerve biopsy: conventional paraffin sections, teased fibers, and epoxy-embedded sections for light and electron microscopy. Each has advantages and each may be done on a separate segment of the fixed tissue obtained at biopsy.

CONVENTIONAL PARAFFIN-EMBEDDED TISSUE. Paraffin sections, following routine staining, are useful for assessing cellular infiltrations, blood vessel changes, and Granulomatous and neoplastic infiltrations. Special

LABORATORY
INVESTIGATION
OF PERIPHERAL
NERVE
DISEASE

231

stains for amyloid and *M. leprae* bacilli are sometimes indicated. Subtle changes in axons, myelin, and Schwann cells are not well appreciated in conventional stained tissue.

SINGLE TEASED FIBERS. This technique readily allows the rapid identification of axonal degeneration and segmental demyelination in long lengths of nerve fibers. Quantitative studies of internodal length and diameter are easily performed, and the relationship between length of internodes and myelinated fiber diameter can be expressed graphically or statistically. Normally there is little variation between internodal lengths in a single fiber (see Figure 4, Chapter 1).

EPOXY RESIN-EMBEDDED TISSUE. Light microscope examination of such sections is an especially useful technique for assessing changes in large numbers of axons, Schwann cells, and myelin since all are stained and well preserved by this technique. Both loss of myelinated fibers and the size of fiber affected can be appreciated by casual examination. The exact change in the population and caliber spectrum can be further determined, if necessary, by photographing the sections and assessing quantitatively fiber numbers and diameters. Ultrathin sections may be cut from the same epoxy blocks and processed for electron microscopy. Electron microscopy is useful for determining ultrastructural features in axons, myelin, and Schwann cells (Figure 1, Chapter 1) and identifying both subtle changes and specific pathologic features characteristic of some neuropathies. Electron microscopy of peripheral nerve, although a powerful research tool, is frequently of little help in diagnostic pathology, since many neuropathies are featured by nonspecific axonal degenerative changes.

REFERENCES

1. *The Physiology of Peripheral Nerve Disease,* Sumner, AJ (ed), WB Saunders, Philadelphia, 1980.
2. Goodgold, J and Eberstein, A: *Electrodiagnosis of Neuromuscular Disease,* ed 2, Williams & Wilkins, Baltimore, 1977.
3. Gupta, PR and Dorfman LJ: *Spinal somatosensory conduction in diabetes.* Neurology (Minneap) 31:841, 1981.
4. Thomas, PK et al: *Spinal somatosensory evoked potentials in hereditary spastic paraplegia.* J Neurol Neurosurg Psychiatry 44:243, 1981.
5. Asbury, AK and Johnson, PC: *Pathology of Peripheral Nerve.* WB Saunders, Philadelphia, 1978.
6. Dyck, PJ and Lofgren, EP: *Nerve biopsy: choice of nerve, method, symptoms, and usefulness.* Med Clin North Am 52:885, 1968.

Appendix 1.

CUTANEOUS FIELDS OF PERIPHERAL NERVES— FIGURES 31 and 32

Please see next page.

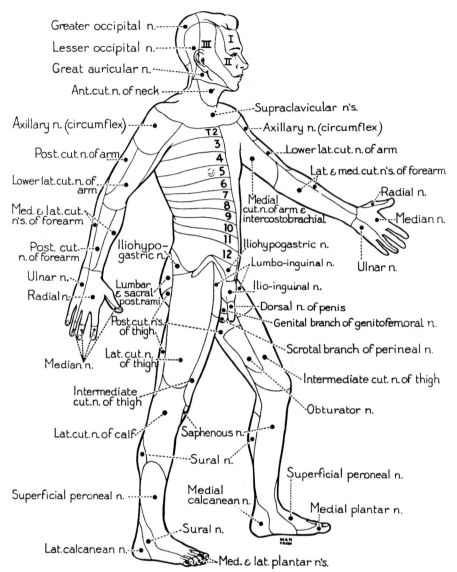

FIGURE 31. Side view of the cutaneous fields of peripheral nerves. (From Haymaker, W and Woodhall, B: *Peripheral Nerve Injuries*, WB Saunders, Philadelphia, 1953, with permission).

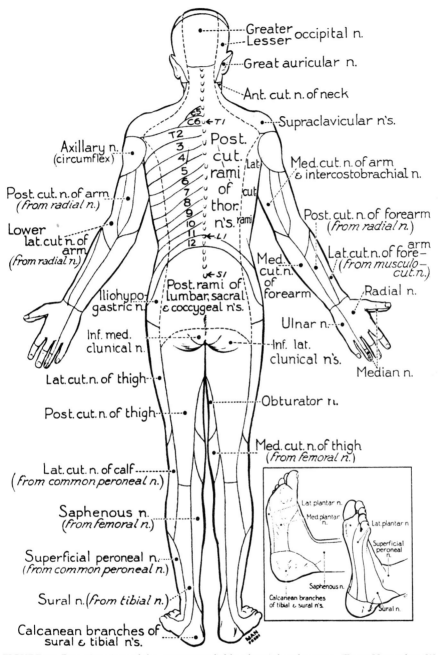

FIGURE 32. Posterior view of the cutaneous fields of peripheral nerves. (From Haymaker, W and Woodhall, B: *Peripheral Nerve Injuries*, WB Saunders, Philadelphia, 1953, with permission.)

Appendix 2.

SEGMENTAL INNERVATION OF SOMATIC MUSCLES— FIGURES 33–35

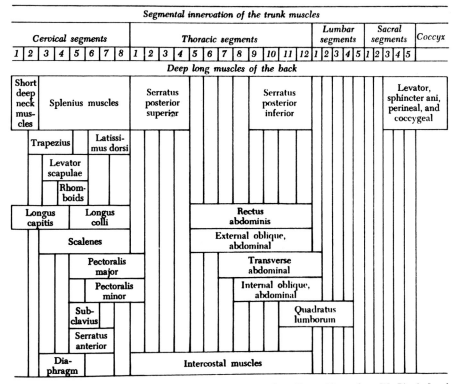

FIGURE 33. Segmental innervation of the trunk muscles. (From Haymaker, W: *Bing's Local Diagnosis in Neurological Disease*, ed 15. CV Mosby, St. Louis, 1969, with permission.)

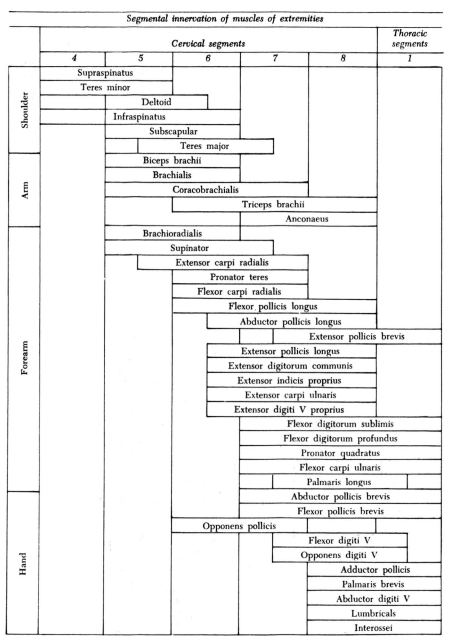

FIGURE 34. Segmental innervation of upper limb muscles. (From Haymaker, W: *Bing's Local Diagnosis in Neurological Disease*, ed 15. CV Mosby, St. Louis, 1969, with permission.)

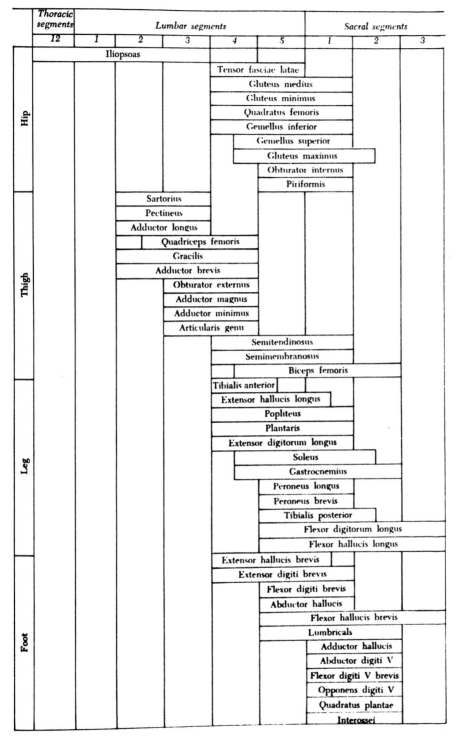

	Thoracic segments	Lumbar segments					Sacral segments		
	12	1	2	3	4	5	1	2	3

Hip
- Iliopsoas
- Tensor fasciae latae
- Gluteus medius
- Gluteus minimus
- Quadratus femoris
- Gemellus inferior
- Gemellus superior
- Gluteus maximus
- Obturator internus
- Piriformis

Thigh
- Sartorius
- Pectineus
- Adductor longus
- Quadriceps femoris
- Gracilis
- Adductor brevis
- Obturator externus
- Adductor magnus
- Adductor minimus
- Articularis genu
- Semitendinosus
- Semimembranosus
- Biceps femoris

Leg
- Tibialis anterior
- Extensor hallucis longus
- Popliteus
- Plantaris
- Extensor digitorum longus
- Soleus
- Gastrocnemius
- Peroneus longus
- Peroneus brevis
- Tibialis posterior
- Flexor digitorum longus
- Flexor hallucis longus

Foot
- Extensor hallucis brevis
- Extensor digiti brevis
- Flexor digiti brevis
- Abductor hallucis
- Flexor hallucis brevis
- Lumbricals
- Adductor hallucis
- Abductor digiti V
- Flexor digiti V brevis
- Opponens digiti V
- Quadratus plantae
- Interossei

FIGURE 35. Segmental innervation of the lower limbs. (From Haymaker, W: *Bing's Local Diagnosis in Neurological Disease*, ed 15. CV Mosby, St. Louis, 1969, with permission.)

INDEX

Diphtheria
  etiology of, 138
  generalized neuropathy, clinical features, 139
  laboratory studies, 140
  local neuropathy, clinical features, 139
  pathology and pathogenesis of, 138–139
Diphtheritic neuropathy. *See* Diphtheria.
Distal axonopathy
  mechanism of, 7–8
  pathologic features of, 8–9
  stocking-glove pattern in, *10*
Distal spinal muscular atrophy, hereditary, 107
Disulfiram, neurotoxicity of, 121
DMAPN intoxication, 136–137. *See also* Toxic neuropathy.
Doriden, neurotoxicity of, 122
Dysproteinemia
  cryoglobulinemia and, 165
  monoclonal gammopathy and, 164–165

ELECTROMYOGRAPHY
  indications and usefulness, 225
  techniques and significance, 225–226
Electron microscopy, biopsy and, 232
Electrophysiology, clinical
  electromyography, 225–226
  nerve conduction studies, 226, t, *227, 228, 229,* 230
  spinal, cortical somatosensory evoked response, 230
Ethionamide, neurotoxicity of, 121
Ethylene oxide neuropathy, 140
FABRY'S disease. *See* Alpha-galactosidase deficiency.
Facial paralysis, idiopathic
  Bell's palsy and, 218–*219*
  clinical features of, 219
  pathology and pathogenesis of, 218–219
  treatment of, 220
Familial dysautonomia. *See* Hereditary sensory neuropathy.
Femoral nerve, 201, *202,* 203
Flagyl, neurotoxicity of, 123
Focal neuropathy
  defined, 5
  ischemia and, 15–17
Focal cranial neuropathy
  idiopathic facial paralysis, 218–*220*
  iodiopathic isolated trigeminal, 218
Friedreich's ataxia, 106, 110
Furadantin, neurotoxicity of, 124

GALACTOSYLCERAMIDE lipidosis
  biochemical abnormality of, 91
  general features of, 91
Globotriosylceramide, 95
Glucocorticoids, use in treatment of CRIP, 36
Glue sniffers, signs and symptoms, 141–142. *See also* Hexacarbon neuropathy.
Glutethimide, neurotoxicity of, 122
Glycosphingolipids, 95
Gold, neurotoxicity of, 121–122

Guillain-Barré syndrome
  case history and comment, 32–33
  conditions associated with, 27
  confusion of, with porphyric neuropathy, 80
  defined, 25
  demyelination and, 11, 26
  differential diagnosis, 31–32
  experimental allergic neuritis and, 26–27
  facial paralysis and, 220
  factors predisposing, 27
  incidence of, 17
  laboratory studies, 29–31
    cerebrospinal fluid, 29–30
    electrodiagnostic, 30
    nerve biopsy, 30
    routine clinical, 29
    special tests, 29
  mortality, 29
  motor and sensory loss in, *13*
  pathogenesis of, 26
  pathology of, 25–26
  prognosis for, 29
  progression of, 29
  recurrences of, 29
  signs and symptoms of, 27–28
  similarity to other autoimmune disorders, 34–35
  treatment of, 30–31
    anti-inflammatory agents, use of, 31
    fluid replacement in, 30
    mechanical ventilation in, 30
    muscle weakness and, 31
    need for hospitalization, 30

HEME biosynthesis, 76, t
Hemodialysis, uremic polyneuropathy and, 71–72
Herpes zoster
  clinical features of, 180
  etiology of, 179
  pathology and pathogenesis of, 179
Hexacarbon neurotoxicity, 140–144
  case history and comment, 143–144
  course and prognosis, 143
  differential diagnosis, 143
  general features, 140
  laboratory studies, 142–143
  pathology and pathogenesis of, 141
  signs and symptoms of, 141–142
High-density lipoprotein deficiency
  biochemical abnormality of, 92–93
  clinical features of, 93–94
  general features of, 93
  pathology and pathogenesis of, 93
Histologic technique, nerve biopsy and, 231
Hodgkin's disease. *See* Lymphoma.
Horner's syndrome, 194, 213
Hydralazine, neurotoxicity of, 122
Hypokalemia, 31
Hypothyroidism
  course, treatment, prognosis, 85
  defined, 83
  differential diagnosis, 85–86
  incidence of, 84